Food Environment and Its Effects on Human Nutrition and Health

Food Environment and Its Effects on Human Nutrition and Health

Editor

Jose M. Miranda

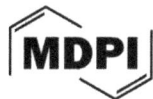

Basel • Beijing • Wuhan • Barcelona • Belgrade • Novi Sad • Cluj • Manchester

Editor
Jose M. Miranda
Departamento de
Química Analítica
Universidade de Santiago
de Compostela
Lugo
Spain

Editorial Office
MDPI AG
Grosspeteranlage 5
4052 Basel, Switzerland

This is a reprint of articles from the Special Issue published online in the open access journal *Nutrients* (ISSN 2072-6643) (available at: https://www.mdpi.com/journal/nutrients/special_issues/0C4Q74BEYU).

For citation purposes, cite each article independently as indicated on the article page online and as indicated below:

Lastname, A.A.; Lastname, B.B. Article Title. *Journal Name* **Year**, *Volume Number*, Page Range.

ISBN 978-3-7258-2025-2 (Hbk)
ISBN 978-3-7258-2026-9 (PDF)
doi.org/10.3390/books978-3-7258-2026-9

© 2024 by the authors. Articles in this book are Open Access and distributed under the Creative Commons Attribution (CC BY) license. The book as a whole is distributed by MDPI under the terms and conditions of the Creative Commons Attribution-NonCommercial-NoDerivs (CC BY-NC-ND) license.

Contents

About the Editor vii

Alicia del Carmen Mondragon Portocarrero and Jose Manuel Miranda Lopez
Food Environment and Its Effects on Human Nutrition and Health
Reprinted from: *Nutrients* **2024**, *16*, 1733, doi:10.3390/nu16111733 1

Bei Zhou, Yupeng Zhang, Michael Hiesmayr, Xuejin Gao, Yingchun Huang, Sitong Liu, et al.
Dietary Provision, GLIM-Defined Malnutrition and Their Association with Clinical Outcome: Results from the First Decade of nutritionDay in China
Reprinted from: *Nutrients* **2024**, *16*, 569, doi:10.3390/nu16040569 6

Man Zhang, Ruixin Chi, Zhenhui Li, Yujie Fang, Na Zhang, Qiaoqin Wan and Guansheng Ma
Different Dimensions of the Home Food Environment May Be Associated with the Body Mass Index of Older Adults: A Cross-Sectional Survey Conducted in Beijing, China
Reprinted from: *Nutrients* **2024**, *16*, 289, doi:10.3390/nu16020289 19

Cindy Needham, Claudia Strugnell, Steven Allender, Laura Alston and Liliana Orellana
BMI and the Food Retail Environment in Melbourne, Australia: Associations and Temporal Trends
Reprinted from: *Nutrients* **2023**, *15*, 4503, doi:10.3390/nu15214503 33

Happy Kurnia Permatasari, Queen Intan Permatasari, Nurpudji Astuti Taslim, Dionysius Subali, Rudy Kurniawan, Reggie Surya, et al.
Revealing Edible Bird Nest as Novel Functional Foods in Combating Metabolic Syndrome: Comprehensive In Silico, In Vitro, and In Vivo Studies
Reprinted from: *Nutrients* **2023**, *15*, 3886, doi:10.3390/nu15183886 46

Laura Sinisterra-Loaiza, Patricia Alonso-Lovera, Alejandra Cardelle-Cobas, Jose Manuel Miranda, Beatriz I. Vázquez and Alberto Cepeda
Compliance with Nutritional Recommendations and Gut Microbiota Profile in Galician Overweight/Obese and Normal-Weight Individuals
Reprinted from: *Nutrients* **2023**, *15*, 3418, doi:10.3390/nu15153418 64

Afshin Zand, Sodbuyan Enkhbilguun, John M. Macharia, Ferenc Budán, Zoltán Gyöngyi and Timea Varjas
Tartrazine Modifies the Activity of *DNMT* and *HDAC* Genes—Is This a Link between Cancer and Neurological Disorders?
Reprinted from: *Nutrients* **2023**, *15*, 2946, doi:10.3390/nu15132946 83

Sunmin Park and Meiling Liu
A Positive Causal Relationship between Noodle Intake and Metabolic Syndrome: A Two-Sample Mendelian Randomization Study
Reprinted from: *Nutrients* **2023**, *15*, 2091, doi:10.3390/nu15092091 95

Fahrul Nurkolis, Nurpudji Astuti Taslim, Dionysius Subali, Rudy Kurniawan, Hardinsyah Hardinsyah, William Ben Gunawan, et al.
Dietary Supplementation of *Caulerpa racemosa* Ameliorates Cardiometabolic Syndrome via Regulation of PRMT-1/DDAH/ADMA Pathway and Gut Microbiome in Mice
Reprinted from: *Nutrients* **2023**, *15*, 909, doi:10.3390/nu15040909 115

Eva Valenčič, Emma Beckett, Clare E. Collins, Barbara Koroušić Seljak and Tamara Bucher
SnackTrack—An App-Based Tool to Assess the Influence of Digital and Physical Environments on Snack Choice
Reprinted from: *Nutrients* **2023**, *15*, 349, doi:10.3390/nu15020349 134

Elisa Martino, Nunzia D'Onofrio, Anna Balestrieri, Antonino Colloca, Camilla Anastasio, Celestino Sardu, et al.
Dietary Epigenetic Modulators: Unravelling the Still-Controversial Benefits of miRNAs in Nutrition and Disease
Reprinted from: *Nutrients* **2024**, *16*, 160, doi:10.3390/nu16010160 147

Zahra A. Padhani, Bernadette Cichon, Jai K. Das, Rehana A. Salam, Heather C. Stobaugh, Muzna Mughal, et al.
Systematic Review of Management of Moderate Wasting in Children over 6 Months of Age
Reprinted from: *Nutrients* **2023**, *15*, 3781, doi:10.3390/nu15173781 169

Aroa Lopez-Santamarina, Alicia del Carmen Mondragon, Alejandra Cardelle-Cobas, Eva Maria Santos, Jose Julio Porto-Arias, Alberto Cepeda and Jose Manuel Miranda
Effects of Unconventional Work and Shift Work on the Human Gut Microbiota and the Potential of Probiotics to Restore Dysbiosis
Reprinted from: *Nutrients* **2023**, *15*, 3070, doi:10.3390/nu15133070 187

Timothy D. Nelson and Eric Stice
Contextualizing the Neural Vulnerabilities Model of Obesity
Reprinted from: *Nutrients* **2023**, *15*, 2988, doi:10.3390/nu15132988 206

Shahrzad Ezzatpour, Alicia del Carmen Mondragon Portocarrero, Alejandra Cardelle-Cobas, Alexandre Lamas, Aroa López-Santamarina, José Manuel Miranda and Hector C. Aguilar
The Human Gut Virome and Its Relationship with Nontransmissible Chronic Diseases
Reprinted from: *Nutrients* **2023**, *15*, 977, doi:10.3390/nu15040977 222

About the Editor

Jose M. Miranda

Associate professor at Universidad de Santiago de Compostela (Spain). After years as a public health inspector, he began teaching veterinary medicine, nutrition and dietetics at the University of Santiago de Compostela. A researcher in the field of gut microbiota and food safety, he has published more than 150 SCI articles, with him being among the 6000 most cited researchers in the world according to Clarivate Analytics between the years 2021–2024.

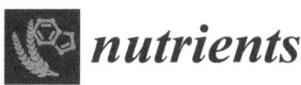

Editorial

Food Environment and Its Effects on Human Nutrition and Health

Alicia del Carmen Mondragon Portocarrero and Jose Manuel Miranda Lopez *

Laboratorio de Higiene, Inspección y Control de Alimentos, Departamento de Química Analítica, Nutrición y Bromatología, Campus Terra, Universidade da Santiago de Compostela, 27002 Lugo, Spain; alicia.mondragon@usc.es
* Correspondence: josemanuel.miranda@usc.es

Citation: Mondragon Portocarrero, A.d.C.; Miranda Lopez, J.M. Food Environment and Its Effects on Human Nutrition and Health. Nutrients 2024, 16, 1733. https://doi.org/10.3390/nu16111733

Received: 9 April 2024
Revised: 22 April 2024
Accepted: 17 May 2024
Published: 1 June 2024

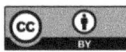

Copyright: © 2024 by the authors. Licensee MDPI, Basel, Switzerland. This article is an open access article distributed under the terms and conditions of the Creative Commons Attribution (CC BY) license (https://creativecommons.org/licenses/by/4.0/).

1. Introduction

The concept of a healthy diet is not a static definition; over the years, it has been molded to scientific knowledge. Recently, international organizations have updated their concept of a healthy diet, defining it as one that promotes all dimensions of health and individual well-being; has low environmental pressure and impact; is accessible, affordable, safe, and equitable; and is also culturally acceptable [1], as consumers are generally reluctant to change their eating habits [2]. Therefore, the ways in which food is produced, processed, packaged, distributed, labeled, priced, consumed, or wasted represent areas that, while not included in the traditional concept of human nutrition, affect human health, and need to be considered [3]. Thus, an ideal diet should aim to achieve optimal growth and development for all individuals and promote physical, mental, and social well-being at different stages of life, reducing the risk of diet-related noncommunicable diseases and supporting the preservation of biodiversity and environmental health [4].

Therefore, in addition to the proportions of foods that can be included in the human diet, there are other conditioning factors that can affect human health [5]. Thus, the dietary contributions of bacteria [6], viruses [7], fungi [8,9], food additives [10], chemical substances [11,12], or exosomes can exert important effects on human health [13]. Similarly, lifestyle factors, such as meal timing, cuisine, and type of work, also have an important effect on human health. It should not be forgotten that through nutrition, we can alleviate or cure diseases that affect organs far away from the digestive system, as in the case of nonfood allergies [14], respiratory viral infections [7], heart diseases [15], diseases of the nervous system, and neurological disorders [16,17].

In view of this, the objective of this Special Issue was to provide an update of knowledge on those environmental factors that play an essential role in human nutrition and, therefore, in the health of individuals, especially about metabolic diseases. A total of nine research articles and five reviews covering numerous topics of great interest and topicality in human nutrition and dietetics were included. Articles investigating the influence of food outlets, the workplace of schedules, and the intake of traditional Asian foods or functional foods, including aspects related to epigenetics or metagenomics, were included. In addition, the information published included different stages of life, such as infant nutrition, the prevention of metabolic diseases in adults, and the prevention and monitoring of malnutrition in the elderly population.

2. An Overview of the Published Articles

Zhou et al. (Contribution 1) present an interesting paper investigating malnutrition rates and their relationship to the length and quality of hospital stay in a total of 5821 hospitalized adult patients. The effect of a nutrition intervention program carried out by volunteers in China called *Nutrition Day* was evaluated in these patients. A malnutrition rate of 22.8% was found, and the results showed that after the implementation of *nutrition* day, the diet and nutritional status of hospitalized patients improved, which had important effects on the length and quality of hospital stay.

In another article, Zhang et al. (Contribution 2) assessed the home eating environment of elderly people, analyzed its association with their body mass index (BMI), and provided recommendations for improving the home eating environment for a total of 1764 elderly people. The results showed that senior people living alone had a greater BMI than those who did not live alone, and highlighted the impact of the home environment, living conditions, and availability of canned food on the BMI of senior people.

Regarding the influence of food sales channels on human nutrition, two interesting papers have been included in this Special Issue. On the one hand, Valenčič et al. (Contribution 3) developed and tested a mobile application (called *SnackTrack*) to investigate the association between physical and digital environments on snack choice, which was tested by 188 users. The results showed that the time at which the snack was obtained did not have a relevant effect on the health of the snacks chosen. In contrast, unhealthy background images seemed to encourage the choice of healthier snacks, thus showing that environmental cues have a strong influence on consumers' food choices. In another article, Needham et al. (Contribution 4) developed a new comprehensive method for ranking food retail environments. This method was tested with the aim of assessing its influence on obesity in a total of 47,245 users. The results obtained showed that increasing access and availability to a diverse range of food outlets, particularly healthy foods, improves consumer health.

Permatasari et al. (Contribution 5) investigated the relationship between the consumption of a typical Asian food, edible bird's nest (EBN), and the development of metabolic diseases. This study involved three approaches: in silico, in vitro, and in vivo molecular docking simulations in rats fed with cholesterol- and fat-rich diets. Interestingly, in vivo studies revealed significant improvements in the lipid profile, blood glucose levels, enzyme levels, and inflammatory biomarker levels in rats given a high-dose dietary supplement of EBN. Additionally, dietary supplementation with high-dose EBN increased peroxisome-proliferator-activated receptor-gamma coactivator and reduced β-hydroxy β-methylglutaryl-CoA reductase. Based on these results, EBN may be a potential functional food for people with metabolic syndrome (MS).

Zand et al. (Contribution 6) investigated the effect of the long-term exposure (30 and 90 days) to a commonly used artificial food coloring agent (tartrazine) in mice. The applied dose of tartrazine was termed the human equivalent dose for the acceptable daily intake (ADI). After this intervention, the impact of tartrazine intake on the transcription of epigenetic effectors, members of the DNA methyltransferase and histone deacetylase families, was evaluated. The results revealed a significant upregulation of genes in the analyzed organs in various patterns following tartrazine intake at the ADI.

Park and Liu (Contribution 7) examined the possible causal relationship between noodle consumption and the risk of MS in adult populations from urban (58,701) and rural (13,598) hospitals. In subjects with high noodle consumption, a higher caloric intake was observed, with lower carbohydrate and higher fat, protein, and sodium intakes and lower calcium, vitamin D, vitamin C, and flavonoid intakes. Together, these proportions indicate lower diet quality. The glycemic index and glycemic load of daily meals were much greater in the high noodle intake group than in the low noodle intake group. In conclusion, noodle intake had a positive causal association with MS in Asian adults.

Nurkolis et al. (Contribution 8) investigated the potential effects of an aqueous extract of *Caulerpa racemosa* (AEC) on markers of cardiometabolic syndrome and modulation of the gut microbiome in mice fed a cholesterol- and fat-enriched diet. The administration of high doses of AECs improved blood lipid and glucose profiles and reduced the levels of several markers of endothelial dysfunction. In addition, a correlation between specific gut microbiomes and biomarkers associated with cardiometabolic diseases was obtained. In vitro assays revealed the antioxidant properties of AECs, while in vivo assay found that

AEC intake contributed to the management of MS through the regulation of oxidative stress, inflammation, and endothelial function and the modulation of the gut microbiota (GM).

To investigate the association between the GM and body weight, Sinisterra-Loaiza et al. (Contribution 9) evaluated the dietary intake of 108 individuals with different weight statuses and analyzed their GM profiles to determine their GM composition and functionality, as well as their associations with BMI and diet. Correlation analysis revealed that adequate nutritional recommendations for fiber were associated with increased abundances of *Prevotella copri*, *Faecalibacterium prausnitzii*, *Bacteroides caccae*, and *Roseburia faecis*, which, together, can be considered an improvement in the GM profile. Benefits were also found at the GM level when subjects ingested amounts of monosaturated fatty acids within current recommendations.

This Special Issue also included a total of five review articles which, like the experimental articles, covered a wide variety of topics. Martino et al. (Contribution 10) reviewed nutrient-driven epigenetic alterations induced by miRNAs derived from food absorbed into the circulatory system that potentially contribute to the modulation of health and disease. The results showed that the absorption of foods carrying exogenous miRNAs modifies redox homeostasis and inflammatory conditions underlying pathological processes, such as type 2 diabetes mellitus (T2D), insulin resistance, MS, and cancer.

Padhani et al. (Contribution 11) reviewed five studies covering 3387 participants that evaluated the effectiveness of specially formulated foods (SFFs) compared to non-food-based approaches for managing malnutrition in children >6 months old. The main conclusion of the review is that SFFs may be a useful tool that can be beneficial for children with moderate wasting, which occurs on a frequent basis in humanitarian contexts.

López-Santamarina et al. (Contribution 12) reviewed the effects of the work environment on the composition and functionality of workers' GM, focusing especially on unconventional work schedules and environments. They also analyzed whether probiotic supplements, through modulation of the GM, can moderate the effects of sleep disturbances on the immune system, as well as restore the dysbiosis caused by unusual work schedules. The results showed that rotating shift work is associated with an increased risk of various metabolic diseases, such as obesity, MS, and T2D. In addition, sleep disturbances induce both physiological and psychological stress responses and alter the healthy functioning of the GM, thus triggering an inflammatory state.

Nelson and Stice (Contribution 13) reviewed neural vulnerability factors that increase the risk of unhealthy weight gain. In conclusion, their review found potential to create novel, comprehensive, multicomponent intervention approaches that address all components of the contextualized neural vulnerability model of obesity. Understanding unique risk pathways may also create opportunities to personalize prevention efforts by identifying combinations of risk factors and tailoring intervention components to the unique needs of the individual.

Finally, Ezzatpour et al. (Contribution 14) reviewed the potential effect and influence of the gut virome, which interacts with the bacterial microbiota. The effectiveness, applicability, and potential of virome-rectification-based therapies for different diseases, including metabolic diseases, were also investigated. As the main conclusion of this review, stool metagenomic investigations should include the identification of bacteria and phages, as well as their correlation networks, to better understand gut microbiota activity in metabolic disease progression.

Author Contributions: Writing—original draft preparation, A.d.C.M.P.; writing—review and editing, J.M.M.L. All authors have read and agreed to the published version of the manuscript.

Conflicts of Interest: The authors declare no conflicts of interest.

List of Contributions

1. Zhou, B.; Zhang, Y.; Hiesmayr, M.; Gao, X.; Huang, Y.; Liu, S.; Zhao, Y.; Cui, Y.; Zhang, L.; Wang, X.; Nutrition Day Chinese Working Goup. Dietary provision, GLIM-defined malnutrition and their association with clinical outcome: Results from the first decade of nutrition Day in China. *Nutrients* **2024**, *16*(4), 569. https://doi.org/10.3390/nu16040569.
2. Zhang, M.; Chi, Q.; Li, Z.; Fang, Y.; Zhang, N.; Wan, Q.; Ma, G. Different dimensions of the home food environment may be associated with the body mass index of older adults: A cross-sectional survey conducted in Beijing, China. *Nutrients* **2024**, *16*(2), 289. https://doi.org/10.3390/nu16020289.
3. Valenčič, E.; Beckett, E.; Collins, C.E.; Seljak, B.K.; Bucher, T. SnackTrack—An app-based tool to assess the influence of digital and physical environments on snack choice. *Nutrients* **2023**, *15*(2), 349. https://doi.org/10.3390/nu15020349.
4. Needham, C.; Strugnell, C.; Allender, S.; Alston, L.; Orellana, L. BMI and the food retail environment in Melbourne, Australia: Associations and temporal trends. *Nutrients* **2023**, *15*(21), 4503. https://doi.org/10.3390/nu15214503.
5. Permatasari, H.K.; Permatasari, Q.I.; Taslim, N.A.; Subali, D.; Kurniawan, R.; Surya, R.; Qhabibi, F.R.; Tanner, M.J.; Batubara, S.C.; Mayulu, N.; Gunawan, W.B.; Syauki, A.Y.; Salindeho, N.; Park, M.N.; Jeremis Maruli Nura Lele, J.A.; Tjandrawinata, R.R.; Kim, B.; Nurkolis, F. Revealing edible bird nest as novel functional foods in combating metabolic syndrome: Comprehensive in silico, in vitro, and in vivo studies. *Nutrients* **2023**, *15*(18), 3886. https://doi.org/10.3390/nu15183886.
6. Zand, A.; Enkhbilguun, S.; Macharia, J.M.; Budán, F.; Gyöngyi, Z.; Varjas, T. Tartrazine modifies the activity of DNMT and HDAC genes—is this a link between cancer and neurological disorders? *Nutrients* **2023**, *15*(13), 2946. https://doi.org/10.3390/nu15132946.
7. Park, S.; Liu, M. A positive causal relationship between noodle intake and metabolic syndrome: A two-sample mendelian randomization study. *Nutrients* **2023**, *15*(9), 2091. https://doi.org/10.3390/nu15092091.
8. Nurkolis, F.; Taslim, N.A.; Subali, D.; Kurniawan, R.; Hardinsyah, H.; Gunawan, W.B.; Kusuma, R.J.; Mayulu, N.; Syauki, A.Y.; Tallei, T.E.; Tsopmo, A.; Kim, B. Dietary supplementation of *Caulerpa racemosa* ameliorates cardiometabolic syndrome via regulation of PRMT-1/DDAH/ADMA pathway and gut microbiome in mice. *Nutrients* **2023**, *15*(4), 909. https://doi.org/10.3390/nu15040909.
9. Sinisterra-Loaiza, L.; Alonso-Lovera, P.; Cardelle-Cobas, A.; Miranda, J.M.; Vazquez, B.I.; Cepeda, A. Compliance with nutritional recommendations and gut microbiota profile in Galician overweight/obese and normal-weight individuals. *Nutrients* **2023**, *15*(15), 3418. https://doi.org/10.3390/nu15153418.
10. Martino, E.; D'Onofrio, N.; Balestrieri, A.; Colloca, A.; Anastasio, C.; Sardu, C.; Marfella, R.; Campanille, G.; Balestrieri, M.L. Dietary epigenetic modulators: Unravelling the still-controversial benefits of miRNAs in nutrition and disease. *Nutrients* **2024**, *16*(1), 160. https://doi.org/10.3390/nu16010160.
11. Padhani, Z.A.; Cichon, B.; Das, J.K.; Salam, R.A.; Stobaugh, H.C.; Mughal, M.; Rutishauser-Perera, A.; Black, R.E.; Bhutta, Z.A. Systematic review of management of moderate wasting in children over 6 months of age. *Nutrients* **2023**, *15*(17), 3781. https://doi.org/10.3390/nu15173781.
12. Lopez-Santamarina, A.; Mondragon, A.C.; Cardelle-Cobas, A.; Santos, E.M.; Porto-Arias, J.J.; Cepeda, A.; Miranda, J.M. Effects of unconventional work and shift work on the human gut microbiota and the potential of probiotics to restore dysbiosis. *Nutrients* **2023**, *15*(13), 3070. https://doi.org/10.3390/nu15133070.
13. Nelson, T.D.; Stice, E. Contextualizing the neural vulnerabilities model of obesity. *Nutrients* **2023**, *15*(13), 2988. https://doi.org/10.3390/nu15132988.
14. Ezzatpour, S.; Mondragon Portocarrero, A.D.C.; Cardelle-Cobas, A.; Lamas, A.; López-Santamarina, A.; Miranda, J.M.; Aguilar, H.C. The human gut virome and its relationship with nontransmissible chronic diseases. *Nutrients* **2023**, *15*, 977. https://doi.org/10.3390/nu15040977.

References

1. FAO; WHO. *Sustainable Healthy Diets: Guiding Principles*; FAO: Rome, Italy; WHO: Geneva, Switzerland, 2019. [CrossRef]
2. Ibsen, D.B.; Laursen, A.S.D.; Wuürtz, A.M.L.; Dahm, C.C.; Rimm, E.B.; Partner, E.T.; Overvad, K.; Jakobsen, M.U. Food substitution models for nutritional epidemiology. *Am. J. Clin. Nutr.* **2021**, *113*, 294–303. [CrossRef] [PubMed]
3. Fanzo, J.; Drewnowski, A.; Blumberg, J.; Miller, G.; Kraemer, K.; Kennedy, E. Nutrients, foods, diets, people: Promoting healthy eating. *Curr. Dev. Nutr.* **2020**, *4*, nzaa069. [CrossRef] [PubMed]

4. Burgaz, C.; Gorasso, V.; Achten, W.M.J.; Batis, C.; Castronuovo, L.; Diouf, A.; Asiki, G.; Swinburn, B.A.; Unar-Mungia, M.; Deveesschauwer, B.; et al. The effectiveness of food system policies to improve nutrition, nutrition-related inequalities and environmental sustainability: A scoping review. *Food Policy* **2023**, *15*, 1313–1344. [CrossRef]
5. Kaspar, D.; Hastreiter, S.; Irmler, M.; Hrabé de Angelis, M.; Beckers, J. Nutrition and its role in epigenetic inheritance of obesity and diabetes across generations. *Mamm. Genome* **2020**, *31*, 119–133. [CrossRef] [PubMed]
6. Singh, R.K.; Chang, H.W.; Yan, D.; Lee, K.M.; Ucmak, D.; Wong, K.; Abrouk, M.; Farahnik, B.; Nakamura, M.; Zhu, T.H.; et al. Influence of diet on the gut microbiome and implications for human health. *J. Transl. Med.* **2017**, *15*, 73. [CrossRef] [PubMed]
7. Lopez-Santamarina, A.; Lamas, A.; Mondragon, A.C.; Cardelle-Cobas, A.; Regal, P.; Rodriguez-Avila, J.A.; Miranda, J.M.; Franco, C.M.; Cepeda, A. Probiotic effects against virus infections: New weapons for an old war. *Foods* **2021**, *10*, 130. [CrossRef] [PubMed]
8. Baxi, S.N.; Portnoy, J.M.; Larenas-Linnemann, D.; Phipatanakul, W.; Barnes, C.; Grimes, C.; Horner, W.E.; Kennedy, K.; Levetin, E.; Miller, J.D.; et al. Exposure and health effects of fungi on humans. *J. Allergy Clin. Immunol. Pract.* **2016**, *4*, 396–404. [CrossRef] [PubMed]
9. Dufossé, L.; Fouillaud, M.; Caro, Y. Fungi and fungal metabolites for the improvement of human and animal nutrition and health. *J. Fungi* **2021**, *7*, 274. [CrossRef] [PubMed]
10. Roca-Saavedra, P.; Mendez-Vilabrille, V.; Miranda, J.M.; Nebot, C.; Cardelle-Cobas, A.; Franco, C.M.; Cepeda, A. Food additives, contaminants and other minor components: Effects on human gut microbiota-a review. *J. Physiol. Biochem.* **2018**, *74*, 69–83. [CrossRef] [PubMed]
11. Huang, Y.; Fang, M. Nutritional and environmental contaminant exposure: A tale of two co-existing factors for disease risks. *Environ. Sci. Technol.* **2020**, *54*, 14793–14796. [CrossRef] [PubMed]
12. Sharma, B.M.; Bharat, G.K.; Chakraborty, P.; Martinik, J.; Audy, O.; Kukucka, P.; Pribylová, P.; Kukreti, P.K.; Sharma, A.; Kalina, J.; et al. A comprehensive assessment of endocrine-disrupting chemicals in an Indian food basket: Levels, dietary intakes, and comparison with European data. *Environ. Pollut.* **2021**, *288*, 117750. [CrossRef] [PubMed]
13. Melnik, B.C.; Stremmel, W.; Weiskirchen, R.; John, S.M.; Schmitz, G. Exosome-derived micrornas of human milk and their effects on infant health and development. *Biomolecules* **2021**, *11*, 851. [CrossRef] [PubMed]
14. Lopez-Santamarina, A.; Gonzalez, E.G.; Lamas, A.; Mondragon, A.C.; Regal, P.; Miranda, J.M. Probiotics as a possible strategy for the prevention and treatment of allergies: A narrative review. *Foods* **2021**, *10*, 701. [CrossRef] [PubMed]
15. Zhang, Y.J.; Li, S.; Gan, R.Y.; Zhou, T.; Xu, D.P.; Li, H.B. Impacts of gut bacteria on human health and diseases. *Int. J. Mol. Sci.* **2015**, *16*, 7493–7519. [CrossRef] [PubMed]
16. Chen, Y.; Xu, J.; Chen, Y. Regulation of neurotransmitters by the gut microbiota and effects on cognition in neurological disorders. *Nutrients* **2021**, *13*, 2099. [CrossRef] [PubMed]
17. Panida, S.; Choi, J.; Lee, S.; Lee, Y.K. The function of gut microbiota in immune-related neurological disorders: A review. *J. Neuroinflammation* **2022**, *19*, 154. [CrossRef] [PubMed]

Disclaimer/Publisher's Note: The statements, opinions and data contained in all publications are solely those of the individual author(s) and contributor(s) and not of MDPI and/or the editor(s). MDPI and/or the editor(s) disclaim responsibility for any injury to people or property resulting from any ideas, methods, instructions or products referred to in the content.

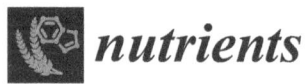

Article

Dietary Provision, GLIM-Defined Malnutrition and Their Association with Clinical Outcome: Results from the First Decade of nutritionDay in China

Bei Zhou [1,2,†], Yupeng Zhang [1,†], Michael Hiesmayr [3], Xuejin Gao [1], Yingchun Huang [1], Sitong Liu [1], Ruting Shen [1], Yang Zhao [4], Yao Cui [5], Li Zhang [1,‡], Xinying Wang [1,*,‡] and on behalf of the nutritionDay Chinese Working Group [§]

1. Department of General Surgery, Jinling Hospital, Medical School of Nanjing University, 305 East Zhongshan Road, Nanjing 210002, China; zhoubei_198@njucm.edu.cn (B.Z.); zhangyupeng@smail.nju.edu.cn (Y.Z.); 522023350251@smail.nju.edu.cn (X.G.)
2. Department of Nutrition, Acupuncture, Moxibustion and Massage College, Health Preservation and Rehabilitation College, Nanjing University of Chinese Medicine, 138 Xianlin Road, Nanjing 210023, China
3. Center for Medical Data Science, Section for Medical Statistics, Medical University Vienna, Spitalgasse 23, A-1090 Vienna, Austria; michael.hiesmayr@meduniwien.ac.at
4. Department of Biostatistics, School of Public Health, Nanjing Medical University, 101 Longmian Avenue, Nanjing 211166, China; yzhao@njmu.edu.cn
5. Department of Nutrition, Pizhou Hospital, Xuzhou Medical University, Xuzhou 221004, China; 760020240003@xzhmu.edu.cn
* Correspondence: wangxinying@nju.edu.cn
† These authors contributed equally to this work.
‡ These authors contributed equally to this work.
§ Membership of the Group Name is provided in the Acknowledgments.

Citation: Zhou, B.; Zhang, Y.; Hiesmayr, M.; Gao, X.; Huang, Y.; Liu, S.; Shen, R.; Zhao, Y.; Cui, Y.; Zhang, L.; et al. Dietary Provision, GLIM-Defined Malnutrition and Their Association with Clinical Outcome: Results from the First Decade of nutritionDay in China. *Nutrients* 2024, 16, 569. https://doi.org/10.3390/nu16040569

Academic Editors: Jose M. Miranda and Miguel Mariscal-Arcas

Received: 4 January 2024
Revised: 4 February 2024
Accepted: 16 February 2024
Published: 19 February 2024

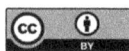

Copyright: © 2024 by the authors. Licensee MDPI, Basel, Switzerland. This article is an open access article distributed under the terms and conditions of the Creative Commons Attribution (CC BY) license (https:// creativecommons.org/licenses/by/ 4.0/).

Abstract: Malnutrition is a common and serious issue that worsens patient outcomes. The effects of dietary provision on the clinical outcomes of patients of different nutritional status needs to be verified. This study aimed to identify dietary provision in patients with eaten quantities of meal consumption and investigate the effects of dietary provision and different nutritional statuses defined by the GLIM criteria on clinical outcomes based on data from the nutritionDay surveys in China. A total of 5821 adult in-patients from 2010 to 2020 were included in this study's descriptive and Cox regression analyses. Rehabilitation and home discharge of 30-day outcomes were considered a good outcome. The prevalence of malnutrition defined by the GLIM criteria was 22.8%. On nutritionDay, 51.8% of all patients received dietary provisions, including hospital food and a special diet. In multivariable models adjusting for other variables, the patients receiving dietary provision had a nearly 1.5 higher chance of a good 30-day outcome than those who did not. Malnourished patients receiving dietary provision had a 1.58 (95% CI [1.36–1.83], $p < 0.001$) higher chance of having a good 30-day outcome and had a shortened length of hospital stay after nutritionDay (median: 7 days, 95% CI [6–8]) compared to those not receiving dietary provision (median: 11 days, 95% CI [10–13]). These results highlight the potential impacts of the dietary provision and nutritional status of in-patients on follow-up outcomes and provide knowledge on implementing targeted nutrition care.

Keywords: dietary provision; GLIM criteria; hospitalized patients; nutritionDay; nutritional status

1. Introduction

Hospital malnutrition has been gaining attention due to its increased incidence. Malnutrition may be related to in-patients' disease stage, economic situation, or other health problems [1–3]. China has participated in the nutritionDay initiative to fight malnutrition in hospital settings since 2010 [4]. nutritionDay is an annual single-day, multinational, cross-sectional audit with 30-day follow-up outcomes [5,6]. With the inspirational global call to action and increasing awareness of malnutrition, the voluntary participation of hospitals in nutritionDay has been expanding. The Chinese nutritionDay Working Group has been established for 10 years and concentrates on real-world studies of in-patients' nutritional status and nutrition intake.

The early identification of malnutrition, followed by timely and appropriate intervention, can significantly improve clinical outcomes and benefit in-patients [1,7,8]. To promote the global use of standardized diagnostic criteria, the Global Leadership Initiative on Malnutrition (GLIM) developed a two-step approach of risk screening and diagnostic assessment to identify malnutrition [9]. The GLIM considered reduced food intake as one of the etiologic criteria for malnutrition. In addition, nutrition intake, including dietary provision and artificial nutrition, is more complicated during nutrition management.

On the one hand, dietary provision is the basis of medical interventions focusing on patients' daily lives [10]. As reported in previous studies, dietary sources of omega-3 fatty acids were recommended instead of supplements in patients with ulcerative colitis [11]; plant-based diets were associated with decreased risk of metabolic syndrome [12,13]; a higher frequency of maternal Mediterranean-style diet was associated with a lower likelihood of neurodevelopmental disabilities in offspring [14]. On the other hand, artificial nutrition should be properly provided to supplement daily metabolic nutrition requirements, particularly in malnourished patients with inadequate dietary intakes [15,16]. However, previous studies on China nutritionDay surveys in single years have highlighted an inappropriate level of nutritional therapy and indicated that patients who needed artificial nutrition were associated with a prolonged length of hospital stay (LOS) [4,17]. Therefore, more attention should be paid to whether adequate food or diet is available in daily nutritional care, especially in malnourished patients. Although the meal consumption of in-patients on nutritionDay was revealed to be negatively associated with mortality [18], evidence on the effect of dietary provision with meal intake is limited [5,18]. Moreover, the effects of dietary provision and different nutritional status on clinical outcomes remain unknown.

Therefore, based on data from the nutritionDay surveys in China, the present study aimed to (1) identify dietary provision in patients with different quantities of meal consumption and (2) investigate the effects of dietary provision and different nutritional statuses defined by the GLIM criteria on clinical outcomes.

2. Materials and Methods

2.1. Study Population

By the end of 2020, 20 Chinese tertiary referral hospitals had participated in the multicenter nutritionDay study. In-hospital patients (excluding patients in the ICU) were prospectively registered for the survey day every November. Patients were excluded if they were under 18 years of age or had missing information on age or the majority of items; participating departments with less than 80% of 30-day outcome records were also excluded (Figure 1). The nutritionDay project was conducted in accordance with the Declaration of Helsinki and approved by the Institutional Review Board (or Ethics Committee) of the Medical University of Vienna (EK407/2005). In accordance with national regulations, this study was also approved by the Ethics Committee of the Jinling Hospital (a Chinese host hospital) and amended annually (approval code 2022DZKY-067-01; date of approval 22 June 2022). All patients provided signed informed consent and were informed of their right to refuse to participate before the survey.

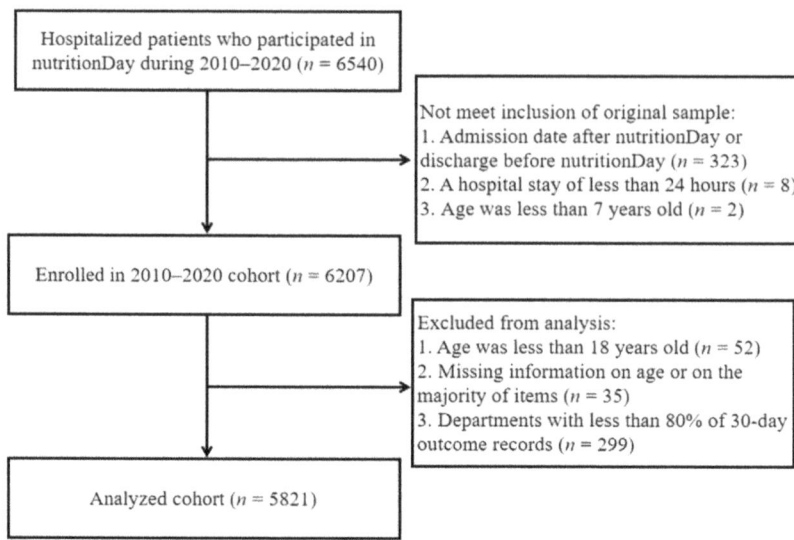

Figure 1. Flowchart describing the selection of study subjects (2010–2020 nutritionDay in China).

2.2. Data Collection

Patient nutritional status and clinical outcomes from 2010 to 2020 were obtained from the nutritionDay dataset of China. Data were collected separately through standardized questionnaires from the nutritionDay website https://www.nutritionday.org/en/-35-.languages/languages.html (accessed on 2 February 2024) for each survey year, categorized into three parts. Part 1 reflected the general situation of the hospital and unit. Part 2 described the patients' characteristics, the clinical information, and the outcome recorded by clinical staff. Part 3 consisted of medical history, nutrition intake, and health status from the patient's perspective. Patients reported their mobility, weight change, food intake history, and meal consumption on nutritionDay, while hospital staff (including caregivers and health care professionals) reported on patient demographics, nutritional provision, and 30-day clinical outcomes. In the present study, nutritional provision was classified as dietary provision (regular hospital food, fortified/enriched hospital food, and special diet), non-dietary provision (protein/energy supplement, enteral nutrition, and parenteral nutrition), as well as multi-form of food and artificial nutrition.

2.3. Nutritional Status Evaluation

Nutritional risk and malnutrition were evaluated through questions regarding weight loss, disease condition, and dietary intake in the nutritionDay questionnaires. Risk screening was assessed using the Malnutrition Universal Screening Tool (MUST) [19], which has been extended to hospital settings because of its validity, as supported by previous studies [20–22]. The MUST score (Supplementary Table S1a) was calculated based on the patient's BMI, weight loss, and acute disease effects. A total MUST score of ≥ 1 is defined as nutritionally at-risk.

Nutritional status was evaluated according to the GLIM criteria [9] for malnutrition. The GLIM system relies on the presence of nutritional risk as the basis for diagnosing malnutrition, including the presence of at least one phenotype (unintentional weight loss, low BMI, or reduced muscle mass) and one etiologic criterion (reduced food intake/assimilation or disease burden/inflammatory condition). In this study, the phenotypic criteria were derived from the patient's weight loss and BMI, and the etiologic criteria were assessed from information about food intake in the week before admission or on the survey day and diagnosis at admission or presence of chronic disease-related comorbidities (Supplementary Table S1b) [23].

2.4. Outcomes

The 30-day outcomes were dichotomized as good or poor according to the outcome codes in the nutritionDay survey. Rehabilitation and home discharge were considered a good outcome, and the remaining outcomes, including still in the hospital, transfer to another hospital, transfer to long-term care, and death, were considered poor outcomes. The LOS before and after the nutritionDay were calculated for each patient. The clinical outcome parameters in this study mainly focused on the good 30-day outcome.

2.5. Statistical Analysis

Patient characteristics were analyzed using descriptive statistics. Continuous variables not normally distributed were expressed as a median with interquartile range (IQR), while categorical variables were expressed as counts and percentages. We used the Wilcoxon rank sum test, Chi-square test, or Fisher's exact tests to compare differences between different groups divided by clinical outcomes or nutritional status where appropriate (Supplementary Tables S2 and S4). Among these, significant variables with $p < 0.05$ and the variables of sex and surgical status [18] were further analyzed to evaluate their association with good 30-day outcomes using Cox regression analysis individually. If significant ($p < 0.05$), these variables were included in three multivariable Cox regression models of dietary provision and malnutrition diagnosis associated with a good 30-day outcome. Model I was used to identify the association between dietary provision and good outcomes, adjusted for departments, survey year, hospital location, sex, BMI, weight change within the last 3 months, major lesion types, comorbidity, food intake in the previous week, eating on nutritionDay, previous ICU stay, mobility, self-rated health, surgical status, LOS before nutritionDay, and number of drugs before admission. Model II was used to identify the association between GLIM-defined malnutrition and good outcome, adjusted for departments, survey year, hospital location, sex, previous ICU stay, mobility, self-rated health, surgical status, LOS before nutritionDay, dietary provision, and the number of drugs before admission. Model III was used to identify the association between malnutrition diagnosis and dietary provision and good outcomes, adjusted for departments, survey year, hospital location, sex, previous ICU stay, mobility, self-rated health, surgical status, LOS before nutritionDay, and the number of drugs before admission. Cumulative incidence curves of good 30-day outcomes were plotted for dietary provision and different nutritional status categories defined by the GLIM criteria. Log-rank tests were used to compare the differences between groups. These results were expressed as median or hazard ratios (HR) with their 95% confidence intervals (CI). Statistical analyses were performed using R version 4.2.1. Statistical significance was set at a p-value < 0.05.

3. Results

3.1. Demographic Characteristics of the Hospitalized Patients

As presented in Table 1, a total of 5821 in-patients from 20 hospitals within various departments were analyzed in this study. Of the total subjects, 40.4% were female, the median age was 58 years (IQR 45–67), and the median BMI was 22.8 kg/m^2 (IQR 20.2–25.2). Approximately 30.9% of all patients were surgical patients. Weight loss in the previous three months was reported by 2246 patients (38.6%). Approximately 19.8% of all patients reported less than half of normal food intake in the previous week. On nutritionDays, dietary provision (in the form of food or diet) was given to 3015 in-patients (51.8%), the majority of whom received hospital food (n = 2699, 46.4%). Screening identified 33.1% of patients who are nutritionally at-risk according to the MUST (MUST score $\geq$ 1, n = 1924), and malnutrition based on the GLIM criteria was diagnosed in 1328 patients (22.8%). The median LOS after nutritionDay was 6 days (IQR 3.0–12.0). A good 30-day outcome, including rehabilitation and home discharge, was recorded in 5093 (87.5%) patients.

Table 1. Demographic data of hospitalized patients, n = 5821.

	Median (IQR) or n (%)
Age, years, median (IQR)	58.0 (45.0–67.0)
Sex [female/male/unknown, n (%)]	2352 (40.4%)/3461 (59.5%)/8 (0.1%)
BMI, kg/m^2, median (IQR)	22.8 (20.2–25.2)
BMI < 18.5 kg/m^2, n (%)	710 (12.2%)
Surgical patients, n (%)	1797 (30.9%)
Weight loss within the last 3 months, n (%)	2246 (38.6%)
Less than half of normal food intake in the previous week, n (%)	1152 (19.8%)
Dietary provision [hospital food/special diet/both, n (%)]	3015 (51.8%)/ 2699 (46.4%)/239 (4.1%)/77 (1.3%)
Full meal eaten on nutritionDay, n (%)	2173 (37.3%)
Full meal not eaten on nutritionDay, n (%)	3372 (57.9%)
Full meal not eaten due to not being allowed to eat, n (%)	968 (16.6%)
Full meal not eaten due to decreased appetite, n (%)	930 (16.0%)
At risk of malnutrition defined by MUST, MUST ≥ 1, n (%)	1924 (33.1%)
Malnutrition defined by GLIM, n (%)	1328 (22.8%)
LOS after nutritionDay, days, median (IQR)	6.0 (3.0–12.0)
Good 30-day outcome, n (%)	5093 (87.5%)

IQR, interquartile range; BMI, body mass index; LOS, length of stay in hospital; MUST, Malnutrition Universal Screening Tool; GLIM, Global Leadership Initiative on Malnutrition.

3.2. Dietary Provision with Meal Consumption on nutritionDay

Notably, the percentage of patients receiving dietary provision and who consumed a meal on nutritionDay were not equivalent: although 51.8% of all in-patients received dietary provision, only 37.3% of patients finished their meals. The main reason for patients eating less or nothing was that they were not allowed to eat (n = 968, 16.6%), followed by decreased appetite (n = 930, 16.0%) (Table 1). Dietary provision, including hospital food (46.4%), special diet (4.1%), and a combination of the two (1.3%), was the main source of nutritional provision for patients, whereas patients without dietary provision mainly received artificial nutrition (23.2%) and nothing else (3.3%). In patients who self-reported eating a full meal, 71.0% received dietary provisions. However, in patients eating nothing but who were allowed to eat, nearly 30% received no dietary provision, which increased to 70.3% in patients eating nothing due to not being allowed to eat (Table 2).

Table 2. Nutritional provision and meal consumption on nutritionDay.

Eating on nutritionDay	n	Type of Nutritional Provision (Row Percentages)						
		Food/Diet			Multi-form of Food and Artificial Nutrition	No Food/Diet		Unsure/Missing
		Hospital food (regular and fortified/enriched hospital food)	Special diet	Multi-form of food and diet		Artificial nutrition [a]	Nothing	
All	5821	46.4%	4.1%	1.3%	10.5%	23.2%	3.3%	11.2%
Eaten all	2173	64.5%	4.8%	1.7%	10.3%	8.2%	2.0%	8.4%
Eaten half	1176	56.5%	5.6%	1.9%	12.9%	12.3%	2.9%	7.8%
Eaten quarter	558	37.8%	6.1%	1.8%	17.2%	26.5%	2.0%	8.6%
Eaten nothing but allowed to eat	721	36.9%	3.6%	1.0%	8.7%	25.2%	4.7%	19.8%
Eaten nothing due to not being allowed to eat	917	9.9%	0.5%	0%	5.1%	63.8%	6.5%	14.1%
Missing data	276	23.2%	1.1%	0%	11.6%	40.6%	2.9%	20.7%

[a] Artificial nutrition includes protein/energy supplements (e.g., ONS drinks), enteral nutrition, and parenteral nutrition.

3.3. GLIM Diagnostic Flow Chart with Dietary Provision and Good 30-Day Outcome

A diagnostic flowchart of the GLIM criteria regarding dietary provision and good 30-day outcomes is presented in Figure 2. In terms of dietary provision, more than half of the non-malnourished patients received food/diet, whereas 41.7% of the malnourished patients did not receive dietary provisions. Furthermore, of the patients with GLIM-defined malnutrition ($n = 1328$, 22.8%), 85.5% of the 455 patients with dietary provision had a good outcome, whereas 72.2% of the 554 patients without dietary provision had a good outcome. In contrast, in the 2249 non-malnourished patients with dietary provision, the frequency of a good outcome increased to 91.9%.

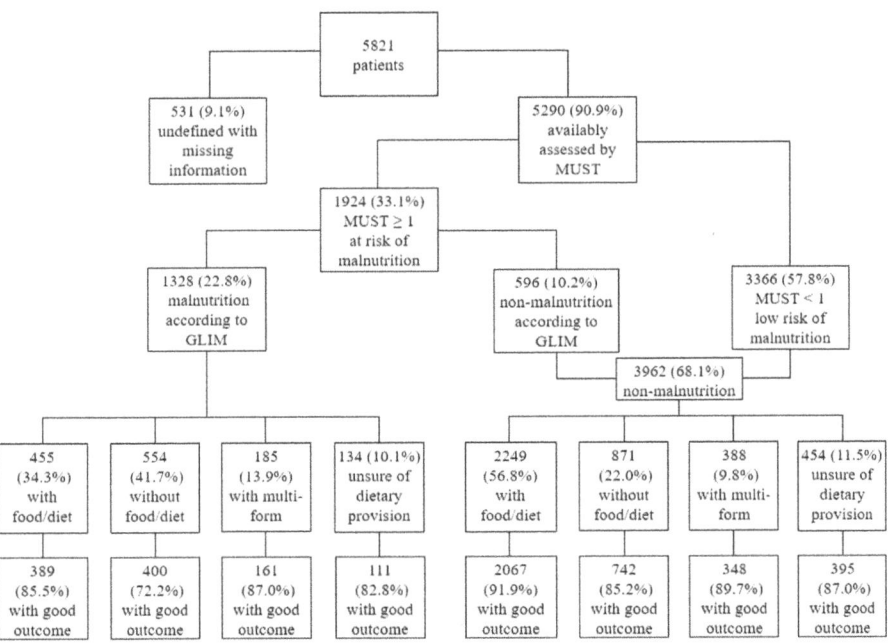

Figure 2. GLIM diagnostic flowchart with dietary provision and good 30-day outcome. MUST, Malnutrition Universal Screening Tool; GLIM, Global Leadership Initiative on Malnutrition.

3.4. Dietary Provision and Malnutrition Diagnosis Associated with Good 30-Day Outcome

Cox regression models were used to determine the association of dietary provision and malnutrition diagnosis with a good 30-day outcome (Table 3). In the univariate analysis shown in Supplementary Table S3, the HR for a good 30-day outcome was 1.55 (95% CI [1.45–1.66], $p < 0.001$) for patients with dietary provision, compared with patients not receiving food/diet. Similar trends between patients with dietary provision and a good 30-day outcome were also found in the multivariable analyses of model I (HR 1.47, 95% CI [1.35–1.60], $p < 0.001$) and model II (HR 1.49, 95% CI [1.38–1.61], $p < 0.001$). Model II revealed a negative relationship between malnutrition defined by the GLIM criteria (HR 0.83, 95% CI [0.77–0.89], $p < 0.001$) and a good 30-day outcome. However, when malnutrition combined with dietary provision was included in model III, it was found that compared with malnourished patients without dietary provision, malnourished patients receiving food/diet (HR 1.58, 95% CI [1.36–1.83], $p < 0.001$), malnourished patients receiving multi-form of food and artificial nutrition (HR 1.34, 95% CI [1.11–1.63], $p = 0.003$), and non-malnourished patients receiving food/diet (HR 1.86, 95% CI [1.64–2.11], $p < 0.001$) were significantly associated with increased good 30-day outcomes.

Table 3. Cox regression models of dietary provision and malnutrition diagnosis associated with good 30-day outcomes.

Variable	Category	Model I HR [95% CI]	Model II (Including GLIM) HR [95% CI]	Model III (Including Malnutrition Diagnosis with Dietary Provision) HR [95% CI]
Dietary provision	No food/diet	Reference	Reference	
	Food/diet	1.47 [1.35–1.60] ***	1.49 [1.38–1.61] ***	
	Multi-form of food and artificial nutrition	1.26 [1.13–1.41] ***	1.29 [1.16–1.43] ***	
	Unsure or missing	1.43 [1.28–1.60] ***	1.44 [1.29–1.61] ***	
Malnutrition defined by GLIM	No		Reference	
	Yes		0.83 [0.77–0.89] ***	
	Undefined		0.97 [0.88–1.08]	
Malnutrition diagnosis with dietary provision	Malnutrition without food/diet			Reference
	Malnutrition with food/diet			1.58 [1.36–1.83] ***
	Malnutrition with multi-form of food and artificial nutrition			1.34 [1.11–1.63] **
	Non-malnutrition without food/diet			1.29 [1.13–1.46] ***
	Non-malnutrition with food/diet			1.86 [1.64–2.11] ***
	Non-malnutrition with multi-form of food and artificial nutrition			1.56 [1.33–1.81] ***

Model I: Multivariable analysis with individual variables included in nutritionDay questionnaires. Model II: GLIM added to multivariable analysis without defined variables, including BMI, age, weight change within the last 3 months, major lesion types, food intake in the previous week, eaten on nutritionDay, and comorbidity. Model III: Malnutrition diagnosis with a dietary provision added to the multivariable analysis. All data are presented as HR and 95% CI. ** $p < 0.01$, *** $p < 0.001$. HR, hazard ratio; CI, confidence interval; LOS, length of stay in hospital; GLIM, Global Leadership Initiative on Malnutrition.

3.5. Cumulative Incidence of Good Outcome within 30 Days after nutritionDay

The good 30-day outcomes in patients with different nutritional status and dietary provisions are visualized using cumulative incidence curves in Figure 3. Patients with malnutrition defined using the GLIM criteria had a median LOS of 8 days after nutritionDay, whereas non-malnourished patients had a median LOS of 6 days after nutritionDay ($p < 0.001$). Similar correlations can be observed for the association between dietary provision and good 30-day outcomes. Moreover, malnourished patients provided with food/diet had a significantly shortened median LOS after nutritionDay compared with those not receiving food/diet (7 days vs. 11 days, $p < 0.001$). Likewise, non-malnourished patients receiving food/diet also had a significantly shortened median LOS after nutritionDay compared with those not receiving dietary provision (5 days vs. 7 days, $p < 0.001$).

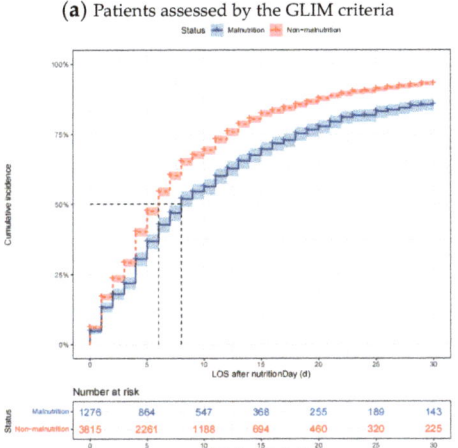
(**a**) Patients assessed by the GLIM criteria

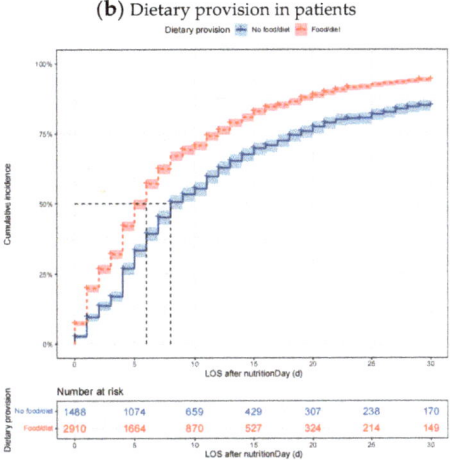
(**b**) Dietary provision in patients

LOS after nutritionDay: median (95% CI)

Malnourished patients vs. Non-malnourished patients: 8 days (8–9) vs. 6 days (6–6), $p < 0.001$.

LOS after nutritionDay: median (95% CI)

Patients without food/diet vs. Patients with food/diet: 8 days (8–9) vs. 6 days (5–6), $p < 0.001$.

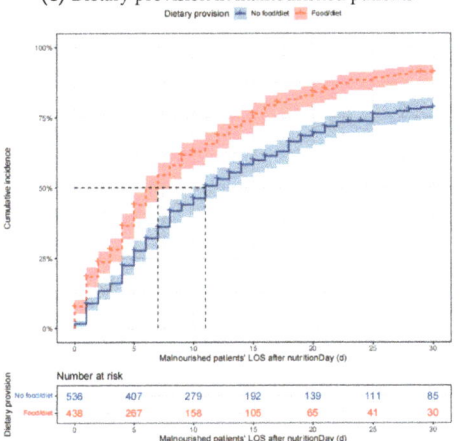
(**c**) Dietary provision in malnourished patients

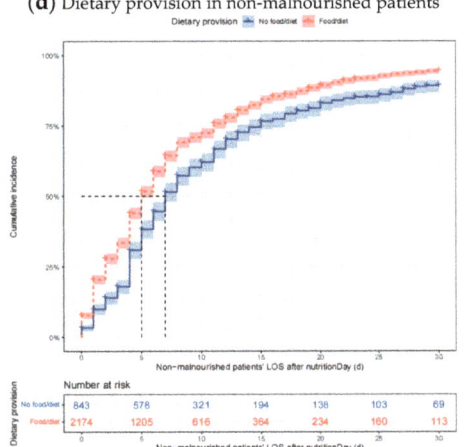
(**d**) Dietary provision in non-malnourished patients

LOS after nutritionDay: median (95% CI)

Malnourished patients without food/diet vs. Malnourished patients with food/diet: 11 days (10–13) vs. 7 days (6–8), $p < 0.001$.

LOS after nutritionDay: median (95% CI)

Non-malnourished patients without food/diet vs. Non-malnourished patients with food/diet: 7 days (7–8) vs. 5 days (5–6), $p < 0.001$.

Figure 3. Cumulative incidence of good outcomes within 30 days after nutritionDay in patients with different nutritional status and dietary provision. Missing data were excluded. Differences in the median LOS after nutritionDay between groups were tested using the log-rank test. Shaded areas indicate 95% CI. LOS, length of stay in hospital; GLIM, Global Leadership Initiative on Malnutrition; CI, confidence interval.

4. Discussion

To our knowledge, this is the first study to focus on the 30-day outcomes of inpatients in association with dietary provision and nutritional status as defined by the GLIM criteria. The results showed that more than half of the patients participating in the Chinese 2010–2020 nutritionDay cohort received dietary provision, especially in patients who reported full meal consumption on nutritionDay. In the multivariable models adjusted for other variables, dietary provision was associated with increased good 30-day outcomes compared to non-dietary provision, even in malnourished patients.

4.1. Dietary Provision with Meal Consumption on nutritionDay

In total, 62.3% of the patients in the Chinese cohort received dietary provisions with any oral diet on nutritionDay compared with 80.9% and 74% in the analyses of Polish results [24] and European data [5], respectively. Moreover, 58% of the patients in Chinese hospitals did not finish their meals, compared with 55% in European hospitals [24]. However, 16.6% of patients who reported eating less in this sample were not allowed to eat, in contrast to 5% of such patients in the European data [24].

The more patients that are allowed to eat and the more dietary provisions administered by hospital staff, the greater number of patients who might at least have some food intake. Among the patients who consumed their full meal on nutritionDay, about 71.0% received dietary provision from hospital food and a special diet, similar to the rate of 75.7% reported in the U.S. [18], but lower than that reported in European hospitals at 84% [5]. The higher rate of dietary provision in Europe might be associated with sustainable nutrition policies and practices [25–27].

Sustainable diets in nutrition policies are reflective of orientation and focus, engagement styles, and modes of leadership [25]. Dietary provision during clinical nutrition management requires careful collaboration across departments and good governance of evidence [28] regarding comparable surveillance data on key indicators and their determinants [26,27]. Evidence-based nutrition policy and approaches to evidence-based practice require the cooperation of nutrition researchers, policymakers, and practitioners to build a flexible scientific framework for dietary provision and monitor dietary intake systems [29].

A cross-sectional study of dietary intakes conducted by Bannerman indicated the need for greater monitoring of patient food consumption [30]. As meal consumption on nutritionDay is considered one of the etiologic criteria in the GLIM criteria assessed from the nutritionDay survey [23], the frequency of dietary provision and clinical outcomes in relation to different nutritional statuses defined by the GLIM criteria are of concern in this study.

4.2. GLIM Diagnostic Flow Chart with Dietary Provision and Good 30-Day Outcome

Nutritional statuses of the 2010–2020 nutritionDay China cohort were systematically evaluated using the GLIM criteria. In the first stage of the malnutrition diagnostic scheme, we found that at least one of every three hospitalized patients was nutritionally at-risk, similar to previous studies in Brazil (32.8%) [31] and Vietnam (30.1%) [32], using the MUST as the risk screening tool. More than 20% of in-patients were defined as malnourished using the GLIM criteria, consistent with a cross-sectional study in elderly in-patients [33] and a reanalysis of a published prospective observational study [34]. However, the lowest frequency of good 30-day outcomes among the clusters of patients was observed in malnourished patients not receiving dietary provision, drawing attention to the association of dietary provision and malnutrition diagnosis with good 30-day outcomes.

4.3. Dietary Provision and Malnutrition Diagnosis Associated with Good 30-Day Outcome

The positive relationship between dietary provision and good 30-day outcomes was consistent in the univariate and multivariable analyses. In the multivariable models adjusting for other variables, patients receiving dietary provision had a nearly 1.5 times higher chance of obtaining a good 30-day outcome compared with those not receiving dietary provision. Dietary provision may, therefore, promote improved clinical outcomes. Moreover, compared with malnourished patients without dietary provision, malnourished and non-malnourished patients receiving dietary provision had a nearly 1.6 to 1.9 higher chance of achieving a good 30-day outcome, highlighting the potential impacts of dietary provision on in-patients. Notably, observational studies such as the nutritionDay surveys mainly show an association between dietary provision and good 30-day outcomes because some unmeasured factors, such as muscle mass and specific laboratory results [35–37], may have improved the prognosis of less severely ill patients who could receive dietary provision. Due to the potential prevention and treatment of dietary interventions on chronic diseases [11–14], hospital staff should take into account the impact of nutrition provision throughout medical care [38,39] on a good prognosis. This consideration could probably affect the nutritional choices of in-patients [40], who could be encouraged to eat meals with dietary provisions during hospitalization [41,42], especially among patients who are allowed to eat.

4.4. Cumulative Incidence of Good Outcome within 30 Days after nutritionDay

In terms of good outcomes, the non-malnourished patients had a significantly shortened median LOS after nutritionDay of 2 days compared with the malnourished patients; a similar trend was observed between the patients receiving and not receiving dietary provision. However, when combined with nutritional status and dietary provision, the malnourished patients receiving dietary provision had a significantly shortened median LOS after nutritionDay of 4 days compared to those not receiving dietary provision. Additionally, the non-malnourished patients receiving dietary provision had a median LOS after nutritionDay of 5 days, which was significantly shorter than the non-malnourished patients not receiving dietary provision. These findings reveal the importance of dietary provision during hospital stays. Tailored dietary provision needs to be delivered precisely while evaluating the nutritional status of in-patients to obtain better clinical outcomes [43]. Hospital staff should keep this in mind and carry it out flexibly as part of the nutrition management process for patients [44], even though they are malnourished with poor meal intake [45]. Specifically, the nutrition education framework should be created for patients, and the availability of a dietary provision practice platform for healthcare professionals should be increased in a benchmarking program designed for nutrition care [46,47].

4.5. Strengths and Limitations

The strengths of this study were that it validated the assessment of malnutrition according to the GLIM criteria using a large number of in-patients from the first decade of nutritionDay surveys in China and determined a relationship between dietary provision and clinical outcomes that can be compared to findings from other studies. However, several limitations in this study need to be noted. Firstly, observational data cannot determine a causal relationship between dietary provision and clinical outcome in a cross-sectional study. Secondly, the evaluations of nutritional status and intervention were based on self-reported data from a single-day cross-snapshot survey and are, therefore, prone to measurement errors due to a lack of periodic monitoring using objective measures, such as muscle mass and laboratory data. Thirdly, this study included participating hospitals that tend to be concerned about nutrition care, which might have introduced selection bias. Fourth, the LOS after nutritionDay in this study was calculated and analyzed instead of total LOS due to its length bias [6]. Fifth, we dichotomized the 30-day outcomes instead of one of the specific outcomes in the nutritionDay survey. Additionally, the 30-day clinical outcomes were limited. Further research on patients' nutritional status would be worthwhile, including more body composition information and biochemical evaluations with long-term follow-up.

5. Conclusions

The results from nutritionDay surveys conducted in China from 2010 to 2020 provide evidence on dietary provision and GLIM-defined malnutrition associated with the 30-day clinical outcomes of in-patients. The results indicate a higher dietary provision in patients who consumed a full meal on nutritionDay. Importantly, dietary provision was associated with increased good 30-day outcomes compared to non-dietary provision, even in patients defined as malnourished according to the GLIM criteria. These results highlight the potential impacts of the dietary provision and nutritional status of in-patients on follow-up outcomes. Further nutrition care campaigns targeting specific dietary interventions are needed to translate this knowledge into action.

Supplementary Materials: The following supporting information can be downloaded at: https://www.mdpi.com/article/10.3390/nu16040569/s1, Table S1: Nutritional status evaluation for nutritionDay 2010–2020 China survey; Table S2: Variables and median LOS after nutritionDay in patients between 30-day poor outcomes and good outcomes; Table S3: Cox regression analysis of 30-day good outcome; Table S4: Demographic characteristics in malnourished patients and non-malnourished patients.

Author Contributions: Conceptualization, X.W., M.H., L.Z. and B.Z.; methodology, X.W. and M.H.; validation, L.Z., Y.Z. (Yupeng Zhang) and B.Z.; formal analysis, X.W., Y.Z. (Yang Zhao) and M.H.; investigation, Y.Z. (Yupeng Zhang), X.G., Y.H., S.L., R.S., Y.C. and The nutritionDay Chinese Working Group; data curation, L.Z., Y.Z. (Yang Zhao) and B.Z.; writing—original draft preparation, B.Z.; writing—review and editing, X.W., M.H., L.Z., Y.Z. (Yang Zhao), Y.Z. (Yupeng Zhang) and B.Z.; visualization, B.Z., Y.Z. (Yang Zhao) and M.H.; supervision, X.W.; project administration, L.Z.; funding acquisition, X.W. All authors have read and agreed to the published version of the manuscript.

Funding: This research was funded by the National Science and Technology Research Funding for Public Welfare Medical Projects (201502022), the National Natural Science Foundation of China (81770531, 82170575), the Science Foundation of Outstanding Youth in Jiangsu Province (BK20170009) and "The 13th Five-Year Plan" Foundation of Jiangsu Province for Medical Key Talents (ZDRCA2016091 Jiangsu Province science and technology program social development-Clinical frontier technology project (BE2022822).

Institutional Review Board Statement: The nutritionDay project was conducted in accordance with the Declaration of Helsinki and approved by the Institutional Review Board (or Ethics Committee) of the Medical University of Vienna (EK407/2005). In accordance with national regulations, this study was also approved by the Ethics Committee of the Jinling Hospital (a Chinese host hospital) and amended annually (approval code 2022DZKY-067-01; date of approval 22 June 2022).

Informed Consent Statement: Informed consent was obtained from all subjects involved in the study.

Data Availability Statement: The raw data supporting the conclusions of this article will be made available by the authors on request. The data are not publicly available as the authors are currently engaged in further exploration and analysis of these data, and hence have chosen not to disclose them publicly at this stage.

Acknowledgments: The authors thank the European Society of Clinical Nutrition and Metabolism (ESPEN) and the Medical University of Vienna for supporting the nutritionDay project. We gratefully acknowledge the nutritionDay International Office and all the members of the nutritionDay Chinese Working Group: Wei Zhou, Lianzhen Chen, Xiaojie Bian, Hengfang Zhao, Xiaolan Zhang, Junying Nie, Jielian Xu, Guifang Deng, Xiaosun Liu, Feng Tian, Xue Jing, Xuqi Li, Wei Chen, Shuli Guo, Leilei Wang, Yinghua Liu, Xianghua Wu, Yongmei Shi, and Yanjin Chen. We thank the cooperation of all centers, hospital staff, and patients participating in the nutritionDay surveys throughout the years.

Conflicts of Interest: The authors declare no conflicts of interest. The funders had no role in the design of the study; in the collection, analyses, or interpretation of data; in the writing of the manuscript; or in the decision to publish the results.

References

1. Schuetz, P.; Seres, D.; Lobo, D.N.; Gomes, F.; Kaegi-Braun, N.; Stanga, Z. Management of disease-related malnutrition for patients being treated in hospital. *Lancet* **2021**, *398*, 1927–1938. [CrossRef]
2. Cass, A.R.; Charlton, K.E. Prevalence of hospital-acquired malnutrition and modifiable determinants of nutritional deterioration during inpatient admissions: A systematic review of the evidence. *J. Hum. Nutr. Diet* **2022**, *35*, 1043–1058. [CrossRef]
3. Steiber, A.; Hegazi, R.; Herrera, M.; Zamor, M.L.; Chimanya, K.; Pekcan, A.G.; Redondo-Samin, D.C.; Correia, M.I.; Ojwang, A.A. Spotlight on Global Malnutrition: A Continuing Challenge in the 21st Century. *J. Acad. Nutr. Diet* **2015**, *115*, 1335–1341. [CrossRef] [PubMed]
4. Zhang, L.; Wang, X.; Huang, Y.; Gao, Y.; Peng, N.; Zhu, W.; Li, N.; Li, J. NutritionDay 2010 audit in Jinling hospital of China. *Asia Pac. J. Clin. Nutr.* **2013**, *22*, 206–213.

5. Hiesmayr, M.; Schindler, K.; Pernicka, E.; Schuh, C.; Schoeniger-Hekele, A.; Bauer, P.; Laviano, A.; Lovell, A.D.; Mouhieddine, M.; Schuetz, T.; et al. Decreased food intake is a risk factor for mortality in hospitalised patients: The NutritionDay survey 2006. *Clin. Nutr.* **2009**, *28*, 484–491. [CrossRef] [PubMed]
6. Frantal, S.; Pernicka, E.; Hiesmayr, M.; Schindler, K.; Bauer, P. Length bias correction in one-day cross-sectional assessments—The NutritionDay study. *Clin. Nutr.* **2016**, *35*, 522–527. [CrossRef] [PubMed]
7. Barker, L.A.; Gout, B.S.; Crow, T.C. Hospital malnutrition: Prevalence, identification and impact on patients and the healthcare system. *Int. J. Environ. Res. Public Health* **2011**, *8*, 514–527. [CrossRef]
8. Jensen, G.L.; Compher, C.; Sullivan, D.H.; Mullin, G.E. Recognizing malnutrition in adults: Definitions and characteristics, screening, assessment, and team approach. *J. Parenter. Enter. Nutr.* **2013**, *37*, 802–807. [CrossRef] [PubMed]
9. Cederholm, T.; Jensen, G.L.; Correia, M.I.T.D.; Gonzalez, M.C.; Fukushima, R.; Higashiguchi, T.; Baptista, G.; Barazzoni, R.; Blaauw, R.; Coats, A.; et al. GLIM criteria for the diagnosis of malnutrition—A consensus report from the global clinical nutrition community. *Clin. Nutr.* **2019**, *38*, 1–9. [CrossRef]
10. Volpp, K.G.; Berkowitz, S.A.; Sharma, S.V.; Anderson, C.A.M.; Brewer, L.C.; Elkind, M.S.V.; Gardner, C.D.; Gervis, J.E.; Harrington, R.A.; Herrero, M.; et al. Food Is Medicine: A Presidential Advisory from the American Heart Association. *Circulation* **2023**, *148*, 1417–1439. [CrossRef]
11. Reznikov, E.A.; Suskind, D.L. Current Nutritional Therapies in Inflammatory Bowel Disease: Improving Clinical Remission Rates and Sustainability of Long-Term Dietary Therapies. *Nutrients* **2023**, *15*, 668. [CrossRef]
12. Castro-Barquero, S.; Ruiz-León, A.M.; Sierra-Pérez, M.; Estruch, R.; Casas, R. Dietary Strategies for Metabolic Syndrome: A Comprehensive Review. *Nutrients* **2020**, *12*, 2983. [CrossRef]
13. Kahleova, H.; Levin, S.; Barnard, N. Cardio-Metabolic Benefits of Plant-Based Diets. *Nutrients* **2017**, *9*, 848. [CrossRef] [PubMed]
14. Che, X.; Gross, S.M.; Wang, G.; Hong, X.; Pearson, C.; Bartell, T.; Wang, X. Impact of consuming a Mediterranean-style diet during pregnancy on neurodevelopmental disabilities in offspring: Results from the Boston Birth Cohort. *Precis. Nutr.* **2023**, *2*, e00047.
15. Lesser, M.N.R.; Lesser, L.I. Nutrition Support Therapy. *Am. Fam. Physician* **2021**, *104*, 580–588.
16. Kaegi-Braun, N.; Mueller, M.; Schuetz, P.; Mueller, B.; Kutz, A. Evaluation of Nutritional Support and In-Hospital Mortality in Patients With Malnutrition. *JAMA Netw. Open* **2021**, *4*, e2033433. [CrossRef]
17. Sun, H.; Zhang, L.; Zhang, P.; Yu, J.; Kang, W.; Guo, S.; Chen, W.; Li, X.; Wang, S.; Chen, L.; et al. A comprehensive nutritional survey of hospitalized patients: Results from nutritionDay 2016 in China. *PLoS ONE* **2018**, *13*, e0194312. [CrossRef]
18. Sauer, A.C.; Goates, S.; Malone, A.; Mogensen, K.M.; Gewirtz, G.; Sulz, I.; Moick, S.; Laviano, A.; Hiesmayr, M. Prevalence of Malnutrition Risk and the Impact of Nutrition Risk on Hospital Outcomes: Results from NutritionDay in the U.S. *J. Parenter. Enter. Nutr.* **2019**, *43*, 918–926. [CrossRef] [PubMed]
19. Stratton, R.J.; Hackston, A.; Longmore, D.; Dixon, R.; Price, S.; Stroud, M.; King, C.; Elia, M. Malnutrition in hospital outpatients and inpatients: Prevalence, concurrent validity and ease of use of the 'malnutrition universal screening tool' ('MUST') for adults. *Br. J. Nutr.* **2004**, *92*, 799–808. [CrossRef] [PubMed]
20. Rabito, E.I.; Marcadenti, A.; da Silva Fink, J.; Figueira, L.; Silva, F.M. Nutritional Risk Screening 2002, Short Nutritional Assessment Questionnaire, malnutrition screening tool, and malnutrition universal screening tool are good predictors of nutrition risk in an emergency service. *Nutr. Clin. Pract.* **2017**, *32*, 526–532. [CrossRef]
21. Kruizenga, H.; van Keeken, S.; Weijs, P.; Bastiaanse, L.; Beijer, S.; Huisman-de Waal, G.; Jager-Wittenaar, H.; Jonkers-Schuitema, C.; Klos, M.; Remijnse-Meester, W.; et al. Undernutrition screening survey in 564,063 patients: Patients with a positive undernutrition screening score stay in hospital 1.4 d longer. *Am. J. Clin. Nutr.* **2016**, *103*, 1026–1032. [CrossRef]
22. Wang, M.; Guo, Q.; Liu, H.; Liu, M.; Tang, C.; Wu, J.; Feng, G.; Wu, W. GLIM criteria using NRS-2002 and MUST as the first step adequately diagnose the malnutrition in Crohn's disease inpatients: A retrospective study. *Front. Nutr.* **2023**, *9*, 1059191. [CrossRef]
23. Moick, S.; Hiesmayr, M.; Mouhieddine, M.; Kiss, N.; Bauer, P.; Sulz, I.; Singer, P.; Simon, J. Reducing the knowledge to action gap in hospital nutrition care—Developing and implementing NutritionDay 2.0. *Clin. Nutr.* **2021**, *40*, 936–945. [CrossRef]
24. Ostrowska, J.; Sulz, I.; Tarantino, S.; Hiesmayr, M.; Szostak-Węgierek, D. Hospital Malnutrition, Nutritional Risk Factors, and Elements of Nutritional Care in Europe: Comparison of Polish Results with All European Countries Participating in the nDay Survey. *Nutrients* **2021**, *13*, 263. [CrossRef]
25. Lang, T.; Mason, P. Sustainable diet policy development: Implications of multi-criteria and other approaches, 2008–2017. *Proc. Nutr. Soc.* **2018**, *77*, 331–346. [CrossRef] [PubMed]
26. Garnica Rosas, L.; Mensink, G.B.M.; Finger, J.D.; Schienkiewitz, A.; Do, S.; Wolters, M.; Stanley, I.; Abu Omar, K.; Wieczorowska-Tobis, K.; Woods, C.B.; et al. Selection of key indicators for European policy monitoring and surveillance for dietary behaviour, physical activity and sedentary behaviour. *Int. J. Behav. Nutr. Phys. Act.* **2021**, *18*, 48. [CrossRef] [PubMed]
27. Fismen, A.S.; Mathisen, J.R.; Vlad, I.; Oldridge-Turner, K.; O'Mara, J.; Klepp, K.I.; Brinsden, H.; Rutter, H.; Kokkorou, M.; Helleve, A. Pilot test of the NOURISHING policy index-Assessing governmental nutrition policies in five European countries. *Obes. Rev.* **2023**, *24* (Suppl. S1), e13532. [CrossRef]
28. Weldon, I.; Parkhurst, J. Governing evidence use in the nutrition policy process: Evidence and lessons from the 2020 Canada food guide. *Nutr. Rev.* **2022**, *80*, 467–478. [CrossRef]
29. Neale, E.P.; Tapsell, L.C. Perspective: The Evidence-Based Framework in Nutrition and Dietetics: Implementation, Challenges, and Future Directions. *Adv. Nutr.* **2019**, *10*, 1–8. [CrossRef] [PubMed]

30. Bannerman, E.; Cantwell, L.; Gaff, L.; Conroy, A.; Davidson, I.; Jones, J. Dietary intakes in geriatric orthopaedic rehabilitation patients: Need to look at food consumption not just provision. *Clin. Nutr.* **2016**, *35*, 892–899. [CrossRef]
31. Lima, J.; Brizola Dias, A.J.; Burgel, C.F.; Bernardes, S.; Gonzalez, M.C.; Silva, F.M. Complementarity of nutritional screening tools to GLIM criteria on malnutrition diagnosis in hospitalised patients: A secondary analysis of a longitudinal study. *Clin. Nutr.* **2022**, *41*, 2325–2332. [CrossRef] [PubMed]
32. Tran, Q.C.; Banks, M.; Hannan-Jones, M.; Do, T.N.D.; Gallegos, D. Validity of four nutritional screening tools against subjective global assessment for inpatient adults in a low-middle income country in Asia. *Eur. J. Clin. Nutr.* **2018**, *72*, 979–985. [CrossRef] [PubMed]
33. Xu, J.Y.; Zhu, M.W.; Zhang, H.; Li, L.; Tang, P.X.; Chen, W.; Wei, J.M. A Cross-Sectional Study of GLIM-Defined Malnutrition Based on New Validated Calf Circumference Cut-off Values and Different Screening Tools in Hospitalised Patients over 70 Years Old. *J. Nutr. Health Aging* **2020**, *24*, 832–838. [CrossRef] [PubMed]
34. Xu, J.Y.; Zhang, X.N.; Jiang, Z.M.; Jie, B.; Wang, Y.; Li, W.; Kondrup, J.; Nolan, M.T.; Andrews, M.; Kang, W.M.; et al. Nutritional support therapy after GLIM criteria may neglect the benefit of reducing infection complications compared with NRS2002: Reanalysis of a cohort study. *Nutrition* **2020**, *79–80*, 110802. [CrossRef] [PubMed]
35. Groothof, D.; Post, A.; Polinder-Bos, H.A.; Hazenberg, B.P.C.; Gans, R.O.B.; Bakker, S.J.L. Muscle mass versus body mass index as predictor of adverse outcome. *J. Cachexia Sarcopenia Muscle* **2021**, *12*, 517–518. [CrossRef] [PubMed]
36. Yugawa, K.; Itoh, S.; Kurihara, T.; Yoshiya, S.; Mano, Y.; Takeishi, K.; Harada, N.; Ikegami, T.; Soejima, Y.; Mori, M.; et al. Skeletal muscle mass predicts the prognosis of patients with intrahepatic cholangiocarcinoma. *Am. J. Surg.* **2019**, *218*, 952–958. [CrossRef] [PubMed]
37. De Giorgi, A.; Marra, A.M.; Iacoviello, M.; Triggiani, V.; Rengo, G.; Cacciatore, F.; Maiello, C.; Limongelli, G.; Masarone, D.; Perticone, F.; et al. Insulin-like growth factor-1 (IGF-1) as predictor of cardiovascular mortality in heart failure patients: Data from the T.O.S.CA. registry. *Intern. Emerg. Med.* **2022**, *17*, 1651–1660. [CrossRef]
38. Thibault, R.; Abbasoglu, O.; Ioannou, E.; Meija, L.; Ottens-Oussoren, K.; Pichard, C.; Rothenberg, E.; Rubin, D.; Siljamäki-Ojansuu, U.; Vaillant, M.F.; et al. ESPEN guideline on hospital nutrition. *Clin. Nutr.* **2021**, *40*, 5684–5709. [CrossRef]
39. Ridley, E.J.; Chapple, L.S.; Chapman, M.J. Nutrition intake in the post-ICU hospitalization period. *Curr. Opin. Clin. Nutr. Metab. Care* **2020**, *23*, 111–115. [CrossRef]
40. Coghlan, B.; Coghlan, S.; Wilson, A. Nutrition education fit for modern health systems. *Lancet* **2019**, *394*, 2071. [CrossRef]
41. van den Berg, G.H.; Huisman-de Waal, G.G.J.; Vermeulen, H.; de van der Schueren, M.A.E. Effects of nursing nutrition interventions on outcomes in malnourished hospital inpatients and nursing home residents: A systematic review. *Int. J. Nurs. Stud.* **2021**, *117*, 103888. [CrossRef]
42. Roberts, H.C.; Pilgrim, A.L.; Jameson, K.A.; Cooper, C.; Sayer, A.A.; Robinson, S. The Impact of Trained Volunteer Mealtime Assistants on the Dietary Intake of Older Female In-Patients: The Southampton Mealtime Assistance Study. *J. Nutr. Health Aging* **2017**, *21*, 320–328. [CrossRef]
43. Downer, S.; Berkowitz, S.A.; Harlan, T.S.; Olstad, D.L.; Mozaffarian, D. Food is medicine: Actions to integrate food and nutrition into healthcare. *BMJ* **2020**, *369*, m2482. [CrossRef]
44. Laur, C.; McCullough, J.; Davidson, B.; Keller, H. Becoming Food Aware in Hospital: A Narrative Review to Advance the Culture of Nutrition Care in Hospitals. *Healthcare* **2015**, *3*, 393–407. [CrossRef]
45. Agarwal, E.; Ferguson, M.; Banks, M.; Vivanti, A.; Batterham, M.; Bauer, J.; Capra, S.; Isenring, E. Malnutrition, poor food intake, and adverse healthcare outcomes in non-critically ill obese acute care hospital patients. *Clin. Nutr.* **2019**, *38*, 759–766. [CrossRef] [PubMed]
46. Khoury, T.; Ilan, Y. Platform introducing individually tailored variability in nerve stimulations and dietary regimen to prevent weight regain following weight loss in patients with obesity. *Obes. Res. Clin. Pract.* **2021**, *15*, 114–123. [CrossRef] [PubMed]
47. Carino, S.; Collins, J.; Malekpour, S.; Porter, J. Harnessing the pillars of institutions to drive environmentally sustainable hospital foodservices. *Front. Nutr.* **2022**, *9*, 905932. [CrossRef] [PubMed]

Disclaimer/Publisher's Note: The statements, opinions and data contained in all publications are solely those of the individual author(s) and contributor(s) and not of MDPI and/or the editor(s). MDPI and/or the editor(s) disclaim responsibility for any injury to people or property resulting from any ideas, methods, instructions or products referred to in the content.

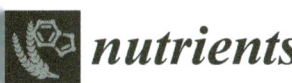 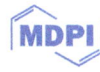

Article

Different Dimensions of the Home Food Environment May Be Associated with the Body Mass Index of Older Adults: A Cross-Sectional Survey Conducted in Beijing, China

Man Zhang [1], Ruixin Chi [2], Zhenhui Li [2], Yujie Fang [2], Na Zhang [2,3], Qiaoqin Wan [1,*] and Guansheng Ma [2,3,*]

1. School of Nursing, Peking University, 38 Xue Yuan Road, Haidian District, Beijing 100191, China; zhangman@bjmu.edu.cn
2. Department of Nutrition and Food Hygiene, School of Public Health, Peking University, 38 Xue Yuan Road, Haidian District, Beijing 100191, China; crx@bjmu.edu.cn (R.C.)
3. Laboratory of Toxicological Research and Risk Assessment for Food Safety, Peking University, 38 Xue Yuan Road, Haidian District, Beijing 100191, China
* Correspondence: qiaoqinwan@bjmu.edu.cn (Q.W.); mags@bjmu.edu.cn (G.M.)

Citation: Zhang, M.; Chi, R.; Li, Z.; Fang, Y.; Zhang, N.; Wan, Q.; Ma, G. Different Dimensions of the Home Food Environment May Be Associated with the Body Mass Index of Older Adults: A Cross-Sectional Survey Conducted in Beijing, China. *Nutrients* **2024**, *16*, 289. https://doi.org/10.3390/nu16020289

Academic Editor: Jose M. Miranda

Received: 27 November 2023
Revised: 9 January 2024
Accepted: 12 January 2024
Published: 18 January 2024

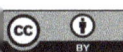

Copyright: © 2024 by the authors. Licensee MDPI, Basel, Switzerland. This article is an open access article distributed under the terms and conditions of the Creative Commons Attribution (CC BY) license (https://creativecommons.org/licenses/by/4.0/).

Abstract: Objective: The objective of this study was to evaluate the home food environment of the elderly in Beijing and analyze its association with the body mass index (BMI) of the elderly, as well as to provide recommendations for improving the home food environment for the elderly. Methods: This study was conducted in Beijing, China, in 2019. The participants were 1764 elderly individuals aged 65 to 80, recruited from 12 communities through a multistage stratified random sampling method. The study involved the use of questionnaire surveys to gather data on participants' demographics, the availability of various foods in their households, and their living conditions. Socioeconomic status (SES) was evaluated based on their educational level, occupation, and income level. Height and weight measurements were taken to calculate BMI. We conducted both univariate analysis and multiple linear regression analysis to evaluate the relationship between the home food environment and BMI. Results: A total of 1800 questionnaires were distributed, of which 1775 were retrieved, resulting in a questionnaire recovery rate of 98.6%. Among these, 1764 questionnaires were deemed valid, corresponding to a questionnaire validity rate of 99.4%. The participants had a mean age of 69.7 ± 4.3 years old, over 40% of whom were overweight or obese. In terms of low-energy/high-nutrient-density foods, the most readily available items were fresh vegetables (95.6%), followed by coarse grains (94.1%), fresh fruits (90.4%), and dairy products (83.6%). Among high-energy/low-nutrient-density foods, preserved foods were the most available (51.9%), followed by salted snacks (40.6%), sugary beverages (28.2%), and fried foods (9.4%). Approximately 7.3% of participants lived alone. Elderly individuals with higher SES had a lower BMI compared to those with medium to low SES (25.9 vs. 26.5, 25.9 vs. 26.4, $p < 0.05$). Those living alone had a higher BMI than those who did not (27.2 vs. 26.2, $p = 0.001$). After controlling for potential confounding variables, older adults with high SES exhibited a BMI reduction of 0.356 kg/m^2 ($p = 0.001$), whereas those living alone exhibited an increase in BMI of 1.155 kg/m^2 ($p < 0.001$). The presence of preserved foods at home was linked to a BMI increase of 0.442 kg/m^2 ($p = 0.008$). Conclusion: This study underscores the significant impact of family SES, living conditions, and the availability of preserved foods on the BMI of elderly individuals.

Keywords: home food environment; body mass index; BMI; older adults

1. Introduction

The world is experiencing a rapid aging phenomenon compared to the past. China transitioned into an aging society in 2000 and currently hosts the largest population of older adults (aged 60 and above) worldwide [1]. The population of individuals aged 65 and above in China had reached 210 million by the end of 2022, accounting for 13.5% of the total population [2]. As the population ages, China has undergone a significant epidemiological shift from infectious diseases to non-communicable diseases (NCDs). Overweight and obesity are closely linked to increased morbidity from NCDs and cardiovascular disease mortality [3]. In recent decades, Chinese residents have undergone a dietary transition characterized by a move towards a diet rich in fats and energy but low in fiber [4]. Concurrently, the issues of overweight and obesity have come to the forefront. Based on the "Report on the Nutrition and Chronic Disease Status of Chinese Residents (2020)", the rate of overweight individuals aged 60 and above increased from 31.9% in 2012 to 36.6% in 2018, and the obesity rate rose from 11.6% to 13.6% [5].

The occurrence and development of obesity are influenced by various factors, including genetic factors, dietary factors, environmental factors, etc. Among these factors, the food environment, as one of the significant influencing factors of obesity, has received increasing attention [6,7]. An ecological framework that illustrates the food environment encompasses individual-level factors, the social environment, the physical surroundings, and macro-level factors [8]. Given that people primarily store and consume food at home, numerous factors within the home food environment have been correlated with dietary behaviors and weight status. Globally, significant evidence has highlighted the associations between the home food environment and body mass index (BMI). However, there is currently no unified concept of the home food environment [9]. Richard R. divides the home food environment into three dimensions: political and economic environments, sociocultural environments, and built and natural environments [10]. As per the ANGELO framework, the obesogenic home environment comprises four dimensions: physical, economic, political, and sociocultural dimensions [11].

Researchers have extensively focused on the physical environment in the home, namely, the availability of food as the primary aspect of the home food environment [12]. While many of these investigations have centered on children, a few have concentrated on adults [12–15]. A study conducted among American adults revealed that a more diverse availability of fruits and vegetables was linked to lower odds of overweight/obesity [12]. Emery reported that homes of obese individuals had a lower availability of healthy food options in comparison to homes of non-obese individuals [13]. Gorin's research similarly revealed that overweight adults had a reduced presence of low-fat snacks and fruits/vegetables but an increased presence of high-fat snacks compared to those with normal weight [14]. In the case of overweight and obese women, the quantity of unhealthy foods within the household was linked to the percentage of calories derived from fat [15]. Home food availability can serve as an effective target for interventions aimed at addressing overweight and obesity.

Socioeconomic status (SES) also has an influence on obesity. A meta-analysis primarily derived from studies conducted in developed countries revealed a correlation between SES and obesity in the female population [16]. In countries with low and middle incomes, individuals with higher SES are more likely to experience obesity [17]. Notably, none of the studies mentioned above were centered on the Chinese population. An investigation targeting Chinese children suggested a potential positive correlation between high SES and childhood obesity [18]. Furthermore, numerous other facets of the home food environment exhibit associations with obesity, including family size and structure, family members dining together, and household dining rules [8,19]. However, there is limited research focusing on these factors.

Currently, most studies in this area are centered on developed countries, with limited studies conducted in China. The distinctive social and cultural context in China may exert different effects on the correlation between the home food environment and the prevalence of overweight and obesity, highlighting the need for more China-specific research to bridge this knowledge gap. The influence of the home food environment may vary significantly based on the dietary habits of specific subgroups. Given the reduced mobility of older adults, their dietary habits and weight status might be more heavily influenced by their home food environment. While most studies have concentrated on children, research on older adults in this regard is notably scarce. Given the increasingly pressing aging demographic in China, prioritizing the health status of elderly individuals is of paramount importance. The incompleteness of current findings, along with the absence of Chinese-specific and older-adult-focused evidence, underscores the necessity for additional research.

In this study, we aimed to comprehensively characterize the home food environment across three dimensions and analyze its association with BMI in the elderly population. Ultimately, our goal was to provide insights and recommendations for the enhancement of the home food environment, thereby improving the health of the elderly.

2. Materials and Methods

2.1. Study Design

Our study employed a cross-sectional design, encompassing both urban and suburban areas of Beijing, China.

2.2. Participants

The participants were from a 2019 cross-sectional survey that focused on the dietary behaviors and factors influencing older adults. The recruitment of participants took place across 12 communities spanning 3 districts in Beijing. A total of 1800 questionnaires were distributed, with participant numbers ranging from 117 to 181 individuals per community. Participants included in the analysis met the criteria of providing complete information on age and gender, in addition to undergoing accurate height and weight measurements. Among these, 1775 were retrieved, resulting in a questionnaire recovery rate of 98.6%. In total, 1764 questionnaires were deemed valid, yielding a questionnaire efficiency rate of 99.4%.

Inclusion criteria for the study encompassed individuals who were between 65 and 80 years old, retired from employment, residing within a single community for at least two years, and functionally independent. Individuals unable to consume food normally and those with cognitive impairment were excluded from the study.

2.3. Sample

2.3.1. Sampling Method

We utilized a multistage stratified random sampling approach. Initially, the survey targeted three districts: Haidian, Shunyi, and Miyun. These districts were selected to represent varying economic statuses and geographical locations within Beijing. Haidian District, positioned in close proximity to Beijing's city center, exhibited the highest level of economic development, succeeded by Shunyi District and, finally, Miyun District. Subsequently, in each district, one urban street and one suburban street were chosen. Following this, two communities within each selected street were identified for study inclusion. Finally, a random selection of older adults residing in each of the chosen communities participated in the survey.

2.3.2. Sample Size Calculation

For sample size calculation, we utilized the obesity rate among older adults in China from previous studies [20,21]. The sample size was determined using the formula $N = Z_{1-\alpha/2}^2 \, p(1-p)/e^2$, where we set $\alpha = 0.05$, $Z_{1-\alpha/2} = 1.96$, and $e = 0.03$. The parameter p denotes the estimated obesity rate among the elderly population in China, which is 0.15.

Considering that we investigated three districts and accounting for a 10% anticipated dropout rate, the determined final sample size for validity was 1800 elderly participants.

2.4. Ethical Review

The study protocol underwent a thorough review and received approval from the Peking University Biomedical Ethics Committee (approval code: IRB00001052-17112). Adherence to the principles outlined in the Declaration of Helsinki was ensured throughout the study. Prior to their participation, all participants were furnished with an informed consent form, and their voluntary commitment to engage in the study was obtained through the act of signing the document. Subsequently, the researchers securely retained the written informed consent from each participant.

2.5. Measurements

2.5.1. Participants' Basic Information

Participant information was gathered via questionnaires, encompassing fundamental details including address; gender; age; educational level; marital status; income; living conditions; occupation; and habits related to exercise, smoking, and drinking. Please refer to Supplementary S1 for the specific content of the questionnaire. The questionnaire was completed individually, with the investigator and each participant filling it out in person.

The economic status of the community was determined based on the address participants filled out in the questionnaire and by querying the Beijing Statistical Zoning Code and Urban Rural Classification Code (2018 Edition) [22]. In this document, all communities in Beijing are coded. The code 111 represents urban areas, 112 represents suburban areas, and 200 represents rural areas. In this study, all communities originated from urban and suburban areas.

2.5.2. Home Food Availability

The questionnaire employed to assess home food availability was derived from a previously published tool [23] and modified based on the results of expert consultation. In this study, a list of eight food items was provided and categorized into two groups based on their nutritional value and caloric density [19]. Among these, four are low-energy/high-nutrient-density foods, which are recommended for sufficient intake in the Dietary Guidelines for Chinese Residents, namely fresh fruits, fresh vegetables, dairy products, and coarse grains; while the other four are high-energy/low-nutrient-density foods, which should be consumed less or avoided, namely salted snacks, sugary beverages, preserved foods, and fried foods. See Table 1 for details of each food item.

Table 1. Food items used to asses home food availability.

Food Item	Concept and Examples
Fresh fruits	Natural, fresh, unprocessed fruits, such as apples, bananas, strawberries, watermelons, oranges, etc.
Fresh vegetables	Natural, fresh, unprocessed vegetables, such as leafy vegetables, fresh beans, rhizomes, melons, eggplant fruits, bacteria, algae, etc.
Dairy products	A variety of dairy products, such as fresh milk, cheese, yogurt, butter, cream, etc.
Coarse grains	Whole grains or cereals that have not been refined, including brown rice, quinoa, barley, oats, millet, buckwheat, etc.
Salted snacks	A category of foods that are typically savory in taste and contain added salt or salt-based flavorings, including potato chips, pretzels, popcorn, crackers, meat snacks like beef jerky, etc.
Sugary beverages	Drinks sweetened with various forms of sugar or sweeteners, including sodas, fruit juices, energy drinks, sweetened teas, flavored coffees, etc.
Preserved foods	Foods typically made by preservation with sugar or salt, including pickled vegetables, salted fish, salted eggs, salted meat, etc.
Fried foods	Various foods that are cooked by being submerged in hot oil or fat, such as French fries, fried chicken, tempura, onion rings, etc.

To evaluate home food availability, participants were asked, "How frequently are the following food items available in your home?" Participants provided responses using a five-point scale, selecting from options including "always", "most of the time", "sometimes", "occasionally", or "never". These response frequencies were further categorized into two groups: "high availability", encompassing "always" and "most of the time", and "low availability", including "sometimes", "occasionally", and "never" [23].

2.5.3. Food Intake Information

The participants' food intake information was collected through a questionnaire. This questionnaire has been applied in many previous studies and proven effective [24–26]. In the questionnaire, the participants were asked to answer the following question: "Have you eaten this kind of food in the past three days?". The food classification was based on the balanced diet pagoda of Chinese residents: cereals, vegetables, fruits, animal meat, fish and shrimp, eggs, milk and dairy products, beans and soy products, and oil and fat. Foods outside these 9 categories, such as carbonated beverages, alcoholic beverages, coffee, candy, etc., were not included in the survey. We only investigated whether the participants had eaten these foods and did not consider the frequency and amount of food intake. The answer options were classified as "yes" or "no". For the 9 types of food we investigated, if the answer was "yes", 1 point was assigned; if the answer was "no", 0 points were assigned. The scores of the 9 food categories were summed to obtain the total DDS score. The minimum score was 0, and the maximum score was 9.

2.5.4. Home Socioeconomic Status (SES)

In this study, we adopted the Programme for International Student Assessment (PISA, 2009) as a reference and integrated methods outlined in the published literature [27–29] to compute the SES of older individuals within their home environments. The specific steps are described as follows.

The initial step involved gathering data on the educational level, occupation, and income level of the elderly via a questionnaire survey. Subsequently, values were assigned to these data points. Educational level was graded in accordance with the criteria used by PISA, with, for instance, 6 points assigned to primary school and 9 points for junior high school. To determine occupation, we considered that the occupational classification within the International Socio Economic Status Occupational Classification Index (ISEI), as used by PISA, was not applicable to China. Consequently, we employed the occupational reputation index developed by Chinese scholar Li Chunling. This index encompasses a total of 161 occupations, each assigned a score ranging from 10.4 to 90 points [30]. Household per capita income in RMB was categorized into discrete points, with "below RMB 2000" earning 2 points, "RMB 2000~3499" earning 3.5 points, "RMB 3500~4999" earning 5 points, "5000~6499" earning 6.5 points, "6500~9999" earning 10 points, and "over RMB 10,000" earning 12 points.

The second step was to address missing values within the three variables. The following principle was used to handle missing data: if two or more variable values were missing within a sample, that sample was classified as missing data. In cases where only one variable value was missing, we utilized the available values of the remaining two variables to conduct regression estimation for the missing variable and subsequently replaced the missing value.

The third step involved calculating the SES score. After transforming the three mentioned variables into standardized scores, we utilized principal component analysis to calculate the SES through the application of the following formula: SES = ($\beta 1 \times$ Z Educational level + $\beta 2 \times$ Z Occupation + $\beta 3 \times$ Z Income level)/εf. In this equation, $\beta 1$, $\beta 2$, and $\beta 3$ represent factor loads, while εf denotes the characteristic root of the first factor. Participants' total scores spanned from -2.89 to 2.98. Higher SES scores reflect a higher objective socioeconomic status of participants' families.

In this study, home SES was categorized into three groups based on SES scores: low, medium, and high.

2.5.5. Physical Measurement

The investigators received prior training. They conducted height and weight measurements using standardized procedures and uniform instruments (RGZ-160; Suheng, Jiangsu, China). Each participant was measured twice. Heights were recorded to the nearest 0.1 cm, and weights were recorded to the nearest 0.1 kg.

For height measurement [31], participants assumed a barefoot, erect posture on the altimeter's floor, ensuring contact of their heel, sacrum, and shoulder blades with the altimeter's base. With the head held upright and eyes looking straight ahead, the upper edge of the tragus and the lower edge of the orbit were aligned horizontally.

For weight measurement [31], participants wore as little clothing as possible and assumed a natural stance at the center of the scale. Data were read once participants achieved a stable stance.

2.6. Variables

2.6.1. Body Mass Index

After determining the mean height and weight, the BMI was calculated and expressed in kg/m^2 to describe the characteristics of the sample. According to The Dietary Guidelines for Chinese Residents (2022) [32], we defined a BMI below 20.0 as underweight, the range from 20.0 to 26.9 as normal weight, and a BMI above 27.0 as overweight or obese.

2.6.2. Home Food Environment Variables

Living conditions were grouped into "living alone" and "not living alone". Socioeconomic status (SES) was classified into three categories: "high", "medium", and "low". Family food availability encompassed a total of eight food items, each classified as binary, indicating "high availability" or "low availability".

2.6.3. Confounders

Confounding variables in our study were identified through a comprehensive literature review and expert discussions. These included individual-level sociodemographic characteristics, such as age, gender, and marital status. Additional behavioral factors were also considered, such as exercise frequency, smoking and drinking habits, dietary diversity score (DDS), and the economic status of the communities.

2.7. Statistical Methods

SPSS Statistics 20.0 (IBM Corp., Armonk, NY, USA) was used for statistical analyses. Descriptive statistics were employed to examine participant and home food environment characteristics. Measurement data are reported as mean and standard deviation, whereas enumeration data are represented in terms of frequency and percentage.

We conducted a univariate analysis of BMI to compare the BMI of older adults with different characteristics. We also used multiple linear regression analysis to investigate the correlation between each home food environment variable and BMI. Model 1 included solely the home food environment variables, while Model 2 incorporated confounders including demographic characteristics, neighborhood socioeconomic level, and behavioral factors. A significance level of $p < 0.05$ was considered statistically significant.

3. Results

3.1. Participant Characteristics

This sample was from the same study as our previously published article. As described in our previous article, a total of 1800 questionnaires were distributed, of which 1775 were retrieved, resulting in a questionnaire recovery rate of 98.6%. Among these, 1764 questionnaires were deemed valid, corresponding to a questionnaire validity rate of 99.4%. Among the participants (n = 1764), the average age was 69.7 ± 4.32 years old, and the male-to-female ratio was approximately 1 to 1.4. The mean BMI was 26.3 ± 3.50 kg/m^2, with over 40% of elderly individuals being overweight or obese. Participants were approximately evenly distributed between urban and suburban areas. Only 17% of the elderly population reported smoking habits, and 24.7% consumed alcohol once a week or more. For a more detailed overview of the participants' basic information, please refer to Table 2 [33].

Table 2. Participant characteristics (*n*, %) [33].

Item	Classification	n	%
BMI (kg/m^2)	Underweight: below 20.0	45	2.6
	Normal: 20–26.9	950	53.8
	Overweight and obese: 27.0 and above	769	43.6
Gender	Male	730	41.4
	Female	1034	58.6
Age	65–69	983	55.7
	70–74	483	27.4
	75–79	298	16.9
Marital status	Unmarried	3	0.2
	Married	1482	84.0
	Widowed	260	14.7
	Separated or divorced	19	1.1
Educational level	Higher education	190	10.8
	Secondary education [1]	923	52.3
	≤Primary education	651	36.9
Income level (RMB) [2]	≤2000	409	23.2
	2000–3500	652	37.0
	3500–5000	376	21.3
	5000–10,000	223	12.6
	≥10,000	24	1.4
	Missing	80	4.5
Neighborhood socioeconomic level	Urban	899	51.0
	Suburban	865	49.0
Frequency of exercise	Never	198	11.2
	1–2 times per week	55	3.1
	3–4 times per week	83	4.7
	5–6 times per week	35	2.0
	Every day	1387	78.6
	Missing	6	0.3
Smoking	No [3]	1464	83.0
	Yes	300	17.0
Drinking	Once a week or more	436	24.7
	Less than once a week	1325	75.1
	missing	3	0.2

[1] Including junior high school, senior high school, and various specialized secondary schools. [2] Per capita monthly income of households in RMB. [3] "No" indicates never smoking or having quit smoking.

3.2. Home Food Availability

Among the four low-energy/high-nutrient-density foods, the highest to lowest availability was fresh vegetables (1686, 95.6%), coarse grains (1660, 94.1%), fresh fruits (1594, 90.4%), and dairy products (1475, 83.6%). Among the four high-energy/low-nutrient-density foods, the availability, ranked from highest to lowest, was preserved foods (915, 51.9%), salted snacks (717, 40.6%), sugary beverages (498, 28.2%), and fried foods (165, 9.4%) (see Figure 1).

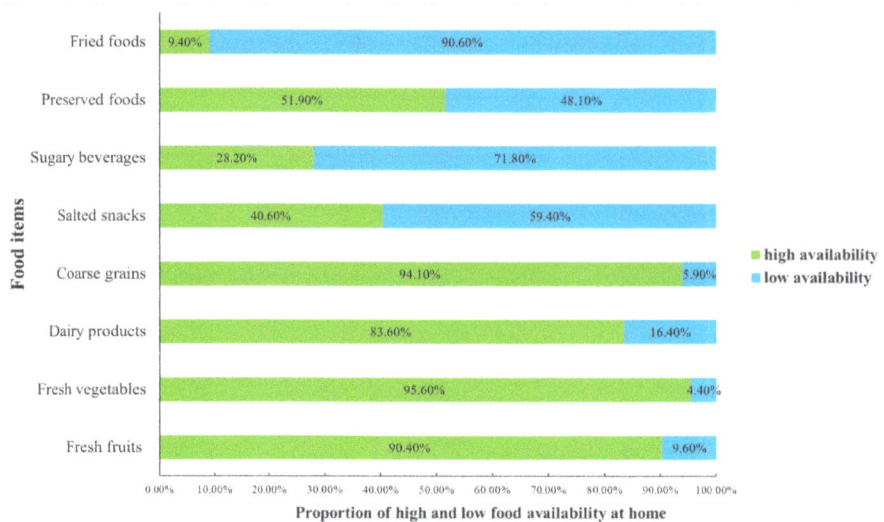

Figure 1. The proportion of high and low food availability of different food items in the home.

3.3. Living Conditions

Among all participants, 7.3% lived alone (see Figure 2).

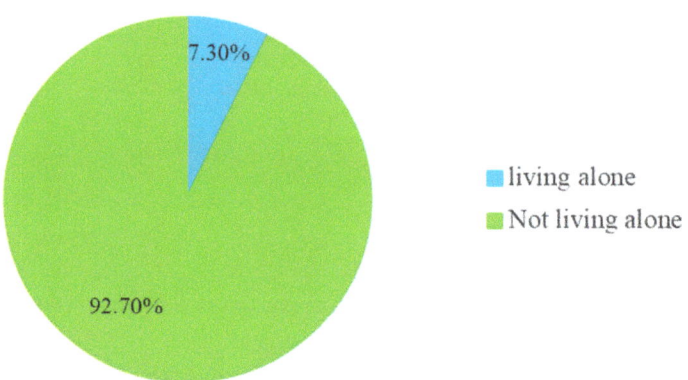

Figure 2. Proportion of older adults with different living conditions.

3.4. Univariate Analysis of BMI

The results of univariate analysis of BMI are presented in Table 3. The BMI of older adults varied with SES. Subsequent pairwise comparisons revealed that elderly individuals with high SES had lower BMI compared to those with medium to low SES (25.9 vs. 26.5, 25.9 vs. 26.4, $p < 0.05$). Older adults living alone exhibited higher BMI values compared to those not living alone (27.2 vs. 26.2, $p = 0.001$). No significant differences in BMI were observed among elderly individuals with either high or low availability of various foods in their homes ($p > 0.05$).

Table 3. Univariate analysis of BMI.

Variables	Group	n	BMI	t/F	p
SES	High	588	25.9 ± 3.4	5.403	0.005
	Medium	588	26.5 ± 3.5		
	Low	588	26.4 ± 3.6		
Living condition	Living alone	128	27.2 ± 3.8	−3.237	0.001
	Not living alone	1636	26.2 ± 3.5		
Availability of fresh fruits	High	1594	26.3 ± 3.5	−1.738	0.082
	Low	170	25.8 ± 3.6		
Availability of fresh vegetables	High	1686	26.2 ± 3.5	1.392	0.164
	Low	78	26.8 ± 3.7		
Availability of dairy products	High	1475	26.2 ± 3.5	1.019	0.308
	Low	289	26.5 ± 3.4		
Availability of coarse grains	High	1660	26.3 ± 3.5	−0.960	0.337
	Low	104	26.0 ± 3.3		
Availability of salted snacks	High	717	26.2 ± 3.5	1.080	0.280
	Low	1047	26.4 ± 3.5		
Availability of sugary beverages	High	498	26.2 ± 3.5	0.446	0.656
	Low	1266	26.3 ± 3.5		
Availability of preserved foods	High	915	26.4 ± 3.4	−1.772	0.076
	Low	849	26.1 ± 3.6		
Availability of fried foods	High	165	26.5 ± 3.7	−0.783	0.433
	Low	1599	26.2 ± 3.5		

3.5. Association between Home Food Environment and BMI

After adjusting for potential confounding factors, our analysis revealed several noteworthy correlations. Specifically, we observed a negative correlation between family SES and BMI. Older adults with higher SES had a reduced BMI of 0.356 kg/m^2 ($p = 0.001$) when compared to those with lower SES. Furthermore, living condition emerged as a key contributor, as older adults living alone experienced an elevation in BMI of 1.155 kg/m^2 ($p < 0.001$) compared to their counterparts who did not live alone. Additionally, we found that the availability of preserved foods was positively associated with BMI, indicating that older adults with higher availability of preserved foods experienced an increase in BMI of 0.442 kg/m^2 ($p = 0.008$) (see Table 4 for more details).

Table 4. Association between home food environment and BMI.

Variable	Model 1 [1]			Model 2 [2]		
	β	SE	p	β	SE	p
SES	−0.280	0.104	0.007	−0.356	0.108	0.001
Living condition	1.053	0.321	0.001	1.155	0.319	<0.001
Fresh fruits	0.865	0.297	0.004	-		
Fresh vegetables	−0.902	0.417	0.031	-		
Dairy products	-			-		
Coarse grains	-			-		
Salted snacks	-			-		
Sugary beverages	-			-		
Preserved foods	-			0.442	0.166	0.008
Fried foods	-			-		

Note. SE: standard error. [1] Model 1 represents the unadjusted model, including solely the home food environment variables. [2] Model 2 is adjusted for age, exercise frequency, smoking habits, and neighborhood socioeconomic level. Covariates are not displayed in the table for conciseness.

4. Discussion

The home serves as the paramount food environment, as the majority of food storage, preparation, and consumption occurs within its confines. Our findings indicate that diverse factors of the home food environment might be linked to BMI among elderly individuals.

According to our results, higher availability of preserved foods within the home was associated with a higher BMI among older adults. In many regions of China, preserved foods constitute an integral part of family diets, including items like preserved vegetables, preserved meat, and preserved fish. Existing research evidence has suggested that frequent consumption of preserved foods may be linked to various health issues, such as overweight, obesity, hypertension, fatty liver, primary liver cancer, and upper gastrointestinal cancer [34–36]. A study involving civil servants aged 30 to 50 also identified frequent consumption of preserved foods as a risk factor for overweight and obesity, while regular intake of fresh vegetables was found to be a protective factor against these conditions [37]. Preserved foods are typically characterized by their high salt content, and older adults may also consume more grains when partaking in such foods, potentially leading to excessive energy intake and an increase in BMI. Consequently, it is advisable to reduce the availability of preserved foods in the home, placing a stronger emphasis on consuming fresh vegetables, meat, and other fresh food items. However, it is worth noting that in this study, preserved foods were not further categorized into subtypes like preserved meat, preserved vegetables, or other preserved foods. Further research is warranted to determine which specific types of preserved foods have a significant impact on BMI.

In this study, a high SES within the household was found to be associated with lower BMI among the elderly. This finding aligns with previous research conducted in developed countries [16] but contrasts with results observed in low-income countries [17]. It is noteworthy that this investigation was conducted in Beijing, the capital of China, which is known for its elevated economic status. To establish a more comprehensive understanding, future research should encompass diverse regions within China. Interestingly, this outcome contradicts prior findings in Chinese children [18], highlighting the potential variability in the influence of SES on BMI across different population groups. This underscores the need for more targeted research specifically focusing on the elderly to better elucidate these dynamics.

Our study revealed that living alone is a contributing factor to increased BMI in older adults—a finding consistent with prior research. In a study involving older Japanese adults, the adjusted prevalence ratios for obesity (BMI $\geq$ 30.0 kg/m^2) indicated that men who exclusively dined alone had a ratio of 1.34 (1.01–1.78) if they lived alone and 1.17 (0.84–1.64) if they lived with others [38]. Additionally, a retrospective cohort study conducted among university students identified living alone as a significant predictor of weight gain and overweight/obesity [39]. Moreover, research involving children and adolescents revealed that those participating in family meals at a frequency of at least three times per week had an increased likelihood of maintaining a normal weight, with a corresponding 12% decrease in the odds of overweight [40]. Individuals living alone face fewer opportunities to dine with others. While intervening in older adults' living conditions can be challenging, encouraging communal eating rather than solitary dining is a feasible behavioral intervention. Community kitchen tables and food delivery services at the community level can serve as potential solutions. The Chinese government has made commendable efforts to date to establish such facilities and services. However, there remain shortcomings, including limited service variety, suboptimal service quality, constraints in terms of site scale, and suboptimal site layouts [41–43]. It should be noted that in this study, the sample size for individuals living alone was relatively small (7.30%), which may have introduced a certain degree of bias. Moreover, the small sample size may have affected the representativeness and generalizability of the results. Specifically, for the population living alone, this limitation in terms of sample size could have led to an overestimation or underestimation of the impact on BMI. Therefore, future research should include a larger number of individuals living alone to validate our findings and to more accurately investigate the relationship between living alone and BMI. Additionally, given the potential bias introduced by the small sample size, we should exercise caution in drawing conclusions.

Our study contributes valuable insights to the growing body of evidence regarding the possible impact of the home food environment among Chinese older adults. Although our study found that SES and the availability of preserved foods have only a slight impact on BMI, these findings are still meaningful. First, research has shown that even minor weight loss, particularly for individuals who are overweight or obese, can reduce the risk of chronic diseases such as cardiovascular disease and diabetes [44,45]. Second, the current results provide an indication of potential trends, laying a foundation for future health education and intervention measures. This research highlights specific target groups for future health education and interventions, notably individuals living alone and those with lower SES. Enhancing food availability within the homes of the elderly, with a particular emphasis on addressing the presence of preserved foods, should be a priority. Achievement of this goal can be facilitated through educational efforts targeting not only the elderly themselves but also their families and peers; the government can play a pivotal role in addressing this issue by implementing a range of measures. These measures may include improving community kitchen facilities and delivery services; reducing the prices of foods characterized by low energy and high nutrient density, such as fresh vegetables and fruits and dairy products; and providing food vouchers for older adults, among other strategies. The combined implementation of these measures can enhance the home food environment for the elderly, ultimately contributing to better health outcomes in this demographic. Additionally, this study offers directions for future research. Future studies should use standardized research tools and methods to examine the home food environment, delving deeper into the differences in food environments across different countries and their impact on BMI and associated health risks.

Our study boasts several notable strengths across various aspects, including innovation, variable measurements, sampling method, and statistical analysis [46]. (1) Insofar as we know, this is a pioneering exploration investigating the correlation between the home food environment and BMI among elderly individuals within the Chinese context. Our research not only contributes empirical evidence on this association but also lays a scientific foundation for policymakers in China. (2) Within the scope of this research, we comprehensively considered various dimensions of the home food environment, encompassing physical, economic, and social aspects. (3) In our study, we employed standardized procedures to measure participants' height and weight directly, enhancing the accuracy of BMI calculations compared to relying on self-reported data. (4) We imposed no restrictions on participants with existing health conditions or obesity, mitigating the potential for selection bias in our sample. (5) Employing a multistage stratified random sampling method, our study effectively addressed neighborhood self-selection bias. (6) Our statistical model includes a wide array of potential confounding factors, encompassing demographic characteristics such as age, gender, and marital status, as well as neighborhood socioeconomic status and behavioral attributes like drinking, smoking, and exercise frequency. This comprehensive approach enhances the robustness of our findings.

Several limitations are inherent in our study. To begin with, the geographical scope was confined solely to the city of Beijing. Therefore, the findings may not be entirely representative of China as a whole. Despite implementing a multistage stratified random sampling method that encompassed diverse economic strata and geographic locations within Beijing, the study predominantly reflects the conditions specific to this city. Given that Beijing is characterized by a high level of economic development in China, our findings may not be applicable to the broader Chinese context. Thus, it is essential to replicate our findings in other regions, especially in cities with varying economic statuses. Secondly, due to the constrained number of questions in our questionnaire, we included only eight food items in our assessment. Four types of low-energy/high-nutrient-density foods are recommended for adequate intake in the Dietary Guidelines for Chinese Residents, while four types of high-energy/low-nutrient-density foods are advised to be consumed less or avoided. In this study, we used categories rather than individual foods. Although this made the food list less detailed, it also ensured that that important foods were not missed. Thirdly, in the complex home environment, we included indicators from only three dimensions: availability of eight food categories, living conditions, and socioeconomic status (SES). Future research should aim for a more comprehensive assessment by including additional relevant factors. Moreover, there is a need for the development of authoritative home food environment questionnaires tailored to different populations. Lastly, like many studies in this field, our research employed a cross-sectional approach. Therefore, it is important to emphasize that causal inferences should not be drawn from our findings.

5. Conclusions

Our study suggests that socioeconomic status (SES), living conditions, and the availability of preserved foods at home may potentially impact the BMI of older adults. However, the complexity of this relationship necessitates a cautious and detailed approach in any potential intervention measures or policy recommendations. Further research is advised to build upon these preliminary findings, guiding effective and contextually appropriate strategies to support the health of the elderly.

Supplementary Materials: The following supporting information can be downloaded at: https://www.mdpi.com/article/10.3390/nu16020289/s1, Supplementary S1: Questionnaire on basic information and Home food availability.

Author Contributions: Conceptualization, M.Z. and G.M.; methodology, M.Z. and G.M.; formal analysis, M.Z. and Y.F.; investigation, M.Z., R.C., Z.L. and N.Z.; resources, Q.W. and G.M.; data curation, M.Z. and Y.F.; writing—original draft preparation, M.Z.; writing—review and editing, Q.W. and G.M.; supervision, G.M. and N.Z.; project administration, N.Z. and G.M. All authors have read and agreed to the published version of the manuscript.

Funding: This research received no external funding.

Institutional Review Board Statement: The study adhered to the principles outlined in the Declaration of Helsinki and received ethical approval from Peking University Biomedical Ethics Committee (protocol code: IRB00001052-17112; approval date: 26 February 2018).

Informed Consent Statement: Informed consent was obtained from all subjects involved in the study.

Data Availability Statement: The data presented in this study are available on request from the corresponding author. The data are not publicly available as the authors are currently engaged in further exploration and analysis of these data, and hence have chosen not to disclose them publicly at this stage.

Acknowledgments: Our heartfelt thanks go to both the participants and coinvestigators who contributed to the survey. Additionally, we wish to convey our gratitude to the reviewers for their invaluable comments, which have greatly enhanced the quality of this manuscript.

Conflicts of Interest: The authors have no conflicts of interest to declare.

References

1. National Bureau of Statistics. National Data. Available online: https://data.stats.gov.cn/easyquery.htm?cn=C01 (accessed on 26 September 2023).
2. Chen, X.; Iles, J.; Yao, Y.; Yip, W.; Meng, Q.; Berkman, L.; Chen, H.; Chen, X.; Feng, J.; Feng, Z.; et al. The path to healthy ageing in China: A Peking University-Lancet Commission. *Lancet* **2022**, *400*, 1967–2006. [CrossRef] [PubMed]
3. Asia Pacific Cohort Studies Collaboration. The burden of overweight and obesity in the Asia-Pacific region. *Obes. Rev.* **2007**, *8*, 191–196. [CrossRef] [PubMed]
4. Du, S.; Lu, B.; Zhai, F.; Popkin, B.M. A new stage of the nutrition transition in China. *Public Health Nutr.* **2002**, *5*, 169–174. [CrossRef] [PubMed]
5. National Health Commission Disease Prevention and Control Bureau. *Report on Nutrition and Chronic Disease Status of Chinese Residents*; People's Medical Publishing House: Beijing, China, 2020.
6. Swinburn, B.A.; Sacks, G.; Hall, K.D.; McPherson, K.; Finegood, D.T.; Moodie, M.L.; Gortmaker, S.L. The global obesity pandemic: Shaped by global drivers and local environments. *Lancet* **2011**, *378*, 804–814. [CrossRef] [PubMed]
7. Bleich, S.; Cutler, D.; Murray, C.; Adams, A. Why is the developed world obese? *Annu. Rev. Public Health* **2008**, *29*, 273–295. [CrossRef]

8. Story, M.; Kaphingst, K.M.; Robinson-O'Brien, R.; Glanz, K. Creating healthy food and eating environments: Policy and environmental approaches. *Annu. Rev. Public Health* **2008**, *29*, 253–272. [CrossRef] [PubMed]
9. Campbell, K.J.; Crawford, D.A.; Salmon, J.; Carver, A.; Garnett, S.P.; Baur, L.A. Associations between the home food environment and obesity-promoting eating behaviors in adolescence. *Obesity* **2007**, *15*, 719–730. [CrossRef]
10. Rosenkranz, R.R.; Dzewaltowski, D.A. Model of the home food environment pertaining to childhood obesity. *Nutr. Rev.* **2008**, *66*, 123–140. [CrossRef]
11. Swinburn, B.; Egger, G.; Raza, F. Dissecting obesogenic environments: The development and application of a framework for identifying and prioritizing environmental interventions for obesity. *Prev. Med.* **1999**, *29*, 563–570. [CrossRef]
12. Kegler, M.C.; Hermstad, A.; Haardorfer, R. Home food environment and associations with weight and diet among U.S. adults: A cross-sectional study. *BMC Public Health* **2021**, *21*, 1032. [CrossRef]
13. Emery, C.F.; Olson, K.L.; Lee, V.S.; Habash, D.L.; Nasar, J.L.; Bodine, A. Home environment and psychosocial predictors of obesity status among community-residing men and women. *Int. J. Obes.* **2015**, *39*, 1401–1407. [CrossRef] [PubMed]
14. Gorin, A.A.; Phelan, S.; Raynor, H.; Wing, R.R. Home food and exercise environments of normal-weight and overweight adults. *Am. J. Health Behav.* **2011**, *35*, 618–626. [CrossRef] [PubMed]
15. Kegler, M.C.; Alcantara, I.; Haardorfer, R.; Gazmararian, J.A.; Ballard, D.; Sabbs, D. The influence of home food environments on eating behaviors of overweight and obese women. *J. Nutr. Educ. Behav.* **2014**, *46*, 188–196. [CrossRef]
16. Newton, S.; Braithwaite, D.; Akinyemiju, T.F. Socio-economic status over the life course and obesity: Systematic review and meta-analysis. *PLoS ONE* **2017**, *12*, e0177151. [CrossRef] [PubMed]
17. Dinsa, G.D.; Goryakin, Y.; Fumagalli, E.; Suhrcke, M. Obesity and socioeconomic status in developing countries: A systematic review. *Obes. Rev.* **2012**, *13*, 1067–1079. [CrossRef]
18. He, W.; James, S.A.; Merli, M.G.; Zheng, H. An increasing socioeconomic gap in childhood overweight and obesity in China. *Am. J. Public Health* **2014**, *104*, e14–e22. [CrossRef]
19. Su, X.; Liu, T.; Li, N.N.; Sun, J.; Cui, J.M.; Zhu, W.L. Development and Assessment of Home Food Environment Measurement Questionnaire for School-aged Children. *Food Nutr. China* **2020**, *26*, 74–79. [CrossRef]
20. Song, M.N.; Cheng, X.; Kong, J.X.; Wang, H.M. Prevalence and influencing factors of overweight and obesity among middle-aged and elderly people in China. *Chin. J. Dis. Control Prev.* **2018**, *22*, 804–808. [CrossRef]
21. Zhang, M.; Jiang, Y.; Li, Y.; Wang, L.; Zhao, W. Prevalence of overweight and obesity among Chinese elderly aged 60 and above in 2010. *Zhonghua Liu Xing Bing Xue Za Zhi* **2014**, *35*, 365–369. [CrossRef]
22. Beijing Municipal Bureau of Statistics. Beijing Statistical Zoning Code and Urban Rural Classification Code (2018 Edition). Available online: https://tjj.beijing.gov.cn/zwgkai/tjbz_31390/xzqhhcxfl_31391/cxfl_31674/202002/t20200214_1631903.html (accessed on 9 January 2024).
23. Chai, W.; Fan, J.X.; Wen, M. Association of Individual and Neighborhood Factors with Home Food Availability: Evidence from the National Health and Nutrition Examination Survey. *J. Acad. Nutr. Diet* **2018**, *118*, 815–823. [CrossRef]
24. Jin, Y. *Study on Associations of Dietary Diversity with Nutrients Adequacy and Nutrition Related Chronic Disease in Chinese Adults*; China Centre for Disease Control and Prevention: Beijing, China, 2009.
25. Hu, Q.Q.; Han, X.X.; Ma, A.G.; Li, X.L. Investigation and analysis of dietary diversity score and health status of middle-aged and elderly people in rural areas. *Food Nutr. China* **2009**, *12*, 58–61.
26. Jin, Y.; Li, Y.P.; Hu, X.Q.; Cui, Z.H.; He, Y.N.; Ma, G.S. Association between dietary diversity and nutrients adequacy in Chinese adults. *Acta Nutr. Sin.* **2009**, *31*, 21–25. [CrossRef]
27. Zhan, S.L. The Influence of Family Socioeconomic Status on Student Academic Performance from Individual and School Perspectives: Insights from the Programme for International Student Assessment (PISA). *J. Shanghai Educ. Res.* **2009**, 10–13.
28. Chen, Y.H.; Cheng, G.; Guan, Y.S.; Zhang, D.J. The Mediating Effects of Subjective Social Status on the Relations between Self-Esteem and Socioeconomic Status for College Students. *Psychol. Dev. Educ.* **2014**, *30*, 594–600. [CrossRef]
29. Guo, Y.R. *Research on Environmental Influencing Factors of Overweight andObesity of Children and Adolescents in China*; East China Normal University: Shanghai, China, 2020.
30. Li, C.L. Stratification of Reputation in Contemporary Chinese Society: Measurement of Occupational Reputation and Socioeconomic Status Index. *Sociol. Stud.* **2005**, 74–102. [CrossRef]
31. General Administration of Sport of China. *National Physical Fitness Standard Handbook*; Senior Part; People's Sports Publishing House of China: Beijing, China, 2003.
32. Chinese Nutrition Society. *Dietary Guidelines for Chinese Residents*; People's Medical Publishing House: Beijing, China, 2022.
33. Zhang, M.; Guo, W.; Zhang, N.; He, H.R.; Zhang, Y.; Zhou, M.Z.; Zhang, J.F.; Li, M.X.; Ma, G.S. Association between Neighborhood Food Environment and Body Mass Index among Older Adults in Beijing, China: A Cross-Sectional Study. *Int. J. Environ. Res. Public Health* **2020**, *17*, 7658. [CrossRef] [PubMed]
34. Tong, G.X.; Gao, X.; Xu, R.Y.; Qin, Y.; Huang, L.; Wang, X.M.; Song, W.J. Relationship between dietary pattern and risk of suffering from hypertension in physical examinees aged 35 years and above in Haidian District of Beijing. *Pract. Prev. Med.* **2022**, *29*, 906–911.
35. Zhang, R.; Li, H.; Li, N.; Shi, J.F.; Li, J.; Chen, H.D.; Ren, J.S.; Chen, W.Q. Nested Case-control Study of Risk Factors for Upper Gastrointestinal Cancer Based on Population Screening Cohort in Urban Areas of China. *China Cancer* **2021**, *30*, 321–327.

36. Wang, M.X.; Zhang, G.D.; Jiang, H.J.; Liu, X.M.; Peng, Y.H. Meta-analysis of the relationship between intake of pickled food in Chinese population and primary liver cancer. *Clin. Res. Pract.* **2020**, *5*, 1–4. [CrossRef]
37. Li, H. *Study on the Health Status and Related Factors of Civil Servant in Changchun District Government*; Ji Lin University: Changchun, China, 2012.
38. Tani, Y.; Kondo, N.; Takagi, D.; Saito, M.; Hikichi, H.; Ojima, T.; Kondo, K. Combined effects of eating alone and living alone on unhealthy dietary behaviors, obesity and underweight in older Japanese adults: Results of the JAGES. *Appetite* **2015**, *95*, 1–8. [CrossRef]
39. Yamamoto, R.; Shinzawa, M.; Yoshimura, R.; Taneike, M.; Nakanishi, K.; Nishida, M.; Yamauchi-Takihara, K.; Kudo, T.; Moriyama, T. Living alone and prediction of weight gain and overweight/obesity in university students: A retrospective cohort study. *J. Am. Coll. Health* **2023**, *71*, 1417–1426. [CrossRef] [PubMed]
40. Hammons, A.J.; Fiese, B.H. Is frequency of shared family meals related to the nutritional health of children and adolescents? *Pediatrics* **2011**, *127*, e1565–e1574. [CrossRef] [PubMed]
41. Sun, Y.S. *Research on Beijing Community Old Age Table Service Demand*; Capital University of Economics and Business: Beijing, China, 2017.
42. Hou, J. *Research on Supply and Demand Deviation and Optimization Strategy of Catering Service for the Elderly in Xi'an Urban Community from the Perspective of Holistic Governance—Take District X as An Example*; Northwest University: Xi'an, China, 2022.
43. Yu, S.W. *The Research on Service Improvement Planning of Community Canteens for the Elderly in Changsha from the Perspective of Urban Catalyst*; Hunan University: Changsha, China, 2022.
44. Wing, R.R.; Lang, W.; Wadden, T.A.; Safford, M.; Knowler, W.C.; Bertoni, A.G.; Hill, J.O.; Brancati, F.L.; Peters, A.; Wagenknecht, L.; et al. Benefits of modest weight loss in improving cardiovascular risk factors in overweight and obese individuals with type 2 diabetes. *Diabetes Care* **2011**, *34*, 1481–1486. [CrossRef] [PubMed]
45. Klein, S.; Burke, L.E.; Bray, G.A.; Blair, S.; Allison, D.B.; Pi-Sunyer, X.; Hong, Y.; Eckel, R.H.; American Heart Association Council on Nutrition; Physical Activity. Clinical implications of obesity with specific focus on cardiovascular disease: A statement for professionals from the American Heart Association Council on Nutrition, Physical Activity, and Metabolism: Endorsed by the American College of Cardiology Foundation. *Circulation* **2004**, *110*, 2952–2967. [CrossRef]
46. Cobb, L.K.; Appel, L.J.; Franco, M.; Jones-Smith, J.C.; Nur, A.; Anderson, C.A. The relationship of the local food environment with obesity: A systematic review of methods, study quality, and results. *Obesity* **2015**, *23*, 1331–1344. [CrossRef]

Disclaimer/Publisher's Note: The statements, opinions and data contained in all publications are solely those of the individual author(s) and contributor(s) and not of MDPI and/or the editor(s). MDPI and/or the editor(s) disclaim responsibility for any injury to people or property resulting from any ideas, methods, instructions or products referred to in the content.

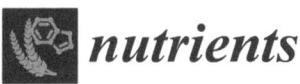

Article

BMI and the Food Retail Environment in Melbourne, Australia: Associations and Temporal Trends

Cindy Needham [1,*], Claudia Strugnell [1,2], Steven Allender [1], Laura Alston [3,4] and Liliana Orellana [5]

1. Global Centre for Preventive Health and Nutrition, Institute for Health Transformation, Deakin University, Geelong, VIC 3220, Australia; claudia.strugnell@deakin.edu.au (C.S.); steven.allender@deakin.edu.au (S.A.)
2. Institute for Physical Activity and Nutrition (IPAN), Deakin University, Geelong, VIC 3220, Australia
3. Colac Area Health, Colac, VIC 3250, Australia; laura.alston@deakin.edu.au
4. Faculty of Health, Deakin Rural Health, Deakin University, Warrnambool, VIC 3280, Australia
5. Faculty of Health, Biostatistics Unit, Deakin University, Geelong, VIC 3220, Australia; l.orellana@deakin.edu.au
* Correspondence: cindy.needham@deakin.edu.au

Abstract: Research into the link between food environments and health is scarce. Research in this field has progressed, and new comprehensive methods (i.e., incorporating all food retail outlets) for classifying food retail environments have been developed and are yet to be examined alongside measures of obesity. In this study, we examine the association and temporal trends between the food environment and BMI of a repeated cross-sectional sample of the adult population between 2008 and 2016. Methods: Food retail data for 264 postal areas of Greater Melbourne was collected for the years 2008, 2012, 2014, and 2016, and a container-based approach was used to estimate accessibility to supermarkets, healthy and unhealthy outlets. Data on BMI for postal areas was obtained from the Victorian Population Health Survey (n = 47,245). We estimated the association between the food environment and BMI using linear mixed models. Results indicated that BMI increased as accessibility to healthy outlets decreased by up to -0.69 kg/m^2 (95%CI: -0.95, -0.44). BMI was lower with high and moderate access to supermarkets compared to low access by -0.33 kg/m^2 (-0.63, -0.04) and -0.32 kg/m^2 (-0.56, -0.07), and with high access to unhealthy outlets compared to low access (-0.38 kg/m^2: -0.64, -0.12) and moderate access (-0.54 kg/m^2: -0.78, -0.30). Conclusion: Our results show that increasing access and availability to a diverse range of food outlets, particularly healthy food outlets, should be an important consideration for efforts to support good health. This research provides evidence that Australia needs to follow suit with other countries that have adopted policies giving local governments the power to encourage healthier food environments.

Keywords: food environment; public health nutrition; BMI; obesity; food retail

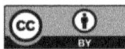

1. Introduction

The World Health Organization's (WHO) Global Action Plan for the Prevention and Control of Noncommunicable Diseases 2023–2030 has a target of halting the rise in the prevalence of people with overweight and obesity by 2030 [1]. To achieve this, the plan highlights the importance of strengthening the capacity of populations to make healthier choices through providing supportive environments [1]. The food environment has the potential to support healthier choices through different elements, including food access and availability, promotion, labelling, and price [2–5]. The food retail environment (FRE), which refers to the accessibility and availability of food retail outlets (i.e., where and what foods can be obtained, respectively) within neighbourhoods, is a key focus for obesity prevention efforts as they have the potential for sustained community-level impact [3–5].

The inclusion of policies that support promoting a healthier FRE is one approach that would assist decision makers in planning healthier urban environments that support healthy choices [2]. Guided by recommendations from the National Institute for Health and Care Excellence [6,7], Public Health England has included within the planning system powers for local authorities to restrict planning permission for takeaways and other food retail outlets in specific areas (i.e., near schools or in areas of deprivation and high obesity prevalence) [8]. Using these planning powers, local authorities in North England have been successful in decreasing the density of unhealthy food outlets (i.e., hot food takeaways) [9]. In Australia, little success has been achieved at the policy level to regulate the healthiness of FRE. Commercial pressures and the absence of strong context-specific evidence to support the need for policy are two barriers to FRE policy development [5].

Lack of investment in nutrition research in Australia may also explain some of the evidence gaps in the link between FRE, diet, and health [10]. A systematic review of studies examining the FRE in Australia identified only 13 of 60 studies (published between 2008 and 2019) that examined the association between the FRE and the prevalence of obesity [11–13]. The majority of studies take a narrow view, examining the FRE cross-sectionally and using only measures of supermarkets or fast-food outlets to represent the FRE [11]. Research in this field has progressed, and new comprehensive methods (i.e., incorporating all food retail outlets) for classifying FRE have been developed and are yet to be examined alongside measures of obesity [14].

The review also brought to the forefront the lack of longitudinal studies examining the FRE alongside health measures [11]. Despite evidence of rapid change in the FRE over time in Australia [15], of five Australian longitudinal studies examining the association between healthy weight and the FRE, only one used time-sensitive measures of the FRE, examining only the top 10 fast-food chains in association with BMI [16]. The remaining four used a single measure of the FRE alongside longitudinal obesity-related measures [17–20]. Studies that use measures of both obesity and the FRE over time have the potential to add value to the research by demonstrating whether relationships remain consistent over time [11,21].

Therefore, this study sought to:

1. Examine the association between the FRE at the postal code level and the BMI of a repeated cross-sectional sample of the adult population residing in those postal codes at four time points (2008, 2012, 2014, and 2016);
2. Examine temporal trends at four time points over eight years in BMI across measures of the FRE.

2. Materials and Methods

2.1. Design

This is a secondary analysis of data from a repeated cross-sectional sample of the Victorian population and an audit of food outlets, both collected in 2008, 2012, 2014, and 2016. BMI data were obtained from the Victorian Population Health Survey (VPHS) [22]. The Victorian Department of Health's Human Research Ethics Committee granted ethics approval for the VPHS [23]. The lead author's institution granted an ethics exemption for the present study.

2.2. Study Region

The setting of the study is Greater Melbourne (Melbourne), Australia. Melbourne is the capital city of Victoria and has experienced rapid population and urban growth at a rate greater than any other Australian city [24,25]. Between 2008 and 2016, Greater Melbourne's population increased from 3.9 million to 4.9 million [24,25]. In 2016, 49% of the population was male and 51% was female [25]. Children (aged 0–14 years) made up 18.3% of the population, and people aged over 65 years made up 14%, with the median age of people being 36 years [25]. The study area included 264 postcodes.

2.3. Victorian Population Health Survey

The VPHS is an annual cross-sectional telephone interview survey [23]. The VPHS collects self-reported data on demographics, health status, behaviours, and risk factors [26].

We used the 2008, 2011–2012, 2014, and 2017 expanded surveys, each including approximately 34,000 participants across Victoria [27].

2.4. Participants

The VPHS collects unidentified individual-level data on the health status of a random sample of adults aged 18 years or more [28] using computer-assisted telephone interviews (CATI) with sampling via random digit dialling [27]. The sample is stratified by local government area (LGA), with a target of 426 interviews per LGA [29]. All data are self-reported and stored within the CATI system [28]. The sampling frame has changed over time to accommodate the increasing proportion of the population that does not have a landline telephone (i.e., mobile-phone-only households) [23]. In 2008, 2012, and 2014, the sampling frame only included landline numbers, whereas from 2015 onwards, a dual-frame sampling design was utilised with randomly generated samples of both landline and mobile phone numbers. Using this design, a larger proportion of persons likely to be mobile-only users can be included in the survey [23].

Participants who lived in one of the 264 (excluding the CBD) residential postcodes located in Melbourne in 2008, 2012, 2014, and 2017 were included in the study sample (n = 47,245). The central business district (postcode 3000) was excluded as food outlet data for this area was not collected.

2.5. Exposure Variables—Food Retail Environment

2.5.1. Data Collection and Definition of Measures

Food outlet data (food outlet name, type, and address) were extracted retrospectively from hard copy business directories (Yellow and White Pages) for the years 2008, 2012, 2014, and 2016 to align with the available expanded population health data from the VPHS. A copy of the Yellow Pages was not available for the year 2017. As such, food outlet data from 2016 was used to represent food retail environment exposure variables for 2017 VPHS participants (referred to as 2016 data from hereon). Melbourne's central business district has a very large number of food outlets, predominantly servicing workers and visitors, and therefore was not collected [30]. The methods used to classify food outlets have been described elsewhere [15]. In short, we adapted an Australian [31] food outlet classification tool to classify outlets into one of 17 types [15] and allocated a score representing healthiness using a 21-point scoring system ranging between −10 (least healthy) and +10 (most healthy) (Supplementary Table S1) [15,31]. Outlets were classified as (1) healthy (healthiness score: +5 to +10), including supermarkets, fruiterers and greengrocers, butchers, fish and poultry shops, and salad/sandwich/sushi bars; (2) less healthy (healthiness score: −4 to +4), including cafes and restaurants (independent and franchise), bakers, and delis; and (3) unhealthy (healthiness score: −10 to −5), including fast-food outlets, independent takeaways, pubs, general stores, and specialty extra.

2.5.2. Geographical Area Level Definition

The addresses of the food outlets were mapped against the 2016 postal area (POA) boundaries of the Australian Bureau of Statistics (ABS) [32]. Food outlet exposure measures (outlets per km^2 and relative healthy food availability) were then calculated for the 264 postal areas that were entirely within Melbourne. In this study, the POA is considered the 'activity space' in which the majority of food retail exposure and purchasing occurs [33].

2.5.3. Food Retail Environment Measures of Accessibility and Availability

We used the most common approach, referred to as the 'container-based method' or 'statistical index approach', to estimate food outlet accessibility [34,35]. In this method, the number of food retail outlets within a geographic unit is summarised (e.g., the number and total area of density within a specific geographic unit) [35]. The approach was selected due to its suitability for comparison across regions and over time [34]. Using this method, the FRE of each POA was characterised using four food retail accessibility measures (FRAMs) and a measure of relative healthy food availability (RHFA) [3,18]. FRAMS represent accessibility defined as the number of food outlets within a POA (the container) per km^2 for: (1) supermarkets; (2) healthy; (3) less healthy; and (4) unhealthy outlets [14]. Supermarkets were considered independently given that they account for the bulk of food retail purchases (68% in 2019) in Australia [36]. Each FRAM measure was then categorised into three levels (Table 1). Less healthy outlets and RHFA were used to inform typology (outlined below), but their association with BMI was not assessed, as less healthy outlets are not considered highly influential on health in the Australian literature [11], and RHFA alone does not reflect the potential accessibility of outlets [37]. RHFA was calculated as the number of food outlets classified as supermarkets, and fruiterers and greengrocers (as a proxy for healthy food outlets) relative to the number of supermarkets, greengrocers plus fast-food franchise and independent takeaway outlets (considered a proxy for unhealthy outlets) [3,18]. The RHFA was categorised into four levels [18] (Table 1). The FRE of POAs was also classified into nine typologies based on the FRAM measures and RHFA, following the approach described by Needham et al. [14]. For POAs with zero food outlets, the FRAMS for the Statistical Area 2 (i.e., suburbs and residential districts) in which the POA was located was used to calculate 'Typology' [38,39].

Table 1. Classification of food retail environment accessibility measures.

Measures		Classification
Relative healthy food availability (RHFA)	**Proportion healthy food resources**	**Availability**
	No food retail *	Low
	≤25%	
	>25 to-≤50%	Moderate
	>50%	High
Food retail accessibility measures (FRAMs)	**Count per km^2**	**Access**
Healthy, less healthy, unhealthy	<1	Low
	≥1 to <2	Moderate
	≥2	High
Supermarkets	<0.625	Low
	0.625 to <1.25	Moderate
	≥1.25	High
**Food environment typology ** **	**FRAMs *** **	**RHFA**	**Typology**
	Low	≤25%	Low access—Low % healthy
	Low	>25% to ≤50%	Low access—Moderate % healthy
	Low	>50%	Low access—High % healthy
	Moderate	≤25%	Moderate access—Low % healthy
	Moderate	>25% to ≤50%	Moderate access—Moderate % healthy
	Moderate	>50%	Moderate access—High % healthy
	High	≤25%	High access—Low % healthy
	High	>25% to ≤50%	High access—Moderate % healthy
	High	>50%	High access—High % healthy

RHFA represents the percentage (%) of the food environment that is composed of healthy (supermarkets and greengrocers) food outlets within each postal area boundary. * Postal areas with no food retail outlets were classified into one of the RHFA categories using a measure of a larger geographical unit (Statistical Area 2). ** Food environment typology measures drawn from Needham et al.'s [14] cluster analysis of the food environment data; these measures represent potential typology classifications that could be found in the data at the POA level. *** Using a combination of FRAMs overall accessibility was defined as: 'Low' if all FRAMs were 'Low'; 'Moderate' where ≥1 FRAMs were 'Moderate'; and 'High' were ≥1 FRAM were 'High'.

2.6. Outcome Measure and Potential Confounders

The outcome measure was BMI (weight (kg)/height^2 (m^2)) determined from VPHS participant self-reported height and weight. Several potential confounders (age, gender, education, annual household income, and employment status) of the relationship between FRE and BMI were considered based on previous literature [11] (Table 2). The variable 'length of time the participant had lived in the current neighbourhood/area/council/local government area (LGA)' (categorical) was used as a proxy for duration of exposure to the local FRE.

Table 2. Characteristics of the Greater Melbourne population sample from the Victorian Population Health Survey (2008, 2011–2012, 2014, and 2017).

Characteristics	Categories	Year			
		2008 (n = 12,526)	2012 (n = 11,246)	2014 (n = 11,760)	2017 (n = 11,713)
Age (%)	18–30	12.9	9.0	5.6	15.3
	31–40	17.6	14.2	10.2	15.1
	41–50	19.9	20.3	17.0	15.4
	51–60	18.7	21.2	20.8	17.4
	61–70	16.5	19.4	23.7	19.6
	71+	14.4	16.0	22.8	17.2
Gender (%)	Male	39.8	40.5	41.9	47.1
	Female	60.2	59.6	58.1	52.9
Education (%)	Primary school/some-high school/other	27.2	21.9	20.7	14.8
	Completed High school/TAFE */trade	37.1	39.3	39.9	36.2
	Tertiary	35.7	38.9	39.4	49.0
Household income (%)	<$20,000	13.2	11.1	9.8	4.4
	≥$20 to <$40,000	17.1	15.3	17.0	16.4
	≥$40 to <$60,000	12.9	12.0	12.0	11.6
	≥$60 to <$80,000	11.6	9.7	8.8	9.3
	≥$80 to <$100,000	8.1	9.5	8.3	8.6
	≥$100,000+	19.8	25.3	18.3	32.8
	Unknown/not reported	17.4	17.1	25.8	17.0
Employment status (%)	Employed **	55.6	56.1	49.2	58.0
	Unemployed	3.1	3.4	3.3	3.7
	Home duties	8.8	6.5	5.0	4.4
	Student	3.3	3.1	2.4	3.8
	Retired	25.7	28.2	37.0	26.8
	Unable to work	3.4	2.6	2.7	2.7
	Other	0.3	0.1	0.5	0.7
Length of time lived in (%) neighbourhood/area/council/ local government area.	<5 years	27.3	17.4	17.3	32.2
	5–10 years	18.2	17.9	15.9	14.7
	10+ years	54.5	64.8	66.8	53.2
BMI mean (standard deviation)		26.0 (5.3)	26.5 (5.3)	26.6 (5.2)	26.5 (5.4)

BMI = body mass index. * TAFE: technical and further education—courses in technical and vocational subjects. ** Regarding employment status, 'employed' reflects participants that were either employed, self-employed, or reported 'other-working'.

2.7. Statistical Analysis

Participants were assigned the FRE exposure measures calculated based on their residential POA in the corresponding calendar year. Linear mixed models were fitted to estimate the mean BMI of participants across exposure levels and study years. All models included the year (categorical), the exposure measure (categorical), the interaction exposure by year, and the potential confounders as fixed effects. The models also included POA as a random effect. Where the interaction exposure by time was non-significant, Sidak-adjusted pairwise comparisons were reported between levels of each factor (exposure and year). Stata version 15.0 was used for all statistical analyses.

3. Results

3.1. Food Environment Characteristics

Supermarket and healthy outlet accessibility was low for most POAs and decreased over time. Almost half of the POAs had high access to unhealthy and less healthy outlets in 2008, increasing across the study period. Of the nine potential typologies, seven were identified across POAs. The two more frequent typologies were High access—Low % healthy and Low Access—Low % healthy. Across study years, forty-three POAs had zero food outlets in at least one of the years (2008: N = 38, 2012: N = 37, 2014: N = 31, 2016: N = 31). Twenty-one SA2's housed the forty-three POAs with zero food retail.

Supplementary Table S2 presents the proportion of POAs that are within each food retail classification. Supplementary Table S3 presents the descriptive statistics for each FRE typology. Supplementary Table S4 presents the proportion of participants within each FRE measure classification.

3.2. Sample Characteristics

The four waves of the VPHS included 52,498 participants residing in Melbourne. Cases were excluded due to missing data for height (n = 1585), weight (n = 3070), education (n = 368), employment status (n = 134), or length lived in the local area (n = 44). A further 52 participants were excluded due to implausible height or weight measures, or where BMI was extreme (BMI $\geq$ 70). The final analysis sample included 47,245 participants. Characteristics of the sample are provided in Table 2.

3.3. Relationship between BMI and Food Retail Environment Measures

The mean BMI profile across the study period was the same for different levels of FRE measures (Figure 1). Sidak-adjusted pairwise comparisons ($p < 0.05$) between exposure levels and between years are reported in Figure 1a–d and Supplementary Tables S5 and S6. There was a significant difference in mean BMI across levels of accessibility to healthy food outlets, with BMI progressively increasing as accessibility to healthy outlets decreased (Figure 1a). BMI was lower in areas with high access to healthy food outlets compared to low access (-0.68 kg/m^2, 95%CI: -0.94, -0.43) and moderate access (-0.34 kg/m^2; -0.60, -0.80); BMI was also lower in areas with moderate access compared to low access (-0.34 kg/m^2; -0.57, -0.12). BMI was lower for people living in POAs with high and moderate access to supermarkets when compared to low access by -0.32 kg/m^2 (-0.64, -0.12) and 0.33 kg/m^2 (-0.63, -0.04) (Figure 1b). BMI was lower in POAs with high access to unhealthy outlets compared to low access (-0.38 kg/m^2; -0.64, -0.12) and moderate access (-0.54 kg/m^2; -0.78, -0.30) (Figure 1c).

The mean BMI was significantly different across FRE typologies (Figure 1.d). BMI was lower in POAs classified High access–Moderate % healthy (-0.73 kg/m^2; -1.08, -0.39) and High access–Low % healthy (-0.84 kg/m^2; -1.2, -0.47) when compared to Low access–Low % healthy. Mean BMI was also lower in High access–Low % healthy (-0.73 kg/m^2; -1.2, -0.27) and Moderate % healthy (-0.63 kg/m^2; -1.08, -0.19) when compared to Low access–Moderate % healthy. This was also the case when High access–Moderate % healthy (-0.57 kg/m^2; -0.94, -0.2) and High access–High % healthy (-0.67 kg/m^2; -1.05, -0.29) were compared to Moderate access—Low % healthy.

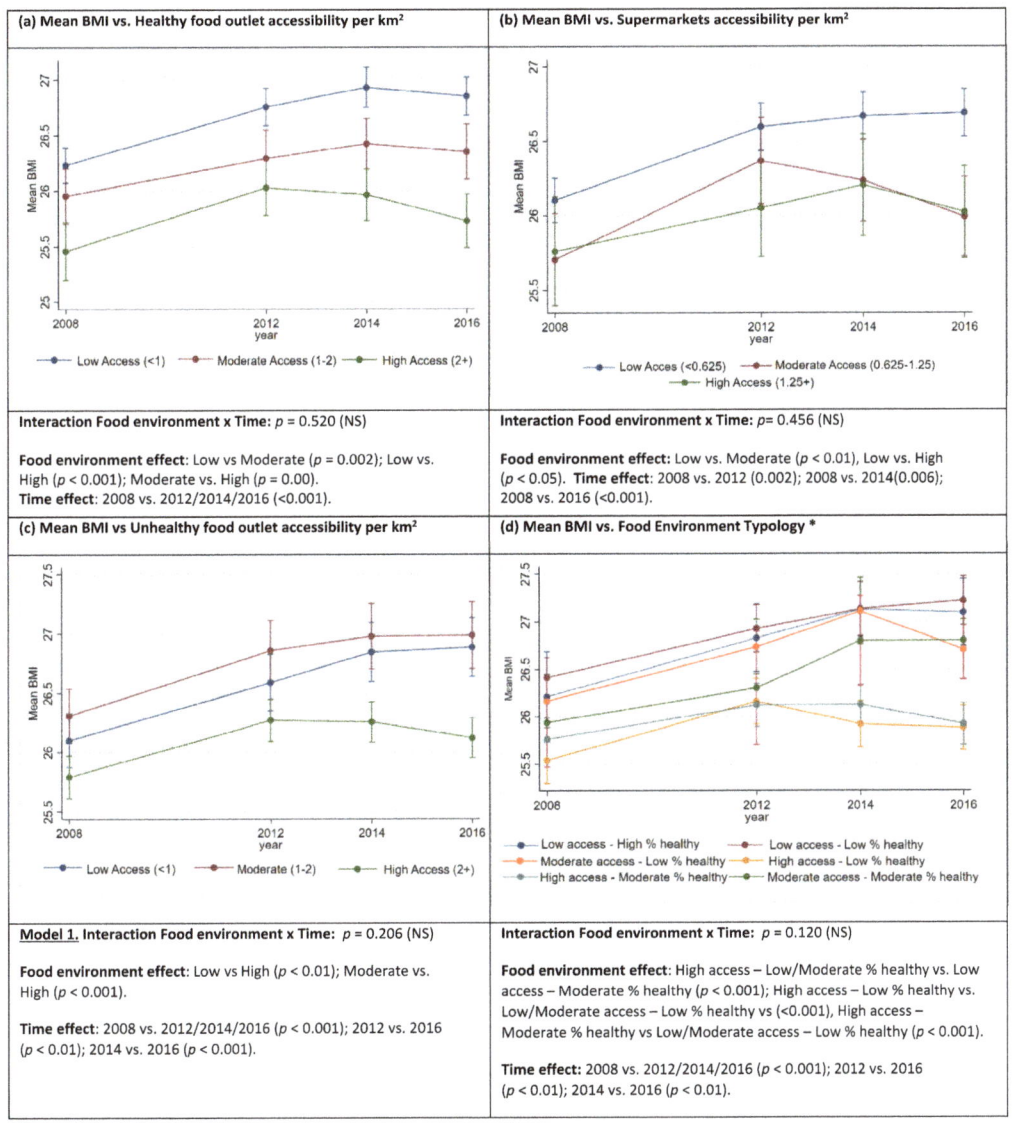

Figure 1. (**a**–**d**). Mean body mass index over the period 2008–2016 across postal areas grouped by food environment exposure variables. Mean BMI estimates and 95% confidence intervals were obtained under linear mixed models including postal area as a random effect, and the food environment measure (healthy, supermarkets, unhealthy food outlets, and combined measure of all outlets 'Typology'), year, interaction food environment measure by year adjusted by age, gender, education, employment status, household income, and length of time lived in the local area. Only pairwise comparisons where $p \leq 0.05$ are reported. * Food environment typology reflects postcodes grouped by similarities across relative healthy food availability (RHFA); and food retail accessibility measures to supermarkets, healthy, less healthy, and unhealthy food outlets per km². RHFA: represents the proportion (%) of the food environment that is composed of supermarkets and greengrocers (as a proxy for healthy food) from the sum of supermarkets, greengrocers, independent takeaway, and fast-food franchise outlets within each postal area boundary. Body mass index (BMI) = weight (kg)/height² (m²)).

3.4. Temporal Trends in BMI

The mean BMI of participants increased across all measures of the food retail environment over the study period by as much as 0.73 kg/m^2 (0.51, 0.95) (Figure 1a–d, Supplementary Tables S5 and S6).

4. Discussion

This study provides the first evidence of a temporal relationship between self-reported BMI and the FRE. A lower BMI was consistently associated with higher access to supermarkets, healthy and unhealthy outlets over the 8-year study period. Using the combined measure 'typology' demonstrated that over half of the postal areas had less than 25% healthy outlets and that access tended to be similar (i.e., where access was high, it was high for all outlets). Findings suggest that having more than 50% healthy outlets in low-access POAs and more than 25% healthy outlets in moderate-access POAs may play some role in facilitating the healthier weight of residents.

Our findings are consistent with earlier studies reporting a relationship between a lower adult BMI and access to healthy outlets in Sydney, Australia [18]. In this study, a higher BMI was associated with FRE, where unhealthy outlets made up more than 25% of all outlets (healthy and unhealthy outlets) within 1.6 and 3.2 km from home [18]. For children in Perth (Australia), decreasing BMI with increasing access to healthy outlets was also reported, with every additional healthy outlet within an 800 m and 3 km buffer from home corresponding with a reduction in risk of being overweight or obese by 19% and 2%, respectively [40]. Our findings are also supported by earlier evidence that suggests good access to supermarkets is associated with a lower BMI for adults, significant within 2 km from home [41].

An inverse relationship between access to unhealthy outlets and BMI is also reflected in earlier studies examining dietary behaviours among women, with results indicating women reporting that they never consume fast food had a higher density and variety of fast food near home in Melbourne (measured as proximity and density within 3 km) [42]. In this 2010 study, access to both fast-food and healthy outlets was highly correlated, and increased fruit and vegetable consumption was also associated with increased access to supermarkets and greengrocers [42]. Another earlier Australian study reported an inverse relationship between the density of fast food near home (2 km) and healthy weight (BMI) in both children and their male parent [43]. The finding that greater access to unhealthy food is associated with a lower BMI should be interpreted with caution. Not least because, evidence from other studies reports a positive association between unhealthy food access, consumption, and unhealthy weight [19,44,45].

An explanatory pathway as to why there is a relationship with a lower BMI where healthy and unhealthy food outlets are more plentiful is that residents have fewer barriers to accessing healthier food and a lower time–cost associated with purchasing food, resulting in more time available for food preparation and a decreased reliance on unhealthy convenience foods [46,47]. This is supported by qualitative studies that suggest those with poor access to food retail develop adaptive shopping behaviours, purchasing food in bulk and selecting products with a longer shelf life (i.e., fewer fresh items, more non-perishable/frozen items), with car ownership and food insecurity further found to accentuate these adaptive behaviours [47,48].

These findings highlight a need to further unpack the drivers of consumption patterns and healthy weight from within the complex FRE using measures, like that used in our study, that take into consideration the full breadth of food outlet types to examine the potential confounding factors at play within the FRE.

4.1. Strengths

This is the first repeated cross-sectional study examining the relationship between BMI and comprehensive longitudinal measures of the FRE alongside BMI. Our findings are strengthened by removing potentially confounding variables, adjusting for socioeconomic differentials, and using a large, comprehensive, and representative sample. Despite some reported discrepancies, correlations between self-reported and measured height and weight were strong in adults (aged ≥ 45) [49].

4.2. Limitations

The duel-frame sampling design introduced in 2015 may have caused some variability in sample selection over the study period [28]. While the VPHS aims to capture a representative sample of the population from each LGA, the differential self-selection of those willing to participate in the survey cannot be ruled out. As a consequence, the samples may not have been representative of the broader population, which may limit the generalizability of the findings. We were also unable to account for other dynamic factors that could influence BMI trends, such as population shifts in dietary preferences, economic conditions, or public health campaigns that may have occurred over the study period. Self-reported height is often overreported, and self-reported weight is often underreported, leading to an overall, but likely uniform, underestimation of BMI [49]. De-identification of the VPHS data meant that the geocoded location of each participant household was not available, and as such, only broad measures of accessibility to food outlets (count per km^2) within each POA could be calculated. Our measure of access assumes food resources and people are evenly spread across POAs; it is likely that food resources cluster around residential areas within POAs and not all residents have the same accessibility. The use of POA in this sample and in geographical research broadly can be subject to a modifiable areal unit problem [50], where the size and shape of different areas can change the picture that the data conveys [50]. Finally, this study does not take into account FRE outside of the residential POA, such as at work, school, or in transit, nor does it include other potential confounders such as physical activity levels and available physical activity infrastructure or other neighbourhood characteristics, or participants' health conditions, which may also influence BMI [51]. While the findings from this study do not imply causation, the comprehensive measures used in the study at the residential POA level provide for a more accurate representation of FRE exposure than reported in earlier studies, and the consistency of results at multiple time points suggests there may be a relationship between population-level estimations of the FRE and BMI.

4.3. Implications for Population Health Policy and Research

This study is of international significance to countries experiencing rapid population growth and urban expansion, providing insight into the higher mean BMI of residents in areas with lower accessibility to a diverse range of food outlets. Future research on longitudinal health and anthropometric (i.e., weight and height) data from a large-scale sample of the population, alongside comprehensive repeated measures of the FRE such as in this study, would provide stronger evidence of the link between the FRE and health. However, given the relationship between healthier BMI and high access to healthier food retail outlets, the findings provide a rationale for policies that aim towards the development of compact cities to support health and encourage increasing accessibility to healthier (healthy and less healthy) food outlets over unhealthy outlets. For policy and planning to gain traction, 'health' needs to be included as a consideration within planning legislation, a central issue raised in an earlier study (December 2016 and August 2017), which undertook interviews with government, non-government, and private stakeholders in Melbourne [52]. Evidence, along with international progress, supports incorporating standards into urban planning guidelines that seek to encourage access to healthy outlets within 1 km of most homes [53]. Where this is not economically viable, facilitating transport opportunities to existing healthy food resources and investing in diverse healthy food retail opportunities (e.g., healthy food delivery services or greengrocer pop-up stores) for residents, particularly those without vehicle access, needs to be explored [48]. Results also suggest that having unhealthy outlets make up no more than 25% of outlets in moderate-access areas and no more than 50% in low-access areas may mitigate the effects of lower accessibility to food retail overall. Future research would benefit from understanding how individuals interact with their FRE, their decision making around the use of one food retailer over others, their purchasing patterns, and how this translates to actual dietary intake [5,40]. Finally, reliable longitudinal FRE data (i.e., routine monitoring) examining all food outlets within neighbourhoods is needed; this will provide for further linkage opportunities with population health data, which will support future research and decision making [11].

5. Conclusions

A consistent relationship exists between self-reported BMI and healthier FRE characteristics. Our results show that increasing access and availability to a diverse range of food outlets, particularly healthy food outlets, should be an important consideration for efforts to support the evolution of healthy weight environments. This research provides evidence that Australia needs to follow suit with other countries that have adopted policies that give local governments the power to encourage healthier FRE. To further understand what the moderators and mediators of healthy weight are from within the FRE, further exploration into the lived experience of the FRE across geographic and socioeconomic differentials over time is required.

Supplementary Materials: The following supporting information can be downloaded at: https://www.mdpi.com/article/10.3390/nu15214503/s1, Table S1: Food outlet descriptions and healthiness scores; Table S2: Proportion of postal areas within each classification of food retail environment measures; Table S3: Summary of food retail environment measures of relative healthy food availability within each food environment typology by postal area in Greater Melbourne between 2008 and 2016; Table S4: Proportion of the Melbourne population sample within each food retail environment measure defined at the postcode level. Table S5: Sidak-adjusted pairwise comparisons of the mean BMI between years and between levels of healthy food outlet accessibility defined at the postcode level in Greater Melbourne, Australia. Table S6: Sidak-adjusted pairwise comparisons of the mean BMI between levels of food environment typology defined at the postcode level in Greater Melbourne, Australia.

Author Contributions: Conceptualisation, C.N., C.S. and S.A.; methodology, C.N., L.A. and C.S.; validation, C.N.; formal analysis, C.N. and L.O.; data curation, C.N. and L.O; writing—original draft preparation, C.N.; writing—review and editing, all authors; visualisation, C.N.; funding acquisition, C.N., C.S. and S.A. All authors have read and agreed to the published version of the manuscript.

Funding: This study was supported by a VicHealth Innovation Grant (IR27123).

Institutional Review Board Statement: The study was conducted in accordance with the Declaration of Helsinki, and an exemption for Ethics Review was granted for research undertaken by the Deakin University Human Research Ethics Committee (reference number 2018-310) on 19 December 2018.

Informed Consent Statement: Not applicable.

Data Availability Statement: The authors were permitted to use the Victorian Population Health Survey data by the Victorian State Government (Australia), which is the custodian of these data. The food environment data used in this study is presented on the Australian Food Retail Environment Monitoring Tool: https://foodenvironmentdashboard.com.au/food-retail/australian-food-retail-environment-monitoring-tool/ (accessed on 16 June 2021).

Conflicts of Interest: The authors declare no conflict of interest. The funders had no role in the design of the study; in the collection, analyses, or interpretation of data; in the writing of the manuscript; or in the decision to publish the results.

References

1. World Health Organization. *Development of an Implementation Roadmap 2023–2030 for the Global Action Plan for the Prevention and Control of NCDS 2013–2030*; World Health Organization: Geneva, Switzerland, 2003.
2. Swinburn, B.; Vandevijvere, S.; Kraak, V.; Sacks, G.; Snowdon, W.; Hawkes, C.; Barquera, S.; Friel, S.; Kelly, B.; Kumanyika, S.; et al. Monitoring and benchmarking government policies and actions to improve the healthiness of food environments: A proposed Government Healthy Food Environment Policy Index. *Obes. Rev.* **2013**, *14* (Suppl. S1), 24–37. [CrossRef]

3. Glanz, K.; Sallis, J.F.; Saelens, B.E.; Frank, L.D. Healthy nutrition environments: Concepts and measures. *Am. J. Health Promot.* **2005**, *19*, 330–333. [CrossRef]
4. World Health Organization. *Diet, Nutrition and the Prevention of Chronic Diseases*; World Health Organization: Geneva, Switzerland, 2003.
5. Swinburn, B.A.; Sacks, G.; Hall, K.D.; McPherson, K.; Finegood, D.T.; Moodie, M.L.; Gortmaker, S.L. The global obesity pandemic: Shaped by global drivers and local environments. *Lancet* **2011**, *378*, 804–814. [CrossRef] [PubMed]
6. National Institute for Care Excellence. *Cardiovascular Disease Prevention*; Public Health Guideline (PH25); National Institute for Care Excellence: London, UK, 2010.
7. MHCLG. Planning Practice Guidance: Healthy and Safe Communities 2019. Available online: https://www.gov.uk/guidance/health-and-wellbeing (accessed on 13 October 2022).
8. Public Health England. Using the planning system to promote healthier weight environments. In *Guidance and Supplementary Planning Document Template for Local Authority Public Health and Planning Teams*; Public Health England: London, UK, 2020.
9. Brown, H.; Xiang, H.; Albani, V.; Goffe, L.; Akhter, N.; Lake, A.; Sorrell, S.; Gibson, E.; Wildman, J. No new fast-food outlets allowed! Evaluating the effect of planning policy on the local food environment in the North East of England. *Soc. Sci. Med.* **2022**, *306*, 115126. [CrossRef] [PubMed]
10. Alston, L.; Raeside, R.; Jia, S.S.; Partridge, S.R. Underinvestment in nutrition research for atrisk populations: An analysis of research funding awarded in Australia from 2014 to 2021. *Nutr. Diet.* **2022**, *79*, 438–446. [CrossRef] [PubMed]
11. Needham, C.; Sacks, G.; Orellana, L.; Robinson, E.; Allender, S.; Strugnell, C. A systematic review of the Australian food retail environment: Characteristics, variation by geographic area, socioeconomic position and associations with diet and obesity. *Obes. Rev.* **2019**, *21*, e12941. [CrossRef] [PubMed]
12. Cobb, L.K.; Appel, L.J.; Franco, M.; Jones-Smith, J.C.; Nur, A.; Anderson, C.A.M. The relationship of the local food environment with obesity: A systematic review of methods, study quality, and results. *Obesity* **2015**, *23*, 1331–1344. [CrossRef] [PubMed]
13. Gamba, R.J.; Schuchter, J.; Rutt, C.; Seto, E.Y.W. Measuring the food environment and its effects on obesity in the United States: A systematic review of methods and results. *J. Community Health* **2015**, *40*, 464–475. [CrossRef]
14. Needham, C.; Strugnell, C.; Allender, S.; Orellana, L. Beyond food swamps and food deserts: Exploring urban Australian food retail environment typologies. *Public Health Nutr.* **2022**, *25*, 1140–1152. [CrossRef]
15. Needham, C.; Orellana, L.; Allender, S.; Sacks, G.; Blake, M.R.; Strugnell, C. Food Retail Environments in Greater Melbourne 2008–2016: Longitudinal Analysis of Intra-City Variation in Density and Healthiness of Food Outlets. *Int. J. Environ. Res. Public Health* **2020**, *17*, 1321. [CrossRef]
16. Lamb, K.E.; Thornton, L.E.; Olstad, D.L.; Cerin, E.; Ball, K. Associations between major chain fast-food outlet availability and change in body mass index: A longitudinal observational study of women from Victoria, Australia. *BMJ Open* **2017**, *7*, e016594. [CrossRef]
17. Baldock, K.L.; Paquet, C.; Howard, N.J.; Coffee, N.T.; Taylor, A.W.; Daniel, M. Are Perceived and Objective Distances to Fresh Food and Physical Activity Resources Associated with Cardiometabolic Risk? *Int. J. Environ. Res. Public Health* **2018**, *15*, 224. [CrossRef]
18. Feng, X.; Astell-Burt, T.; Badland, H.; Mavoa, S.; Giles-Corti, B. Modest ratios of fast food outlets to supermarkets and green grocers are associated with higher body mass index: Longitudinal analysis of a sample of 15,229 Australians aged 45 years and older in the Australian National Liveability Study. *Health Place* **2018**, *49*, 101–110. [CrossRef]
19. Paquet, C.; Coffee, N.T.; Haren, M.T.; Howard, N.J.; Adams, R.J.; Taylor, A.W.; Daniel, M. Food environment, walkability, and public open spaces are associated with incident development of cardio-metabolic risk factors in a biomedical cohort. *Health Place* **2014**, *28*, 173–176. [CrossRef]
20. Tseng, M.; Thornton, L.E.; Lamb, K.E.; Ball, K.; Crawford, D. Is neighbourhood obesogenicity associated with body mass index in women? Application of an obesogenicity index in socioeconomically disadvantaged neighbourhoods. *Health Place* **2014**, *30*, 20–27. [CrossRef]
21. Walker, R.E.; Keane, C.R.; Burke, J.G. Disparities and access to healthy food in the United States: A review of food deserts literature. *Health Place* **2010**, *16*, 876–884. [CrossRef]
22. Department of Health and Human Services. Victorian Population Health Survey: Victorian State Government. 2022. Available online: https://www.health.vic.gov.au/population-health-systems/victorian-population-health-survey (accessed on 1 August 2022).
23. Department of Health and Human Services. *Inequalities in the Social Determinants of Health and What It Means for the Health of Victorians: Findings from the 2014 Victorian Population Health Survey*; Victorian State Government: Melbourne, Australia, 2014.
24. Australian Bureau of Statistics. *3218.0—Regional Population Growth, Australia, 2008–2009*; Commonwealth of Australia: Canberra, Australia, 2010. Available online: https://www.abs.gov.au/ausstats/abs@.nsf/Products/3218.0~2008-09~Main+Features~Main+Features?OpenDocument#:~:text=3218.0%20%2D%20Regional%20Population%20Growth%2C%20Australia%2C%202008%2D09&text=Australia\T1\textquoterights%20estimated%20resident%20population%20(ERP,five%20years%20to%20June%202009 (accessed on 1 June 2019).
25. Australian Bureau of Statistics. *Census of Population and Housing: Socio-Economic Index for Areas (SEIFA), Australia, 2016*; Commonwealth of Australia: Canberra, Australia, 2016.

26. Department of Health and Human Services. *Victorian Population Health Survey Victoria*; Victorian State Government: Melbourne, Australia, 2021. Available online: https://www2.health.vic.gov.au/public-health/population-health-systems/health-status-of-victorians/survey-data-and-reports/victorian-population-health-survey (accessed on 12 January 2021).
27. Department of Health and Human Services. *Report 1: Victorian Population Health Survey 2014: Modifiable Risk Factors Contributing to Chronic Disease*; Victorian State Government: Melbourne, Australia, 2014.
28. Department of Health and Human Services. *Victorian Population Health Survey 2016: Selected Survey Findings*; Victorian State Government: Melbourne, Australia, 2018.
29. Department of Health and Human Services. *Victorian Population Health Survey 2008*; State Government of Victoria: Melbourne, Australia, 2008.
30. NBSP; Thornton, L.E.; Lamb, K.E.; Ball, K. Fast food restaurant locations according to socioeconomic disadvantage, urban–regional locality, and schools within Victoria, Australia. *SSM—Popul. Health* **2016**, *2*, 1–9. [CrossRef]
31. Moayyed, H.; Kelly, B.; Feng, X.; Flood, V. Evaluation of a 'healthiness' rating system for food outlet types in Australian residential communities. *Nutr. Diet.* **2017**, *74*, 29–35. [CrossRef]
32. Australian Bureau of Statistics. 1270.055.003—Australian Statistical Geography Standard (ASGS): Volume 2—Non ABS Structures, July 2016 Canberra. Available online: https://www.abs.gov.au/ausstats/abs@.nsf/Lookup/by%20Subject/1270.0.55.003~July%202016~Main%20Features~Postal%20Areas%20(POA)~8 (accessed on 25 May 2020).
33. Raskind, I.G.; Kegler, M.C.; Girard, A.W.; Dunlop, A.L.; Kramer, M.R. An activity space approach to understanding how food access is associated with dietary intake and BMI among urban, low-income African American women. *Health Place* **2020**, *66*, 102458. [CrossRef]
34. Wang, S.; Wang, M.; Liu, Y. Access to urban parks: Comparing spatial accessibility measures using three GIS-based approaches. *Comput. Environ. Urban Syst.* **2021**, *90*, 101713. [CrossRef]
35. Zhang, X.; Lu, H.; Holt, J.B. Modeling spatial accessibility to parks: A national study. *Int. J. Health Geogr.* **2011**, *10*, 31. [CrossRef]
36. Crothers, L. Australia Retail Foods: Retail Food Sector Report 2019. USDA Foreign Agricultural Service: Global Agricultural Information Network. 2019. Available online: https://apps.fas.usda.gov/newgainapi/api/report/downloadreportbyfilename?filename=Retail%20Foods_Canberra_Australia_6-27-2019.pdf (accessed on 18 July 2020).
37. Thornton, L.E.; Lamb, K.E.; White, S.R. The use and misuse of ratio and proportion exposure measures in food environment research. *Int. J. Behav. Nutr. Phys. Act.* **2020**, *17*, 118. [CrossRef]
38. Australian Bureau of Statistics. 1270.0.55.001—Australian Statistical Geography Standard (ADGS): Volume 1—Main Structure and Greater Capital City Statistical Areas, July 2016: Australian Federal Government; 2016 [updated July 2016]. Available online: https://www.abs.gov.au/ausstats/abs@.nsf/Lookup/by%20Subject/1270.0.55.001~July%202016~Main%20Features~Statistical%20Area%20Level%202%20(SA2)~10014 (accessed on 25 May 2019).
39. Australian Bureau of Statistics (ABS). *Estimated Resident Population (ERP) and Components by LGA (ASGS 2018) 2001 to 2018*; Commonwealth of Australia: Canberra, Australia, 2018.
40. Miller, L.J.; Joyce, S.; Carter, S.; Yun, G. Associations between childhood obesity and the availability of food outlets in the local environment: A retrospective cross-sectional study. *Am. J. Health Promot.* **2014**, *28*, e137–e145. [CrossRef]
41. Abbott, G.; Backholer, K.; Peeters, A.; Thornton, L.; Crawford, D.; Ball, K. Explaining educational disparities in adiposity: The role of neighborhood environments. *Obesity* **2014**, *22*, 2413–2419. [CrossRef]
42. Thornton, L.E.; Crawford, D.A.; Ball, K. Neighbourhood-socioeconomic variation in women's diet: The role of nutrition environments. *Eur. J. Clin. Nutr.* **2010**, *64*, 1423–1432. [CrossRef]
43. Crawford, D.A.; Timperio, A.F.; Salmon, J.A.; Baur, L.; Giles-Corti, B.; Roberts, R.J.; Jackson, M.L.; Andrianopoulos, N.; Ball, K. Neighbourhood fast food outlets and obesity in children and adults: The CLAN Study. *Pediatr. Obes.* **2008**, *3*, 249–256. [CrossRef]
44. Burgoine, T.; Sarkar, C.; Webster, C.J.; Monsivais, P. Examining the interaction of fast-food outlet exposure and income on diet and obesity: Evidence from 51,361 UK Biobank participants. *Int. J. Behav. Nutr. Phys. Act.* **2018**, *15*, 71. [CrossRef]
45. De Vogli, R.; Kouvonen, A.; Gimeno, D. 'Globesization': Ecological evidence on the relationship between fast food outlets and obesity among 26 advanced economies. *Crit. Public Health* **2011**, *21*, 395–402. [CrossRef]
46. Wool, J.L.; Walkinshaw, L.P.; Spigner, C.; Thayer, E.K.; Jones-Smith, J.C. A Qualitative Study of Living in a Healthy Food Priority Area in One Seattle, WA, Neighborhood. *Int. J. Environ. Res. Public Health* **2021**, *18*, 12251. [CrossRef]
47. Tach, L.; Amorim, M. Constrained, Convenient, and Symbolic Consumption: Neighborhood Food Environments and Economic Coping Strategies among the Urban Poor. *J. Urban Health* **2015**, *92*, 815–834. [CrossRef]
48. Christian, T.J. Grocery Store Access and the Food Insecurity–Obesity Paradox. *J. Hunger. Environ. Nutr.* **2010**, *5*, 360–369. [CrossRef]
49. Ng, S.P.; Korda, R.; Clements, M.; Latz, I.; Bauman, A.; Bambrick, H.; Liu, B.; Rogers, K.; Herbert, N.; Banks, E. Validity of self-reported height and weight and derived body mass index in middle-aged and elderly individuals in Australia. *Aust. New Zealand J. Public Health* **2011**, *35*, 557–563. [CrossRef]
50. Australian Bureau of Statistics. Statistical Geography Explained: Australian Bureau of Statistics. 2022. Available online: https://www.abs.gov.au/statistics/statistical-geography/statistical-geography-explained (accessed on 7 November 2022).
51. Dornelles, A. Impact of multiple food environments on body mass index. *PLoS ONE* **2019**, *14*, e0219365. [CrossRef] [PubMed]

52. Murphy, M.; Badland, H.; Jordan, H.; Koohsari, M.J.; Giles-Corti, B. Local Food Environments, Suburban Development, and BMI: A Mixed Methods Study. *Int. J. Environ. Res. Public Health* **2018**, *15*, 1392. [CrossRef] [PubMed]
53. Growth Areas Authority. *Precinct Structure Planning Guidelines Part Two: Preparing the Precinct Structure Plan*; Victorian State Government: Melbourne, Australia, 2013.

Disclaimer/Publisher's Note: The statements, opinions and data contained in all publications are solely those of the individual author(s) and contributor(s) and not of MDPI and/or the editor(s). MDPI and/or the editor(s) disclaim responsibility for any injury to people or property resulting from any ideas, methods, instructions or products referred to in the content.

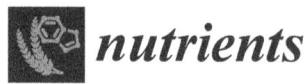 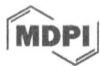

Article

Revealing Edible Bird Nest as Novel Functional Foods in Combating Metabolic Syndrome: Comprehensive In Silico, In Vitro, and In Vivo Studies

Happy Kurnia Permatasari [1,*], Queen Intan Permatasari [2], Nurpudji Astuti Taslim [3], Dionysius Subali [4], Rudy Kurniawan [5], Reggie Surya [6], Faqrizal Ria Qhabibi [7], Melvin Junior Tanner [8], Siti Chairiyah Batubara [9], Nelly Mayulu [10], William Ben Gunawan [11], Andi Yasmin Syauki [3], Netty Salindeho [12], Moon Nyeo Park [13,14], Juan Alessandro Jeremis Maruli Nura Lele [15], Raymond R. Tjandrawinata [16], Bonglee Kim [13,14] and Fahrul Nurkolis [17]

1. Department of Biochemistry and Biomolecular, Faculty of Medicine, University of Brawijaya, Malang 65145, Indonesia
2. Department of Pharmacy, Faculty of Medicine, University of Brawijaya, Malang 65145, Indonesia
3. Division of Clinical Nutrition, Department of Nutrition, Faculty of Medicine, Hasanuddin University, Makassar 90245, Indonesia
4. Department of Biotechnology, Faculty of Biotechnology, Atma Jaya Catholic University of Indonesia, Jakarta 12930, Indonesia
5. Diabetes Connection Care, Eka Hospital Bumi Serpong Damai, Tangerang 15321, Indonesia
6. Department of Food Technology, Faculty of Engineering, Bina Nusantara University, Jakarta 11480, Indonesia
7. Medical School Department, Faculty of Medicine, Brawijaya University, Malang 65145, Indonesia
8. Nutrition Coaching Development, PT. Prima Sehat Makmur Utama, Jakarta 12430, Indonesia
9. Food Technology Department, Sahid University of Jakarta, South Jakarta 12870, Indonesia
10. Department of Nutrition, Faculty of Health Science, Muhammadiyah Manado University, Manado 95249, Indonesia
11. Department of Nutrition Science, Faculty of Medicine, Diponegoro University, Semarang 50275, Indonesia
12. Fishery Products Technology Study Program, Faculty of Fisheries and Marine Sciences, Sam Ratulangi University, Manado 95115, Indonesia
13. Department of Pathology, College of Korean Medicine, Kyung Hee University, Seoul 02447, Republic of Korea; bongleekim@khu.ac.kr (B.K.)
14. Korean Medicine-Based Drug Repositioning Cancer Research Center, College of Korean Medicine, Kyung Hee University, Seoul 02447, Republic of Korea
15. Faculty of Medicine, Universitas Kristen Indonesia, Jakarta 13630, Indonesia
16. Dexa Laboratories of Biomolecular Science, Dexa Medica Group, Cikarang 17530, Indonesia
17. Department of Biological Sciences, Faculty of Sciences and Technology, State Islamic University of Sunan Kalijaga (UIN Sunan Kalijaga), Yogyakarta 55281, Indonesia; fahrul.nurkolis.mail@gmail.com
* Correspondence: happykp@ub.ac.id

Abstract: Metabolic dysfunction, which includes intra-abdominal adiposity, glucose intolerance, insulin resistance, dyslipidemia, and hypertension, manifests into metabolic syndrome and related diseases. Therefore, the discovery of new therapies in the fight against metabolic syndrome is very challenging. This study aims to reveal the existence of an edible bird nest (EBN) as a functional food candidate that may be a new alternative in fighting metabolic syndrome. The study included three approaches: in silico molecular docking simulation, in vitro, and in vivo in rats fed on cholesterol- and fat-enriched diets. Four terpenoids of Bakuchiol, Curculigosaponin A, Dehydrolindestrenolide, and 1-methyl-3-(1-methyl-ethyl)-benzene in EBN have been identified through LCMS/MS-QTOF. In molecular docking simulations, Bakuchiol and Dehydrolindestrenolide are considered very potent because they have higher inhibitory power on the four receptors (iNOS, ROS1 kinase, FTO, and lipase) than standard drugs. In vitro tests also provide insight into the antioxidant, antidiabetic, and antiobesity activities of EBN, which is quite feasible due to the smaller EC_{50} value of EBN compared to standard drugs. Interestingly, in vivo studies also showed significant improvements ($p < 0.05$) in the lipid profile, blood glucose, enzymatic levels, and inflammatory biomarkers in rats given high-dose dietary supplementation of EBN. More interestingly, high-dose dietary supplementation of EBN upregulates PGC-1α and downregulates HMG-CoA reductase. Comprehensively, it has been revealed that EBN can be novel functional foods for combating metabolic syndrome.

Citation: Permatasari, H.K.; Permatasari, Q.I.; Taslim, N.A.; Subali, D.; Kurniawan, R.; Surya, R.; Qhabibi, F.R.; Tanner, M.J.; Batubara, S.C.; Mayulu, N.; et al. Revealing Edible Bird Nest as Novel Functional Foods in Combating Metabolic Syndrome: Comprehensive In Silico, In Vitro, and In Vivo Studies. *Nutrients* 2023, 15, 3886. https://doi.org/10.3390/nu15183886

Academic Editor: Jose M. Miranda

Received: 1 August 2023
Revised: 4 September 2023
Accepted: 5 September 2023
Published: 6 September 2023

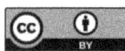

Copyright: © 2023 by the authors. Licensee MDPI, Basel, Switzerland. This article is an open access article distributed under the terms and conditions of the Creative Commons Attribution (CC BY) license (https://creativecommons.org/licenses/by/4.0/).

Keywords: edible bird nest; swallow bird nest; metabolic syndrome; functional food; terpenoids; metabolites; antioxidants; antiobesity; antidiabetic

1. Introduction

Metabolic syndrome is a cluster of interrelated risk factors that reflect overnutrition, sedentary lifestyles, and resultant excess adiposity [1]. It is characterized by a combination of risk factors encompassing obesity, high blood sugar levels, insulin resistance, elevated blood pressure, and non-HDL cholesterol [2,3]. It has been widely accepted that metabolic syndrome significantly increases the likelihood of developing cardiovascular diseases and diabetes mellitus [4]. About one-third of adults in the US have been reported to suffer from metabolic syndrome [2]. Concerning obesity as a risk factor for metabolic syndrome, the World Health Organization (WHO) stated that there were 650 million adults, 340 million adolescents, and 39 million children who were obese [5]. Today, obesity is not even considered a disease of affluence anymore, according to a global survey, since its prevalence has doubled in 73 countries and increased in other countries in the last quarter decade, most of which were countries with low socio-economic index [6]. Since environmental factors play an essential role in the development of metabolic syndrome, adopting a healthy lifestyle is paramount to preventing its prevalence [7]. Therefore, eating in a healthy manner could be adopted to support a healthy lifestyle that would prevent metabolic syndrome, such as by consuming functional food.

Previously, the use of functional foods has been suggested as a potential therapeutic option for treating metabolic syndrome, in particular with regard to its relation to obesity [8]. Edible bird nest (EBN), a renowned Asian delicacy derived from the saliva of swiftlets, has been consumed in many parts of the world for its nutritional and medical values [9], thus suggesting it to be a functional food. EBN is mainly produced in Southeast Asian countries (mainly Indonesia, Thailand, and Malaysia) and has been culturally regarded as a high-grade, expensive health food [10]. The nutritional content of EBN dry matter is mainly constituted of protein (>50%), followed by carbohydrates (40–45%) and ash (5%) with very little fat (<0.5%) [11]. Peptides are the most important protein components in EBN, with the total essential amino acids appreciably greater than in other foods known as sources of protein, such as eggs and milk [12]. Sialic acid is the major component of carbohydrates in EBN (10%) besides mannose, glucosamine, galactosamine, galactose, and fucose [13]. Studies focusing on metabolites such as terpenoids and their biological activity from EBN are limited to date and need further exploration.

Several scientific studies have been conducted to explore the potential of EBN for health promotion. Bioactive peptides and glycoproteins present in EBN are often considered to be the main compounds contributing to the health benefits of EBN [14]. Several recognized health properties of EBN include anti-influenza virus, immunomodulatory, antioxidant, anti-inflammatory, and anti-aging. In addition, EBN has been reported to improve neurodegenerative and cardiovascular diseases [9]. With regard to metabolic syndrome, EBN has been reported to prevent insulin resistance induced by a high-fat diet in rats [15] and ameliorate atherosclerosis in hypercholesterolemic mice [16]. Hydrolyzed bird nests had the potential to regulate pancreatic β-cell function and insulin signaling in diabetic mice [17].

These nutritional characteristics make EBN an intriguing subject for scientific exploration and potential therapeutic applications. Further research is warranted to elucidate the specific bioactive components and mechanisms underlying the potential health benefits associated with the consumption of EBN. The present study aimed to investigate the effects of EBN consumption on cholesterol- and fat-enriched diet animal models. The focus was emphasized on the lipid profile, blood glucose, enzymatic metabolic, and inflammatory biomarkers; more specifically, to complement the current evidence-based EBN, this study also looked at modulatory effects on peroxisome proliferator-activated receptor-gamma coactivator-1 alpha (PGC-1α) and HMG-CoA reductase. The PGC-1α pathway regulates cellular metabolism, energy homeostasis, and aging [18]. Dysregulation of this pathway is implicated in metabolic disorders and age-related diseases [18]. HMG-CoA reductase, as an enzyme regulating the rate of cholesterol biosynthesis, and HMG-CoA reductase inhibitors still need to be explored further to fight metabolic syndrome [18]. By knowing the modulation, there will be a new insight into the evidence base of EBN health benefits.

In addition, the characterization of chemical constituents in EBN and their biological activities were also analyzed using computational molecular docking on the selected receptors. In vitro antioxidant, antidiabetic, and antiobesity activities were also reported in this study to complement the current EBN literature. Understanding the full potential of EBN as a functional food may provide valuable insights into its role in managing metabolic syndrome and improving overall health outcomes.

2. Materials and Methods

2.1. Edible Bird Nest

EBN was obtained by our research team from wallet bird farmers in Pasuruan Regency, East Java, Indonesia, as formally confirmed. The EBN obtained had gone through a cleaning process by certified farmers and was ready to eat. EBN did not go through any extraction process because it aims to see the benefits if consumed as usual (consumption of EBN by the community without any extraction treatment), as the researchers wanted to study the impact directly, which is similar to consumption habits by consumers. Because of their edible and resistant nature, EBN samples were stored in aluminum foil at room temperature before further laboratory tests.

2.2. Metabolites Screening by LCMS/MS-QTOF Analysis

EBN samples were sent to SIG Laboratory (ISO 17025:2017 Accredited LP-184-IDN, Bogor, West Java) for liquid chromatography analysis of mass spectrometry-quadrupole—time of flight (LCMS/MS-QTOF) with a GIS certificate number of LHP. VI.2023.051606162. LCMS/MS-QTOF analysis is performed according to Qiao et al. [19]. The sample preparation involves weighing 1 g of the sample into a 10 mL volumetric flask. Next, suitable methanol or solvent was added and sonicated for 30 min. The mixture was concentrated with suitable methanol or solvent and homogenized. The mixture was then filtered through a GHP/PTFE 0.22-μm membrane filter and injected into the UPLC system. The instrumental measurement conditions were set as follows: LC Column = C18, Column Temperature = 40 °C, Autosampler Temperature = 15 °C, Injection Volume = 10 μL, Mobile Phase = A = 0.1% formic acid in acetonitrile, B = 0.1% formic acid in water, and Flow Rate = 0.6 mL/min, Gradient. MS Settings used were as follows: Mode of Operation = Tof MSE, Ionization = ESI (−)/ESI (+), and Acquisition Range = 50–1200 Da.

Screening for active compounds in natural products is carried out using LCMS/MS-QTOF with UNIFI software (version 1.6), which contains a library of mass spectra of active compounds from the Waters database. The UNIFI software (version 1.6) allows the identification of mass spectra of compounds in the sample, which are then matched with the mass spectra in the library.

2.3. In Silico Molecular Docking Analysis

The research was conducted on an ASUS Vivobook M413ia—Ek502t laptop with a 2.3 GHz AMD Ryzen 5 4500u processor, 8 GB DDR4 memory, and 512 GB SSD M.2 storage. This laptop was equipped with ChemDraw Ultra 12.0, AutoDock tools (version 4.2), and BIOVIA Discovery software (version 20.1), as well as the Windows 10 Home operating system and the AutoDock tools (version 4.2). In addition, the researchers utilized the Protein Data Bank and PubChem structure databases. The study's protocols for molecular coupling simulation were based on previously established methodologies [20].

From the EBN profiles, specific compounds were identified for the test ligands. These compounds were created in 2D with ChemDraw Ultra 12.0, converted to 3D, and optimized using the MM2 algorithm. The focus of the investigation was on four Protein Data Bank-obtained target proteins: human inducible nitric oxide synthase (PDB ID: 3E7G), human reactive oxygen species 1 kinase (PDB ID: 3ZBF), human pancreatic lipase (PDB ID: 1LPB), and fat mass and obesity-associated protein (PDB ID: 3LFM).

To validate the process of molecular docking, redocking was performed. Using precise grid coordinates, AutoDock tools (version 4.2) were used to position the original ligand back into the target binding site. After redocking, the ligand's position was evaluated, and it was required to have a root-mean-square deviation (RMSD) of less than 2.0. Grid and docking parameter adjustments were made based on the results of the docking validation. The final conformation structure of each docking was stored as a *dlg file, and Discovery Studio 2016 was used to analyze the interaction between the ligands and receptors.

2.4. Antioxidant Activity by ABTS and DPPH Radical Scavenging Activity Assays

Following the methodology described in prior investigations [21,22], the scavenging activity of 2,2'-azino-bis(3-ethylbenzothiazoline-6-sulfonic acid) (ABTS+; Sigma-Aldrich, Saint Louis, MO, USA) was determined. To produce the ABTS working solution, 7 mM ABTS, and 2.4 mM potassium persulfate were combined in equal proportions and incubated for 14 h at 22 °C in a dark container. The mixture was then diluted to produce a new working solution with an absorbance of 0.706% at 734 nm. Various concentrations of EBN preparations (50, 100, 150, 200, and 250 µg/mL) were diluted with 1 mL of the ABTS working solution for the ABTS scavenging assay. After a 7-min incubation period, each sample's absorbance at 734 nm was measured. In this investigation, the positive control was Trolox. The procedures detailed in previous investigations were followed [18,21,22].

The 2,2-diphenyl-1-picrylhydrazyl radical-scavenging activity (DPPH) test was performed. Different concentrations of EBN preparations (50, 100, 150, 200, and 250 µg/mL) were added to containers containing 3 mL of DPPH reagent. After 30 min of incubation at ambient temperature, the absorbance of each sample was measured at 517 nm. This assay utilized glutathione (GSH; Sigma-Aldrich, 354102) as the positive control. To assure accurate and reliable results, each sample was subjected to triplicate analysis ($n = 3$) for both the ABTS and DPPH assays. As determined by the experimental procedure, the inhibition of DPPH and ABTS was calculated using the corresponding formula. Inhibition of DPPH and ABTS was determined according to the following formula:

$$Inhibition\ Activity\ (\%) = \frac{A0 - A1}{A0} \times 100\%$$

where $A0$ = absorbance of blank; and $A1$ = absorbance of standard or sample.

The half-maximal effective concentration ratio (EC_{50}) with Trolox for the ABTS test and glutathione for the DPPH assay, the radical-scavenging capacity of EBN (Edible Birds Nest), was expressed. EC_{50} stands for the sample concentration at which the initial radical concentration is reduced by 50%. In other words, the sample's capacity to scavenge free radicals is represented by the EC_{50} value, with lower values indicating greater antioxidant activity. To compare the radical-scavenging capacities of EBN against well-known antioxidants, tronx and glutathione were employed as reference molecules.

2.5. In Vitro Antidiabetic Assay via α-Glucosidase and α-Amylase Inhibition

The researchers performed two different inhibitory activity tests on the EBN samples, as per methodologies described in previous literature [23,24]. The α-amylase inhibition activity of EBN samples was measured based on the previous literature [18,25]. For the α-glucosidase inhibition test, a phosphate buffer solution with a volume of 50 mL (pH 6.9) containing the enzyme was prepared. The enzyme concentration in the solution was 1.52 UI/mL. Maltose and sucrose solutions were added to the mixture, followed by the addition of EBN samples at various concentrations (ranging from 50 µg/mL to 250 µg/mL). Each sample was then mixed and incubated at 37 °C for 20 min. The enzyme was later inactivated by heating the tubes at 100 °C for 2 min. Acarbose was used as a positive control in this experiment. Regarding the α-amylase inhibition activity, diluted EBN samples were incubated at five different concentrations (ranging from 50 µg/mL to 250 µg/mL) along with NaCl (0.006 M), sodium phosphate buffer (pH 6.9), and porcine pancreatic amylase (0.5 mg/mL). Afterward, each mixture was combined with 500 µL of 1% starch solution and incubated at 25 °C for 10 min. Following this, 3,5-dinitro salicylic acid was added to complete the reaction, and the mixture was incubated at 100 °C for 5 min. After cooling at 22 °C, the absorbance of each sample was measured at 540 nm after dilution with distilled water. Acarbose served as the positive control in this case as well.

2.6. In Vitro Antiobesity Evaluation via Lipase Inhibition Assay

The inhibitory data was obtained using the previously described equation [23,24]. Initially, crude pig pancreatic lipase (PPL, 1 mg/mL) was dissolved in a 50 mM phosphate buffer (pH 7) prior to centrifugation at 12,000 g to remove insoluble components. In order to create an enzyme stock (0.1 mg/mL), the supernatant was diluted 10 times with a buffer. Based on prior research [26], a 96-well microplate containing 100 µL of EBN samples was combined with 20 L of 10 mM p-nitrophenyl butyrate (pNPB) in a buffer and incubated at 37 degrees Celsius (C) for 10 min. Orlistat (C29H53NO5, PubChem CID: 3034010), a well-known PPL or lipase inhibitor, was used as a comparison drug. At 405 nm, measurements were taken using a DR-200Bc ELISA microplate reader. Using the yield of the reaction rate of 1 mol of p-nitrophenol (4-nitrophenol, C6H5NO3) per minute at 37 degrees Celsius (C), the unit of activity was calculated. To determine the lipase inhibition activity, the PPL activity in the test mixture was decreased by a predetermined amount. To assure the validity of the study's findings, each sample was verified three times ($n = 3$) or in triplicate.

$$Inhibition\ of\ Lipase\ Activity\ (\%) = 100 - \frac{B - Bc}{A - Ac} \times 100\%$$

where A = Activity without inhibitor; B = Activity with inhibitor; Ac = Negative control (−) without inhibitor; Bc = Negative control (−) with inhibitor.

2.7. In Vivo Study Design on Rats Fed on Cholesterol- and Fat-Enriched Diet

2.7.1. Animal Handling and Ethical Approval

Forty male Rattus norvegicus (*Rattus norvegicus*) rats weighing 204.03 ± 3.68 g were used in the in vivo investigation. The rats came from the Animal Model Farm in Yogyakarta, Indonesia, and were acclimated for 10 days in a controlled environment (27 °C, 50–60% relative humidity, balanced light–dark cycle), with access to regular animal feed and water from PT Citra Ina Feedmill. The study protocol gained ethical approval from the International Register of Preclinical Trial Animal Studies Protocols (preclinicaltrials.eu; https://preclinicaltrials.eu, accessed on 22 March 2023) with registration number PCTE0000371 and complied with the Guidelines for Reporting In Vivo Experiments (ARRIVE).

2.7.2. Study Design of Treatments

The rats were randomly separated into four treatment groups following the acclimation phase. Groups C and D were also fed CFED diets and water ad libitum but with daily supplements of 22.5 (low dose/LD) and 45 (high dose/HD) mg/kg body weight (BW) of EBN, respectively. Group A received a normal diet and water ad libitum. Group B was fed a cholesterol- and fat-enriched (CFED) diet with ad libitum water. The oral EBN doses were given by a professional and administered by oral gavage. Throughout the study, the daily intake of food and water was observed, and there were no changes between the control and experimental groups in this respect.

2.7.3. Feed or Pellet Composition and CFED Production

The typical pellets are purchased from Rat Bio® in Jakarta, Indonesia, and have the following composition percentages: 12% moisture, 20% protein, 4% fat, 14% calcium, 1% fiber, 0.7% phosphorus, 11.5% total ash, 0.3% vitamin C, and 0.1% vitamin E. According to the recommendations of the manufacturer, these pellets were properly stored in a cool, dry location away from direct sunlight.

A technique based on earlier research [26,27] was used to develop the CFED diet. The procedure involves adding certain additives to the dry, standard pellets. These additions comprised 2% powdered cholesterol, 2% maize oil, 20% animal fat, and 1% cholic acid. After homogenizing the mixture, 1 L of distilled water was used to break the mixture pellets into smaller pieces. The pellets were initially dried sterile at ambient temperature before being kept at 4 °C to reduce oxidation. The CFED diet is composed of the following: carbs make up 43.6% of the diet, protein makes up 12.4%, fiber makes up 4.7%, fat makes up 3.2%, cholesterol makes up 2%, cholic acid makes up 1%, animal fat makes up 20%, total ash makes up 4%, maize oil makes up 2%, and the rest is moisture.

2.7.4. Biomedical Analysis of Collected Blood Samples

Blood samples were taken six weeks after the rats received interventional feeding. The animals were fasted overnight and given ketamine as anesthesia prior to the blood collection. Blood was extracted from the venous sinus and put in an unanticoagulated, dry, and sterile tube. The blood was then left to coagulate at room temperature. The serum was collected after 20 min of centrifugation at 3000 rpm. The COBAS Integra® 400 Plus Analyzer (Roche Diagnostics, Basel, Switzerland) was used to conduct biomedical studies of several parameters. Low-density lipoprotein (LDL), triglycerides (TG), high-density lipoprotein (HDL), total cholesterol (TC), and blood glucose (BG) levels were among them. Blood was also drawn from the cardiac tissue in order to evaluate other biomarkers. Using the SOD Assay Kit from Sigma-Aldrich, the superoxide dismutase (SOD) enzyme activity was assessed. The Mouse Pancreatic Lipase ELISA Kit (Merck KGaA, Darmstadt, Germany) was used to assess blood lipase levels, and the Mouse Pancreatic Amylase ELISA Kit to measure serum amylase levels. Using particular ELISA kits, the levels of the inflammatory biomarkers PGC-1 (peroxisome proliferator-activated receptor-gamma coactivator-1 alpha), TNF-alpha (tumor necrosis factor-alpha), and IL-10 (interleukin 10) were measured. PGC-1, TNF-alpha, and IL-10 were evaluated using kits from Sunlong Biotech Co., Ltd. (Zhejiang, China), PGC-1 Mouse ELISA Kit from Abcam, and Mouse Tumor Necrosis Factor-alpha (TNF-alpha) Kit from Sunlong Biotech Co., Ltd. (Zhejiang, China). Additionally, during the investigation, the body weights of the rats were determined using digital scales.

2.8. Data Analysis and Management

Numerous statistical techniques were used in the data analysis and management area to evaluate the experimental outcomes both in vitro and in vivo. The unpaired t-test was utilized to establish the statistical significance of the in vitro investigations, which included antioxidant inhibition of ABTS and DPPH, as well as inhibitory actions for lipase, -amylase, and -glucosidase. In order to ensure reproducibility, these tests were carried out in triplicate. Nonlinear regression methods were utilized to construct each EC_{50} dataset, which helped determine the sample concentration that resulted in a 50% reduction in the starting radical concentration. Several factors for in vivo data processing were investigated. Multivariate analysis of variance (ANOVA) was used to examine the lipid profile (LDL, HDL, TG, TC, and BG), inflammatory biomarkers (IL-10, TNF, and PGC-1), and enzymatic tests (SOD cardio, serum lipase, and serum amylase). This made it possible to look at several variables' connections at once. Pairwise t-tests (or dependent t-tests) were used to determine whether there were any significant differences in body weights (g) within each group between the starting and finishing points. Additionally, a one-way ANOVA was used to find differences between each secondary parameter, including the beginning, final, and daily weight gain (g/day) for each group, water intake (mL), food intake (g), the food efficiency ratio (FER), and water consumption. With a 95% level of confidence, all reported data were given as mean values with a standard error of the mean (SEM). Data analysis on MacBook laptops was done using GraphPad Prism 9.4.1 software.

3. Results

3.1. Terpenoids Observed in EBN

The analysis of compounds in natural products is very important for the basic characterization of potential components in them. In this study, four terpenoid compounds (Bakuchiol, Curculigosaponin A, Dehydrolindestrenolide, and 1-methyl-3-(1-methyl-ethyl)-benzene) have been observed in EBN through LCMS/MS-QTOF analysis, and the data are presented in Table 1, which have met the criteria: Mass error $\leq$ 5 ppm; Isotope match MZ RMS PPM $\leq$ 6 ppm; Isotope match MZ RMS % $\leq$ 10%; Intensity/Response $\geq$ 300; and Fragment match $\geq$ 1 mass fragment. Chromatogram mass spectrum data can be viewed in Supplementary Materials File S1.

Table 1. Confirmed terpenoids component in EBN via LCMS/MS-QTOF analysis.

Component Name	Formula	Observed RT (min)	Mass Error (ppm)	Total Fragments Found	Isotope Match Mz RMS PPM	Isotope Match Mz Intensity y RMS Percent	Response	Adducts
Bakuchiol	$C_{18}H_{24}O$	16.82	0.7	2	0.90	2.93	817	+H
Curculigosaponin A	$C_{36}H_{60}O_9$	17.19	−3.9	19	4.47	2.13	26866	+H
Dehydrolindestrenolide	$C_{15}H_{16}O_2$	16.67	−1.4	17	3.32	3.19	1272	+H
1-Methyl-3-(1-methyl-ethyl)-benzene	$C_{11}H_{16}$	16.72	−1.4	12	1.58	2.41	1493	+H

The four compounds observed in EBN (Table 1) were continued preparation for in silico molecular docking tests.

3.2. In Silico Molecular Docking Simulation in Selected Receptors

The observed metabolites, Bakuchiol, Curculigosaponin A, Dehydrolindestrenolide, and 1-methyl-3-(1-methyl-ethyl)-benzene were then followed by in silico or molecular docking studies on selected receptors for antioxidants and obesity. The molecular docking assay focuses on specific receptors such as human inducible nitric oxide synthase (iNOS), human pancreatic lipase, human reactive oxygen species (ROS) 1 kinase, and fat mass and obesity-associated (FTO) proteins. All these receptors were continued with molecular docking validation tests and obtained an assessment accuracy value of less than 2 Å which indicates they are successfully validated; the data are shown in Table 2.

Table 2. Validation of molecular docking simulation.

No.	Drug Target	PDBID	Docking Site (x;y;z)	Docking Area (x;y;z)	RMSD (Å)	ΔG (kcal/mol)	Numb in Cluster (/100)	Judgment (<2 Å)
1	iNOS	3E7G	55.022, 21.817, 78.677,	40 × 40 × 40	1.789	−6.67	98	Valid
2	ROS1 kinase	3ZBF	42.521, 19.649, 3.987,	40 × 40 × 40	1.216	−7.83	90	Valid
3	Human pancreatic lipase	1LPB	−0.423, 16.723, 26.546,	42 × 40 × 40	1.499	−4.13	26	Valid
4	Fat mass and obesity-associated (FTO) protein	3LFM	29.043, −6.644, −29.329,	42 × 42 × 42	0.715	−6.29	90	Valid

Protein data bank–PDB, Root mean square deviation–RMSD.

After being successfully declared valid, molecular docking simulations were carried out between ligands or identified compounds from EBN against selected receptors, and molecular docking value data, or ΔG (kcal/mol), is presented in Table 3. Based on Table 3, molecular docking results show that the four terpenoids of EBN have higher ΔG values than standard control drugs (orlistat) in terms of antiobesity potential (potential inhibiting FTO protein and human lipase enzymes). Interestingly, Curculigosaponin A has inhibitory activity against three of the four selected receptors and has a higher value than standard drugs as controls, especially being more potent in inhibiting iNOS than S-ibuprofen. More interestingly, Bakuchiol and Dehydrolindestrenolide are considered very potential candidates for antioxidant and antiobesity-related metabolic syndrome because they have higher inhibitory power at all four receptors than standard drugs as controls, including the ROS1 kinase receptor. This proves molecularly that the compound components in EBN have the potential to have antioxidant and antiobesity properties in an in silico molecular docking simulation.

Table 3. Molecular docking parameter of identified terpenoid compounds of two EBNs.

No.	Substance	Number in Cluster (/100)				ΔG (kcal/mol)				K_i			
		3E7G	3ZBF	1LPB	3LFM	3E7G	3ZBF	1LPB	3LFM	3E7G	3ZBF	1LPB	3LFM
	Control												
1	S-ibuprofen	33				−4.73				128.28 μM			
2	Trolox		100				−5.36				85.58 uM		
3	Orlistat			6	5			−2.38	−3.71			5.22 mM	212.83 uM
1	Bakuchiol	74	66	68	89	−5.85	−6.12	−5.94	−6.80	19.90 uM	9.04 uM	386.01 nM	6.14 uM
2	Curculigosaponin A	52	20	23	34	−5.53	−4.70	−6.51	−5.36	15.85 uM	26.89 uM	11.59 uM	10.51 uM
3	Dehydrolindestrenolide	100	100	100	100	−7.34	−6.95	−6.74	−7.04	4.14 uM	7.85 uM	11.38 uM	6.85 uM
4	1-methyl-3-(1-methyl-ethyl)-benzene	100	100	96	77	−4.47	−4.74	−4.47	−4.75	515.43 uM	329.80 uM	525.40 uM	268.68 uM

Visualization of the interaction of amino acids from the active compound EBN against iNOS, ROS1 kinase, FTO, and lipase can be seen in Supplementary File S2. Indeed, in silico studies above have observed the potential of EBN against selected receptors. However, further studies of in vitro biological activity are needed to validate these results. In vitro studies in this study have also been conducted and reported in the sections below.

3.3. In Vitro Study Reveals the Antioxidants, Antidiabetic, and Antiobesity Potential of EBN

The results of the in vitro study presented in Figure 1 are in line with the results of in silico tests described in the previous section, indicating that EBN indeed has potential as a promising antioxidant, antidiabetic, and antiobesity compound. Judging from the EC_{50} value in the antioxidant activity test via ABTS inhibition activity with a value of 77.62 μg/mL, which is smaller than Trolox (78.74 μg/mL), a control, this shows that EBN is more potent in free radical scavenging than Trolox (EC_{50} EBN < EC_{50} Trolox). Furthermore, the EC_{50} value of EBN in α-amylase inhibition activity also shows similar things to the ABTS, EC_{50} EBN < EC_{50} Acarbose or control tests (Figure 1). Interestingly, the EC_{50} EBN in lipase inhibition activity has a value of 59.30 μg/mL, which is more potent in antiobesity candidates than orlistat or control, which has a greater EC_{50} value (61.36 μg/mL). Overall, these in vitro tests are consistent with in silico tests that reveal the health effects of EBN in terms of metabolic syndrome.

To provide comprehensive knowledge of the health benefits of EBN, especially as a functional food candidate that can fight metabolic syndrome, in vivo tests on animal models were also conducted and reported in this study.

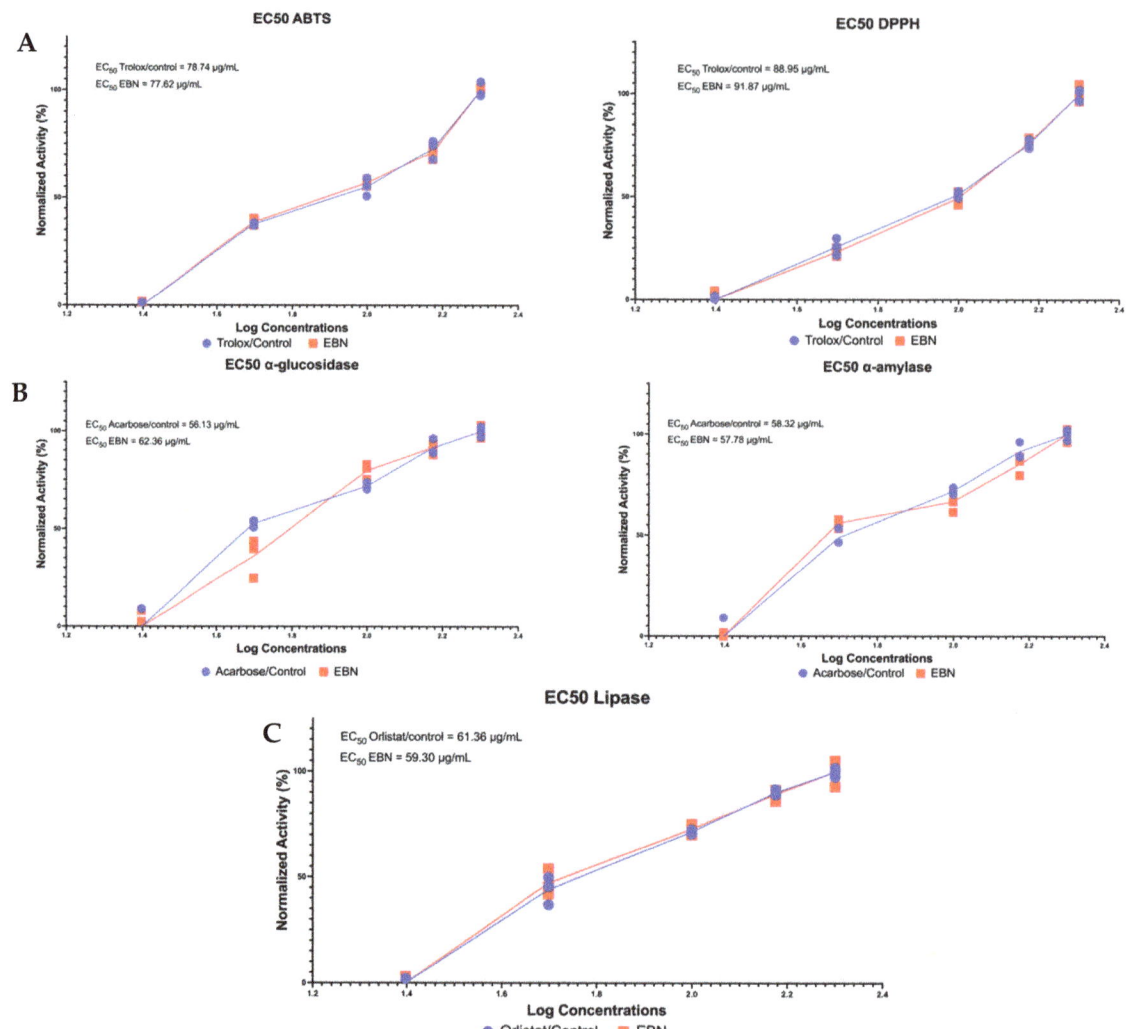

Figure 1. In vitro antioxidants, antidiabetic and antiobesity activities of EBN. (**A**) EC_{50} antioxidants via ABTS and DPPH inhibition activity. (**B**) EC_{50} antidiabetic via α-glucosidase and α-amylase inhibition activity. (**C**) EC_{50} antiobesity via lipase inhibition activity.

3.4. In Vivo Study Reveals Attenuation Metabolic Syndrome by EBN Supplementation

Data characteristics of experimental rats (*R. norvegicus*), including body weight (BW), feed, water intake, and FER, are presented in Table 4. It is clear that the initial BW of all groups is the same, and there is no significant difference. The BW, food intake, and water intake of experimental rats were calculated daily and obtained values that did not differ significantly in each group during treatment. However, interestingly, it was clear that the CFED diet had significantly higher final BW values than both the normal and EBN treatment groups. Furthermore, the group fed the diet with a second dose of EBN had significantly lower final BW values than CFED and even the normal group ($p < 0.05$). The group with a high dose of EBN supplementation had the lowest final BW score of the other groups.

Table 4. Body weight, feed, water intake, and FER characteristics of experimental rats (*R. norvegicus*).

Group	Normal	CFED	CFED + Low Dose EBN	CFED + High Dose EBN	*p* **
Initial BW (g)	203.62 ± 2.99	203.11 ± 2.80	204.19 ± 4.32	205.20 ± 4.53	0.2805
Final BW (g)	244.63 ± 3.19	277.09 ± 6.70	235.48 ± 3.23	230.10 ± 2.01	<0.0001
p *	<0.000001	<0.000001	<0.000001	<0.000001	
Weight gain (g/day)	0.89 ± 0.08	1.61 ± 0.17	0.68 ± 0.08	0.55 ± 0.10	0.8004
Food intake (g)	4.79 ± 0.47	4.89 ± 0.50	4.94 ± 0.69	5.05 ± 0.87	0.9960
Water intake (mL)	5.44 ± 0.63	5.37 ± 0.83	5.26 ± 0.79	5.01 ± 0.61	0.9822
FER (%)	18.74 ± 2.09	33.01 ± 3.15	13.96 ± 2.22	11.39 ± 3.84	0.0004

* Dependent or paired *t*-test CI 95% (0.05). ** ANOVA CI 95% (0.05). Food Efficiency Ratio (FER) was calculated by dividing body weight (BW) gain by food intake.

Improvements in lipid and blood glucose profiles were also observed in the CFED group given EBN supplementation at both doses; the data are presented in Figure 2. In general, high LDL, TG, TC, and BG values and low HDL levels were observed significantly in the CFED group when compared to the normal control group. Both doses of EBN were significantly observed to upregulate levels of HDL and downregulate levels of LDL, TG, TC, and BG. Interestingly, high-dose EBN supplementation was significantly better at reducing levels of LDL, TG, TC, and BG and HDL enhancement when compared to normal and low-dose EBN controls. Overall, high-dose EBN supplementation led to the modulation of both lipid profiles and blood glucose in CFED rats. This is possible because there are two terpenoids, namely Bakuchiol and Dehydrolindestrenolide, which in in silico molecular docking can inhibit lipase and FTO protein (Table 3).

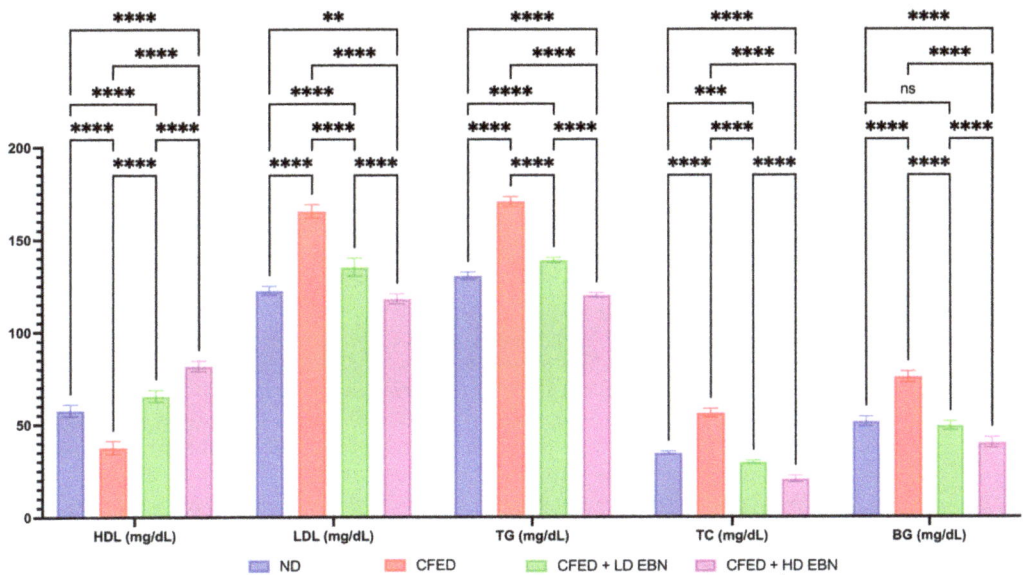

Figure 2. Improvements in lipid profile and blood glucose were observed in experimental rats. **** $p < 0.0001$, *** $p = 0.0004$, ** $p = 0.0011$, and ^{ns} $p > 0.05$.

In addition to improvements in lipid profiles and blood glucose (Figure 2), improvements in the metabolic enzymes HMG-CoA reductase, lipase, and α-amylase were observed in experimental rats supplemented with EBN, and the data can be seen in Figure 3. In general, CFED-only rats had significantly higher levels of HMG-CoA reductase, lipase, and α-amylase when compared to both the normal and EBN intervention groups. Again, it was found that HD of EBN led to improvements in the metabolic enzymes HMG-CoA reductase, lipase, and α-amylase, although both doses of EBN also had a good effect on decreasing these enzymes. Interestingly, serum aspartate transaminase (AST) and alanine transaminase (ALT) were observed within normal limits, and there were no significant differences across treatment groups. This can be a marker of less toxicity for EBN as a candidate for functional food that is already widely consumed by humans.

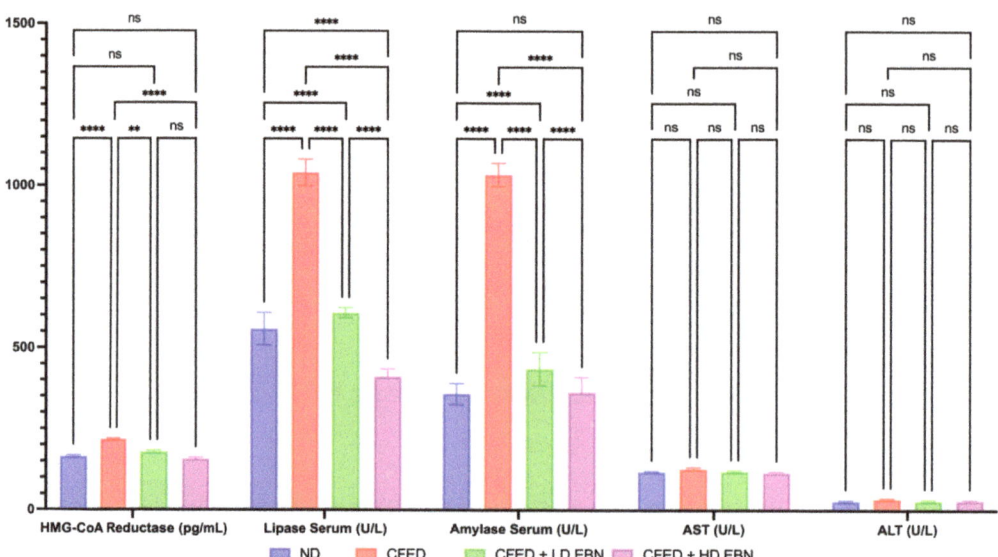

Figure 3. Improvements in metabolic syndrome-related enzymatic levels observed in experimental rats. **** $p < 0.0001$, ** $p = 0.0036$, and ^{ns} $p > 0.05$.

CFED rats supplemented with both doses of EBN had significant improvements in inflammatory biomarkers, including peroxisome proliferator-activated receptor-γ coactivator 1-α Levels (PGC-1α), tumor necrosis factor-alpha (TNF-α), interleukin 10 (IL-10), and superoxide dismutase (SOD) serum levels and can be seen in Figure 4. In addition, it generally appears that the CFED group did have high levels of TNF-α and levels of PGC-1α, IL-10, and SOD that were significantly lower than the normal diet group and the EBN intervention group. HD of EBN continues to lead the way in upregulating levels of PGC-1α, IL-10, and SOD and downregulating TNF-α. This comprehensively shows that EBN, in addition to improving lipid profiles, blood glucose, and metabolic enzymes, can also help modulate inflammatory biomarkers, making it a functional food candidate that also has the potential as an anti-inflammatory related to metabolic syndrome.

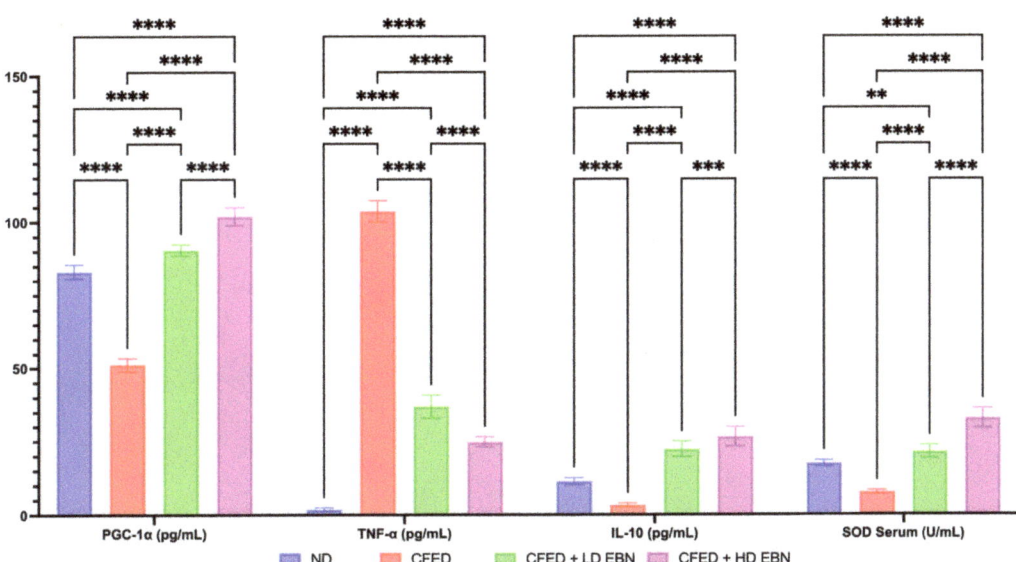

Figure 4. Improvements of metabolic syndrome-related inflammatory biomarkers observed in experimental rats. **** $p < 0.0001$, *** $p = 0.0008$, and ** $p = 0.0024$.

4. Discussion

Edible bird nest (EBN) is consumed in many parts of the world and has been developed into several processed foods; some markets even claim that it is healthy for the body. However, unfortunately, these claims are still poorly supported by evidence-based medicine. In particular, studies of the characterization of metabolite components such as terpenoids and in silico molecular docking analysis of receptors that cause non-communicable diseases such as metabolic syndromes are limited. Furthermore, in vitro and animal model studies regarding the supplementation of EBN are urgently needed to complement the current evidence of its health benefits, especially in fighting metabolic syndrome, and this is the urgency of current research.

Metabolic syndrome is closely related to the incidence of oxidative stress and several related diseases such as obesity and diabetes (Figure 5) [28]. In people with metabolic syndrome, iNOS levels are found to be higher, and this correlates with the incidence of oxidative stress [29]. In addition, lowering and inhibiting ROS1 kinase, FTO protein, and lipase can reduce the incidence of metabolic syndrome in obese people, and inhibiting these receptors can also be an anti-aging approach [20,30,31]. In this current study, four kinds of terpenoid compounds in EBN have been identified, and molecular docking simulations show activity in inhibiting iNOS, ROS1 kinase, FTO protein, and lipase, which has never been reported in similar studies before. Even two of the four compounds observed clearly showed the potential of EBN in inhibiting iNOS receptors, ROS1 kinase, FTO protein, and lipase higher than the control drugs, namely Bakuchiol and Dehydrolindestrenolide. Bakuchiol has been shown to have pharmacological effects, including as an antioxidant, reducing blood glucose and triglycerides, and anti-inflammatory effects [32]. Interestingly, our study complements previous findings that have explored Dehydrolindestrenolide as a new cancer-fighting sesquiterpene [33]. EBN is more complete with the content of Curculigosaponin A, which has been shown by some studies to be a therapeutic alternative in obesity-related metabolic syndrome [34]. Interestingly, the results of this study can provide insight into the pharmaceutical industry to develop and synthesize the observed

Bakuchiol and Dehydrolindestrenolide from EBN to be used as further treatments for metabolic syndrome. A systematic review has further analyzed the nutritional bioactive compounds of EBN, but only focused on bioactive glycopeptides [35]. In addition, the latest study also recently focused on protein profiling of EBN [36]. Therefore, most recent EBN studies have focused on protein profiles and included bioactive peptides. Our study presents the latest findings that provide information on the content of terpenoids in EBN and their molecular activity computationally or in in silico.

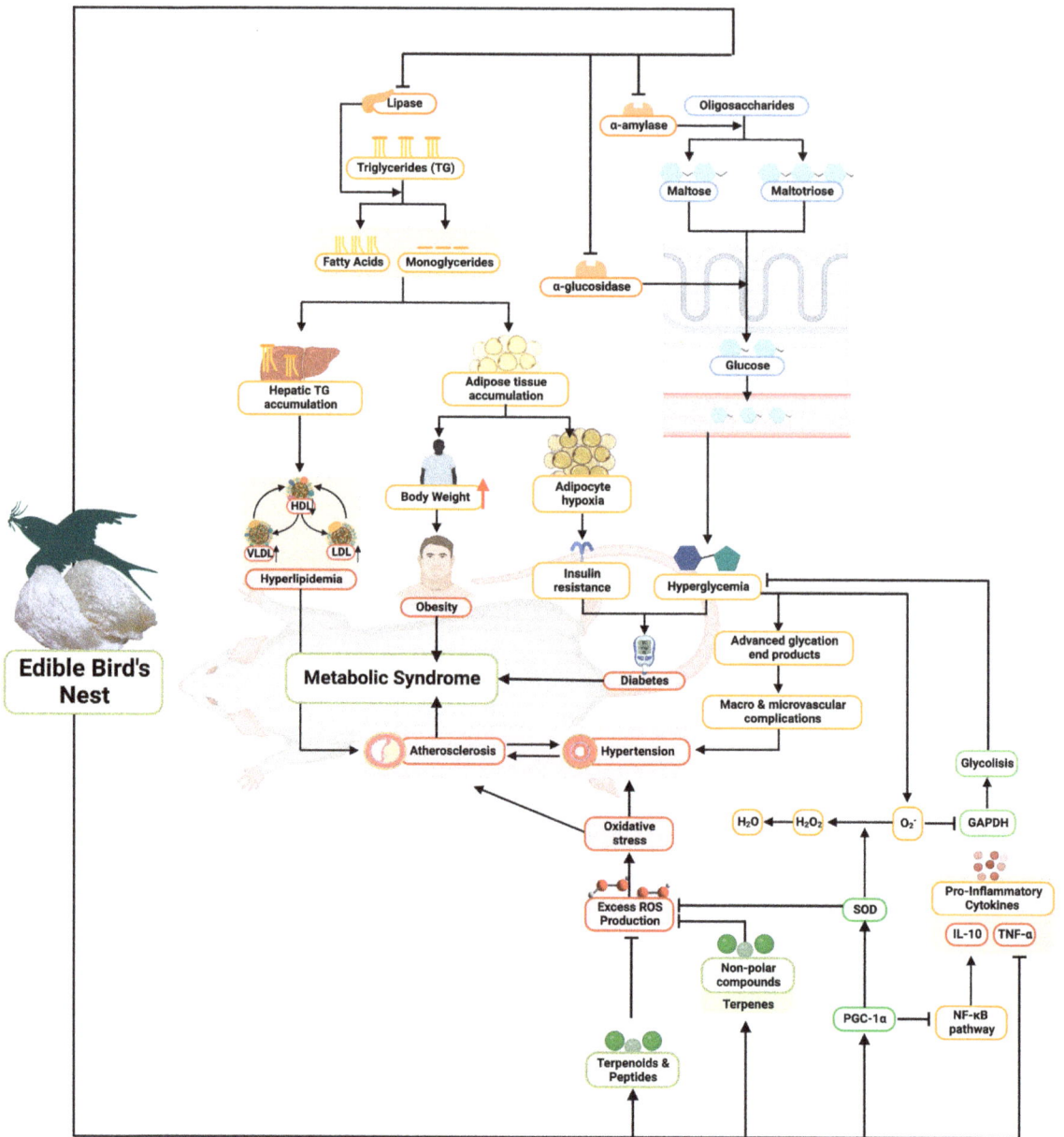

Figure 5. Biomechanism of EBN as novel functional foods in combating metabolic syndrome.

In in vitro studies, the EBN antioxidants in our study complement previous studies. Oxidative stress, which is the result of an imbalance in the homeostasis of the reduction-oxidation reaction between prooxidants and antioxidants, is a major player in the pathogenesis of many diseases such as metabolic, inflammatory, degenerative, and cardio-vascular (Figure 5) [37]. To counteract these pathological mechanisms, exogenous antioxidants are needed that will act interactively and synergistically with endogenous antioxidant defense systems to maintain the homeostasis of reduction-oxidation (redox) reactions [37]. A meta-analysis and systematic review study of randomized clinical controls showed that antioxidant supplementation is essential for the improvement of metabolic disorders in obese patients [38]. The role of pancreatic lipase inhibitors in lipid metabolism is very important in reducing hyperlipidemia, especially in obese patients with metabolic syndrome [39]. Lipase inhibitors from natural ingredients are very important to explore further, like this EBN, which has a higher ability to inhibit lipase than control or orlistat drugs (Figure 1). People with obesity relatively have a higher risk of developing type 2 diabetes [40], and α-amylase inhibitors from natural ingredients are an alternative therapy. In addition, in vitro antidiabetic EBN showed higher potential in inhibiting α-amylase compared to acarbose as a drug or control (Figure 1). Our study complements previous findings showing that EBN has been shown to fight hyperglycemia and oxidative stress [41].

In metabolic syndrome, which is also characterized by inflammation, PGC-1α dysregulation modifies the metabolic properties of tissues by altering mitochondrial function and inducing ROS accumulation (Figure 5) [42]. Hence the importance of maintaining PGC-1α levels and increasing them, for balance and control of mitochondrial DNA replication and cellular oxidative metabolism [43]. Rats supplemented with high doses of EBN were found to have higher levels of PGC-1α than other groups, and this upregulation is an important key role of EBN in modulating metabolic syndrome. In addition, it is important to find new HMG-CoA reductase inhibitors as new alternatives to fight metabolic syndrome because HMG-CoA reductase inhibitors can reduce TC, LDL, and TG concentrations and increase HDL concentrations with various potentials [44,45]. EBN has been clearly significant in modulating or downregulating metabolic enzymes such as HMG-CoA reductase, lipase, and α-amylase serum, decreased blood glucose suppression, lipid profile, and weight loss in EBN-treated rats. The decrease in LDL, TG, TC, and BG is strongly suspected to contribute to the reduction of fat stores and free fatty acids in many organs and/or tissues, which can be seen from the resulting weight loss [46]. Metabolic syndrome is also characterized by an increase in oxidative stress which contributes to impaired inflammation [47]; thankfully, EBN in silico, in vitro, and in vivo can be anti-inflammatory. In this in vivo study, HD of EBN continues to lead in upregulating levels of PGC-1α, IL-10, SOD, and downregulation of TNF-α; which will reduce the complications of metabolic syndrome (Figure 5). Several studies of other natural ingredients also support the potential for improvement of metabolic syndrome, such as green algae (*Caulerpa racemosa*) extract [18,24,27] and *Clitoria ternatea* Kombucha [20,22], which have an improving effect on lipid profiles and inflammation. However, if we compare *C. racemosa* extract and *C. ternatea* with EBN, EBN is the one that is easier to consume and prepare (considering that there are already many on the market).

This study managed to comprehensively uncover the remedial effects of fighting metabolic syndrome through integrated studies in silico, in vitro, and in vivo, which have never been reported before. This study is the first study to successfully identify terpenoid components in EBN and analyze their molecular activity against selected receptors for metabolic syndrome computationally in silico. This in vivo study was also the first to successfully explore the modulation of PGC-1α and HMG-CoA reductase by EBN. However, this research is only at the stage of animal models, which certainly cannot represent the results in human clinical trials. Therefore, further human clinical trials with doses derived from this reported in vivo study are needed. In addition, limited funding has resulted in researchers not being able to conduct fecal microbiota analyses that other studies are expected to do in the future to complement current knowledge about EBN. Furthermore,

EBN is a complex mixture of various components that may vary depending on the origin, processing, and storage of the product; therefore, further research focusing on the basic characterization of EBN from all islands in Indonesia complements current knowledge.

5. Conclusions

Something new and comprehensive related to the health benefits of edible bird nests (EBN) has been reported in this study, especially in the fight against metabolic syndrome. A total of four terpenoids contained in EBN were successfully identified, and two of the four compounds (Bakuchiol and Dehydrolindestrenolide) had great activity in inhibiting iNOS, ROS1 kinase, FTO, and lipase via in silico molecular docking simulation. Interestingly, in vitro studies validated the observed effects of in silico studies and provided insight into antioxidants, antidiabetic, and antiobesity of EBN, which is certainly associated with metabolic syndrome. More interestingly, in vivo tests revealed that improvements in lipid profiles, blood glucose, inflammatory biomarkers, and also enzymatic levels were obtained in rats supplied by EBN with high doses. Finally, this study has revealed the potential of EBN as a new functional food candidate against metabolic syndrome, and of course, clinical trials in humans are needed to see further efficacy.

6. Patents

The preparation method and formulation of edible bird nest as novel functional foods in combating metabolic syndrome resulting from the work reported in this study have been registered as a patent in Indonesia (Fahrul Nurkolis is the patent holder of the EBN Formulation).

Supplementary Materials: The following supporting information can be downloaded at: https://www.mdpi.com/article/10.3390/nu15183886/s1, Supplementary File S1: Chromatogram data from observed compounds in EBN; Supplementary File S2: Visualization of the amino acid interactions of the active compound EBN on iNOS, ROS1 kinase, FTO, and lipase.

Author Contributions: Conceptualization, H.K.P. and F.N.; Data curation, D.S., R.K., R.S., F.R.Q., M.J.T., W.B.G., A.Y.S., J.A.J.M.N.L. and F.N.; Formal analysis, H.K.P., Q.I.P., N.A.T., D.S., R.K., S.C.B., N.S. and F.N.; Funding acquisition, B.K.; Investigation, H.K.P. and F.N.; Methodology, H.K.P., N.A.T., N.M., B.K. and F.N.; Project administration, H.K.P. and F.N.; Resources, H.K.P. and F.N.; Software, F.N.; Supervision, N.A.T., N.M., M.N.P., B.K. and F.N.; Validation, N.A.T., N.M., A.Y.S., R.R.T. and B.K.; Visualization, F.N.; Writing—original draft, H.K.P., N.A.T., D.S., R.K., R.S., W.B.G., J.A.J.M.N.L., R.R.T. and F.N.; Writing—review & editing, Q.I.P., N.A.T., F.R.Q., M.J.T., S.C.B., N.M., W.B.G., A.Y.S., N.S., M.N.P., J.A.J.M.N.L., R.R.T., B.K. and F.N. All authors have read and agreed to the published version of the manuscript.

Funding: This research was supported by Graduate School Innovation office, Kyung Hee University, a grant from Kyung Hee University in 2023 (KHU-20230914), Basic Science Research Program through the National Research Foundation of Korea (NRF) funded by the Ministry of Education (NRF-2020R1I1A2066868), the National Research Foundation of Korea (NRF) grant funded by the Korea government (MSIT) (No. 2020R1A5A2019413), and the innovation network support Program through the INNOPOLIS funded by Ministry of Science and ICT (2022-IT-RD-0205-01-101).

Institutional Review Board Statement: In this animal study conducted in the preclinical stage, the research methodology was designed in accordance with the Guidelines for Reporting In Vivo Experiments (ARRIVE) and was approved by the Integrated Management Information System of Health Research Ethics—Ethics Committee for Health Research and Development of the Ministry of Health of the Republic of Indonesia—Health Research Ethics Committee of RSUP. RD. Kandou with a registration number of 040/EC/KEPK-KANDOU/IV/2023 and has received approval from the ethics board of the International Register of Preclinical Trial Animal Studies Protocols (preclinicaltrials.eu) under the registration number PCTE0000371.

Informed Consent Statement: Not applicable.

Data Availability Statement: The data datasets generated and/or analyzed in this study are available on request from the corresponding author.

Acknowledgments: Thank you to Darmawan Alisaputra for assisting in the computational process of in silico molecular docking simulation. Thank you to the institution of each author who contributed to this manuscript and especially to the Department of Biochemistry and Biomolecular, Faculty of Medicine, University of Brawijaya, Indonesia.

Conflicts of Interest: The authors declare no conflict of interest.

References

1. Grundy, S.M. Metabolic Syndrome Update. *Trends Cardiovasc. Med.* **2016**, *26*, 364–373. [CrossRef]
2. Saklayen, M.G. The Global Epidemic of the Metabolic Syndrome. *Curr. Hypertens. Rep.* **2018**, *20*, 12. [CrossRef] [PubMed]
3. Dobrowolski, P.; Prejbisz, A.; Kuryłowicz, A.; Baska, A.; Burchardt, P.; Chlebus, K.; Dzida, G.; Jankowski, P.; Jaroszewicz, J.; Jaworski, P.; et al. Metabolic Syndrome—A New Definition and Management Guidelines. *Arch. Med. Sci.* **2022**, *18*, 1133–1156. [CrossRef] [PubMed]
4. Haffner, S.M. The Metabolic Syndrome: Inflammation, Diabetes Mellitus, and Cardiovascular Disease. *Am. J. Cardiol.* **2006**, *97*, 3–11. [CrossRef] [PubMed]
5. World Health Organization. World Obesity Day 2022—Accelerating Action to Stop Obesity. Available online: https://www.who.int/news/item/04-03-2022-world-obesity-day-2022-accelerating-action-to-stop-obesity (accessed on 31 July 2023).
6. Afshin, A.; Forouzanfar, M.H.; Reitsma, M.B.; Sur, P.; Estep, K.; Lee, A.; Marczak, L.; Mokdad, A.H.; Moradi-Lakeh, M.; Naghavi, M.; et al. Health Effects of Overweight and Obesity in 195 Countries over 25 Years. *N. Engl. J. Med.* **2017**, *377*, 13–27. [CrossRef]
7. Kuneš, J.; Vaněčková, I.; Mikulášková, B.; Behuliak, M.; Maletínská, L.; Zicha, J. Epigenetics and a New Look on Metabolic Syndrome. *Physiol. Res.* **2015**, *64*, 611–620. [CrossRef]
8. Brown, L.; Poudyal, H.; Panchal, S.K. Functional Foods as Potential Therapeutic Options for Metabolic Syndrome. *Obes. Rev.* **2015**, *16*, 914–941. [CrossRef]
9. Dai, Y.; Cao, J.; Wang, Y.; Chen, Y.; Jiang, L. A Comprehensive Review of Edible Bird's Nest. *Food Res. Int.* **2021**, *140*, 109875. [CrossRef]
10. Lee, T.H.; Wani, W.A.; Lee, C.H.; Cheng, K.K.; Shreaz, S.; Wong, S.; Hamdan, N.; Azmi, N.A. Edible Bird's Nest: The Functional Values of the Prized Animal-Based Bioproduct from Southeast Asia—A Review. *Front. Pharmacol.* **2021**, *12*, 626233. [CrossRef]
11. Hun Lee, T.; Hau Lee, C.; Alia Azmi, N.; Kavita, S.; Wong, S.; Znati, M.; Ben Jannet, H. Characterization of Polar and Non-Polar Compounds of House Edible Bird's Nest (EBN) from Johor, Malaysia. *Chem. Biodivers.* **2020**, *17*, e1900419. [CrossRef]
12. Quek, M.C.; Chin, N.L.; Yusof, Y.A.; Law, C.L.; Tan, S.W. Characterization of Edible Bird's Nest of Different Production, Species and Geographical Origins Using Nutritional Composition, Physicochemical Properties and Antioxidant Activities. *Food Res. Int.* **2018**, *109*, 35–43. [CrossRef] [PubMed]
13. Ling, A.J.W.; Chang, L.S.; Babji, A.S.; Latip, J.; Koketsu, M.; Lim, S.J. Review of Sialic Acid's Biochemistry, Sources, Extraction and Functions with Special Reference to Edible Bird's Nest. *Food Chem.* **2022**, *367*, 130755. [CrossRef] [PubMed]
14. Ma, F.; Liu, D. Sketch of the Edible Bird's Nest and Its Important Bioactivities. *Food Res. Int.* **2012**, *48*, 559–567. [CrossRef]
15. Yida, Z.; Imam, M.U.; Ismail, M.; Ooi, D.-J.; Sarega, N.; Azmi, N.H.; Ismail, N.; Chan, K.W.; Hou, Z.; Yusof, N.B. Edible Bird's Nest Prevents High Fat Diet-Induced Insulin Resistance in Rats. *J. Diabetes Res.* **2015**, *2015*, 760535. [CrossRef]
16. Akmal, M.N.; Intan-Shameha, A.R.; Ajat, M.; Mansor, R.; Zuki, A.B.Z.; Ideris, A. Edible Bird's Nest (EBN) Supplementation Ameliorates the Progression of Hepatic Changes and Atherosclerosis in Hypercholesterolaemic-Induced Rats. *Malays. J. Microsc.* **2018**, *14*, 103–114.
17. Choy, K.W.; Zain, Z.M.; Murugan, D.D.; Giribabu, N.; Zamakshshari, N.H.; Lim, Y.M.; Mustafa, M.R. Effect of Hydrolyzed Bird's Nest on β-Cell Function and Insulin Signaling in Type 2 Diabetic Mice. *Front. Pharmacol.* **2021**, *12*, 632169. [CrossRef]
18. Permatasari, H.K.; Nurkolis, F.; Hardinsyah, H.; Taslim, N.A.; Sabrina, N.; Ibrahim, F.M.; Visnu, J.; Kumalawati, D.A.; Febriana, S.A.; Sudargo, T.; et al. Metabolomic Assay, Computational Screening, and Pharmacological Evaluation of *Caulerpa Racemosa* as an Anti-Obesity with Anti-Aging by Altering Lipid Profile and Peroxisome Proliferator-Activated Receptor-γ Coactivator 1-α Levels. *Front. Nutr.* **2022**, *9*, 939073. [CrossRef]
19. Qiao, L.; Lewis, R.; Hooper, A.; Morphet, J.; Tan, X.; Yu, K. *Using Natural Products Application Solution with UNIFI for the Identification of Chemical Ingredients of Green Tea Extract*; Report No. APNT134775221; Waters Corporation: Milford, MA, USA, 2013.
20. Hardinsyah, H.; Gunawan, W.B.; Nurkolis, F.; Alisaputra, D.; Kurniawan, R.; Mayulu, N.; Taslim, N.A.; Tallei, T.E. Antiobesity Potential of Major Metabolites from *Clitoria ternatea* Kombucha: Untargeted Metabolomic Profiling and Molecular Docking Simulations. *Curr. Res. Food Sci.* **2023**, *6*, 100464. [CrossRef]
21. Sabrina, N.; Rizal, M.; Nurkolis, F.; Hardinsyah, H.; Tanner, M.J.; Gunawan, W.B.; Handoko, M.N.; Mayulu, N.; Taslim, N.A.; Puspaningtyas, D.S.; et al. Bioactive Peptides Identification and Nutritional Status Ameliorating Properties on Malnourished Rats of Combined Eel and Soy-Based Tempe Flour. *Front. Nutr.* **2022**, *9*, 963065. [CrossRef]
22. Permatasari, H.K.; Nurkolis, F.; Gunawan, W.B.; Yusuf, V.M.; Yusuf, M.; Kusuma, R.J.; Sabrina, N.; Muharram, F.R.; Taslim, N.A.; Mayulu, N.; et al. Modulation of Gut Microbiota and Markers of Metabolic Syndrome in Mice on Cholesterol and Fat Enriched Diet by Butterfly Pea Flower Kombucha. *Curr. Res. Food Sci.* **2022**, *5*, 1251–1265. [CrossRef]

23. Nurkolis, F.; Taslim, N.A.; Qhabibi, F.R.; Kang, S.; Moon, M.; Choi, J.; Choi, M.; Park, M.N.; Mayulu, N.; Kim, B. Ulvophyte Green Algae *Caulerpa lentillifera*: Metabolites Profile and Antioxidant, Anticancer, Anti-Obesity, and In Vitro Cytotoxicity Properties. *Molecules* **2023**, *28*, 1365. [CrossRef]
24. Nurkolis, F.; Taslim, N.A.; Subali, D.; Kurniawan, R.; Hardinsyah, H.; Gunawan, W.B.; Kusuma, R.J.; Yusuf, V.M.; Pramono, A.; Kang, S.; et al. Dietary Supplementation of *Caulerpa racemosa* Ameliorates Cardiometabolic Syndrome via Regulation of PRMT-1/DDAH/ADMA Pathway and Gut Microbiome in Mice. *Nutrients* **2023**, *15*, 909. [CrossRef] [PubMed]
25. Jiang, Z.; Yu, G.; Liang, Y.; Song, T.; Zhu, Y.; Ni, H.; Yamaguchi, K.; Oda, T. Inhibitory Effects of a Sulfated Polysaccharide Isolated from Edible Red Alga *Bangia Fusco-Purpurea* on α-Amylase and α-Glucosidase. *Biosci. Biotechnol. Biochem.* **2019**, *83*, 2065–2074. [CrossRef] [PubMed]
26. Permatasari, H.K.; Firani, N.K.; Prijadi, B.; Irnandi, F.D.; Riawan, W.; Yusuf, M.; Amar, N.; Chandra, L.A.; Yusuf, V.; Subali, A.D. Kombucha Drink Enriched with Sea Grapes (*Caulerpa racemosa*) as Potential Functional Beverage to Contrast Obesity: An In Vivo and In Vitro Approach. *Clin. Nutr. ESPEN* **2022**, *49*, 232–240. [CrossRef] [PubMed]
27. Kuswari, M.; Nurkolis, F.; Mayulu, N.; Ibrahim, F.M.; Taslim, N.A.; Wewengkang, D.S.; Sabrina, N.; Arifin, G.R.; Mantik, K.E.K.; Bahar, M.R.; et al. Sea Grapes Extract Improves Blood Glucose, Total Cholesterol, and PGC-1α in Rats Fed on Cholesterol- and Fat-Enriched Diet. *F1000Research* **2021**, *10*, 718. [CrossRef]
28. Piché, M.-E.; Tchernof, A.; Després, J.-P. Obesity Phenotypes, Diabetes, and Cardiovascular Diseases. *Circ. Res.* **2020**, *126*, 1477–1500. [CrossRef] [PubMed]
29. Mahdy, N.E.; Abdel-Baki, P.M.; El-Rashedy, A.A.; Ibrahim, R.M. Modulatory Effect of Pyrus Pyrifolia Fruit and Its Phenolics on Key Enzymes against Metabolic Syndrome: Bioassay-Guided Approach, HPLC Analysis, and In Silico Study. *Plant Foods Hum. Nutr.* **2023**, *78*, 383–389. [CrossRef]
30. Khella, M.S.; Hamdy, N.M.; Amin, A.I.; El-Mesallamy, H.O. The (FTO) Gene Polymorphism Is Associated with Metabolic Syndrome Risk in Egyptian Females: A Case-Control Study. *BMC Med. Genet.* **2017**, *18*, 101. [CrossRef]
31. Nurkolis, F.; Purnomo, A.F.; Alisaputra, D.; Gunawan, W.B.; Qhabibi, F.R.; Park, W.; Moon, M.; Taslim, N.A.; Park, M.N.; Kim, B. In Silico and in Vitro Studies Reveal a Synergistic Potential Source of Novel Anti-Ageing from Two Indonesian Green Algae. *J. Funct. Foods* **2023**, *104*, 105555. [CrossRef]
32. Xin, Z.; Wu, X.; Ji, T.; Xu, B.; Han, Y.; Sun, M.; Jiang, S.; Li, T.; Hu, W.; Deng, C.; et al. Bakuchiol: A Newly Discovered Warrior against Organ Damage. *Pharmacol. Res.* **2019**, *141*, 208–213. [CrossRef]
33. Yang, H.J.; Kwon, E.B.; Li, W. Linderolide U, a New Sesquiterpene from *Lindera aggregata* Root. *Nat. Prod. Res.* **2022**, *36*, 1914–1918. [CrossRef]
34. Zhang, T.; Zhong, S.; Li, T.; Zhang, J. Saponins as Modulators of Nuclear Receptors. *Crit. Rev. Food Sci. Nutr.* **2020**, *60*, 94–107. [CrossRef] [PubMed]
35. Hui Yan, T.; Babji, A.S.; Lim, S.J.; Sarbini, S.R. A Systematic Review of Edible Swiftlet's Nest (ESN): Nutritional Bioactive Compounds, Health Benefits as Functional Food, and Recent Development as Bioactive ESN Glycopeptide Hydrolysate. *Trends Food Sci. Technol.* **2021**, *115*, 117–132. [CrossRef]
36. Mohamad Nasir, N.N.; Mohamad Ibrahim, R.; Abu Bakar, M.Z.; Mahmud, R.; Ab Razak, N.A. Characterization and Extraction Influence Protein Profiling of Edible Bird's Nest. *Foods* **2021**, *10*, 2248. [CrossRef]
37. Abdel-Daim, M.M.; El-Tawil, O.S.; Bungau, S.G.; Atanasov, A.G. Applications of Antioxidants in Metabolic Disorders and Degenerative Diseases: Mechanistic Approach. *Oxid. Med. Cell. Longev.* **2019**, *2019*, 4179676. [CrossRef] [PubMed]
38. Wang, J.; Liao, B.; Wang, C.; Zhong, O.; Lei, X.; Yang, Y. Effects of Antioxidant Supplementation on Metabolic Disorders in Obese Patients from Randomized Clinical Controls: A Meta-Analysis and Systematic Review. *Oxid. Med. Cell Longev.* **2022**, *2022*, 7255413. [CrossRef] [PubMed]
39. Liu, T.-T.; Liu, X.-T.; Chen, Q.-X.; Shi, Y. Lipase Inhibitors for Obesity: A Review. *Biomed. Pharmacother.* **2020**, *128*, 110314. [CrossRef]
40. Shi, Z.; Zhu, Y.; Teng, C.; Yao, Y.; Ren, G.; Richel, A. Anti-Obesity Effects of α-Amylase Inhibitor Enriched-Extract from White Common Beans (*Phaseolus vulgaris* L.) Associated with the Modulation of Gut Microbiota Composition in High-Fat Diet-Induced Obese Rats. *Food Funct.* **2020**, *11*, 1624–1634. [CrossRef]
41. Murugan, D.D.; Md Zain, Z.; Choy, K.W.; Zamakshshari, N.H.; Choong, M.J.; Lim, Y.M.; Mustafa, M.R. Edible Bird's Nest Protects against Hyperglycemia-Induced Oxidative Stress and Endothelial Dysfunction. *Front. Pharmacol.* **2020**, *10*, 1624. [CrossRef]
42. Rius-Pérez, S.; Torres-Cuevas, I.; Millán, I.; Ortega, Á.L.; Pérez, S.; Sandhu, M.A. PGC-1 α, Inflammation, and Oxidative Stress: An Integrative View in Metabolism. *Oxid. Med. Cell. Longev.* **2020**, *2020*, 1452696. [CrossRef]
43. Cheng, C.F.; Ku, H.C.; Lin, H. Pgc-1α as a Pivotal Factor in Lipid and Metabolic Regulation. *Int. J. Mol. Sci.* **2018**, *19*, 3447. [CrossRef] [PubMed]
44. Han, K.H. Functional Implications of HMG-CoA Reductase Inhibition on Glucose Metabolism. *Korean Circ. J.* **2018**, *48*, 951–963. [CrossRef] [PubMed]
45. Wang, K.; Bao, L.; Zhou, N.; Zhang, J.; Liao, M.; Zheng, Z.; Wang, Y.; Liu, C.; Wang, J.; Wang, L.; et al. Structural Modification of Natural Product Ganomycin I Leading to Discovery of a α-Glucosidase and HMG-CoA Reductase Dual Inhibitor Improving Obesity and Metabolic Dysfunction in Vivo. *J. Med. Chem.* **2018**, *61*, 3609–3625. [CrossRef] [PubMed]

46. Brown, J.D.; Buscemi, J.; Milsom, V.; Malcolm, R.; O'Neil, P.M. Effects on Cardiovascular Risk Factors of Weight Losses Limited to 5–10%. *Transl. Behav. Med.* **2016**, *6*, 339–346. [CrossRef] [PubMed]
47. Monserrat-Mesquida, M.; Quetglas-Llabrés, M.; Capó, X.; Bouzas, C.; Mateos, D.; Pons, A.; Tur, J.A.; Sureda, A. Metabolic Syndrome Is Associated with Oxidative Stress and Proinflammatory State. *Antioxidants* **2020**, *9*, 236. [CrossRef]

Disclaimer/Publisher's Note: The statements, opinions and data contained in all publications are solely those of the individual author(s) and contributor(s) and not of MDPI and/or the editor(s). MDPI and/or the editor(s) disclaim responsibility for any injury to people or property resulting from any ideas, methods, instructions or products referred to in the content.

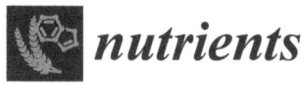 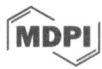

Article

Compliance with Nutritional Recommendations and Gut Microbiota Profile in Galician Overweight/Obese and Normal-Weight Individuals

Laura Sinisterra-Loaiza, Patricia Alonso-Lovera, Alejandra Cardelle-Cobas *, Jose Manuel Miranda, Beatriz I. Vázquez and Alberto Cepeda

Laboratorio de Higiene, Inspección y Control de Alimentos, Departamento de Química Analítica, Nutrición y Bromatología, Campus Terra, Universidade da Santiago de Compostela, 27002 Lugo, Spain; laura.sinisterra@usc.es (L.S.-L.); patricia.alonso.lovera@rai.usc.es (P.A.-L.); josemanuel.miranda@usc.es (J.M.M.); beatriz.vazquez@usc.es (B.I.V.); alberto.cepeda@usc.es (A.C.)
* Correspondence: alejandra.cardelle@usc.es

Abstract: Different research studies have identified specific groups or certain dietary compounds as the onset and progression of obesity and suggested that gut microbiota is a mediator between these compounds and the inflammation associated with pathology. In this study, the objective was to evaluate the dietary intake of 108 overweight (OW), obese (OB), and normal-weight (NW) individuals and to analyze their gut microbiota profile to determine changes and associations with Body Mass Index (BMI) and diet. When individuals were compared by BMI, significant differences in fiber and monounsaturated fatty acids (MUFAs) intake were observed, showing higher adequacy for the NW group. The analysis of gut microbiota showed statistical differences for 18 ASVs; *Anaerostipes* and *Faecalibacterium* decreased in the OW/OB group, whereas the genus *Oscillospira* increased; the genus was also found in the LEFSe analysis as a biomarker for OW/OB. *Roseburia faecis* was found in a significantly higher proportion of NW individuals and identified as a biomarker for the NW group. Correlation analysis showed that adequation to nutritional recommendation for fiber indicated a higher abundance of *Prevotella copri*, linearly correlated with *F. prausnitzii*, *Bacteroides caccae*, and *R. faecis*. The same correlation was found for the adequation for MUFAs, with these bacteria being more abundant when the intake was adjusted to or below the recommendations.

Keywords: gut microbiota; obesity; fiber; monounsaturated fatty acids; BMI

1. Introduction

Western societies have undergone a process that involves major qualitative and quantitative changes in dietary habits. Thus, traditional diets have been replaced by diets characterized by a higher energy load and a decrease in fiber and complex carbohydrates. These changes, in addition to behavioral changes such as less physical activity, have resulted in an increase in worldwide overweight and obesity rates [1]. Obesity is the abnormal or excessive accumulation of fat that can be detrimental to health. It is of multifactorial origin, resulting from pathological processes and deriving from an interrelation between numerous factors [2,3].

According to the European Health Survey in Spain 2020, about 16% of the Spanish population suffers from obesity, while 37.60% of the population is overweight [4]. Other recent monitoring work revealed that Galicia is one of the regions of Spain in which there are higher rates of obesity in adults, reaching 26.7% [5]. Additionally, a study reported that during the COVID-19 confinement, 44% of participants indicated an increase in their body weight, with an average increase of 2.8 kg [6]. Thus, it is probably true that the current overweight rate of Galician people could now be higher than those in the cited reports [4,5].

Several authors have pointed out that the dietary habits of Galician people do not follow the same patterns as in the rest of Spain. However, together with the north of Portugal,

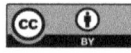

they are included in the dietary model known as the Atlantic Diet [7,8]. Knowledge of the dietary patterns of the population is essential to understanding the potential impact of the strategies implemented to prevent the increase in obesity rates [9].

One approach to treating obesity in recent years involves the study of the gut microbiota, the results of which in both mice and humans describe remarkable differences between the gut microbiota of obese (OB) and normal-weight (NW) subjects. When there is an excess of body fat, colonic concentrations of Firmicutes increase by more than 50%, while those of Bacteroides decrease correlatively compared to NW subjects [10]. The composition of the gut microbiota of obese individuals is characterized by a decrease in genera such as *Akkermansia*, *Alistipes*, *Faecalibacterium*, and *Oscillibacter* [11,12] and an increase in *Staphylococcus* and *Clostridium* [13–16].

In addition, dietary patterns are considered modulators of the gut microbiota; for example, excessive fat consumption induces an imbalance in the gut microbiota, leading to gut barrier dysfunction, increased host body weight, and low-grade inflammation of adipose tissue [17]. A high-protein diet, on the other hand, increases the growth of bile-tolerant bacterial species (*Alistipes*, *Bilophila*, and *Bacteroides*) and decreases bacteria that hydrolyze disaccharides or polysaccharides into simple carbohydrates (*Roseburia*, *Eubacterium rectale*, and *Ruminococcus bromii*) [18].

Although there is available evidence about the differences in gut microbiota composition in both overweight or obese and normal-weight individuals, there is scarce information about potential biomarkers associated with certain dietary compounds. Thus, the hypothesis of the present study is that dietary intake, especially specific dietary components, is associated with different gut microbiota compositions in both overweight or obese and normal-weight subjects. Therefore, the aim of this study was to differentiate the gut microbiota of overweight (OW) and OB subjects from that of NW subjects, in a sample of Galician people, compare the results with previous studies to establish potential biomarkers and determine its association with dietary components potentially diminished or increased in each group under study.

2. Materials and Methods

2.1. Population and Sample Size

This cross-sectional study is part of an international project about the search for novel biomarkers in diabetes and obesity in Iberian-America (CyTED project 918PTE0540). The study population for the present analysis included 108 individuals, ranging in age from 40 to 70 years, with habitual residence in Galicia (a northwest region of Spain). The sample size was estimated based on previous studies [19–21]. The participants were informed of the objectives of the study, and informed consent was obtained from each volunteer to participate in the study, and all data obtained were handled according to Spanish Law 3/2018 on personal data protection. This consent detailed the conditions of the research, highlighting the voluntary nature of participation, the possibility of withdrawing from the study even with the acceptance of the consent, and the anonymous treatment of the data for research purposes only.

The following inclusion criteria were used: age between 40 and 70 years; absence of diagnosed pathologies, not having undergone medical treatment with hormones, corticoids, or having recently consumed any of the following substances: proton pump inhibitors, amphetamines, alpha-adrenergic drugs, alpha-blockers, beta-blockers, opiates, calcium-antagonists, neuroleptics, tricyclic antidepressants, phenothiazines, central nervous system stimulants (cocaine, etc.); not having consumed any supplement containing probiotics or prebiotics during the previous 2 months; in the case of women, not being pregnant

Ethical approval for this study was obtained from The Regional Ethics Committee for Clinical Research (Galician Health Service, SERGAS, n° 2018/270) in compliance with the Declaration of Helsinki of 1964 regarding privacy, confidentiality, and informed consent. All experiments were carried out in accordance with approved guidelines and regulations.

2.2. Anthropometric Measures

Anthropometric measurements were obtained. Weight was determined using an InBody 127 digital scale (InBody, Tokyo, Japan). Height was measured with a portable stadiometer (ADE MZ10042; Hamburg, Germany), with the subject upright and in balance, without bending the knees. Subsequently, the Body Mass Index (BMI) was calculated using the Quetelet formula: BMI = weight (kg)/[height (m)]^2. According to the classification ranges proposed by the Spanish Obesity Society [22], three volunteers were grouped in groups according to their BMI: 18–24.9 kg/m^2 for NW, 25–29.9 kg/m^2 for OW, and $\geq$30 OB kg/m^2.

2.3. Dietary Information

A 72 h dietary record was completed by the volunteers for 3 days (2 workdays and 1 weekend day). The volunteers were given instructions on how to record their dietary intake. They were also asked to provide information on the portions of food consumed, the ingredients and techniques used in cooking, and the type and quantity of beverages consumed.

The mean daily energy and nutrient intake of each volunteer were calculated using the open software "diet calculator", available on the website of the Endocrinology and Clinical Nutrition Research Centre [23], which is based on Spanish foods. Data obtained from the software were compared to the nutritional objectives for the Spanish adult population published by the Spanish Society of Community Nutrition (SENC, 24) to determine their nutritional adequacy. The data obtained were compared by sex and by BMI of volunteers.

Data about micronutrient (minerals and vitamins) intake were compared to Reference Dietary Intakes (RDI) established by the Spanish Federation of Nutrition, Food and Dietetics Societies [24]. The data obtained were compared by sex and BMI of the volunteers.

2.4. Fecal Sample Collection and DNA Extraction

Volunteers received detailed instructions to collect fecal samples and were provided with a sterile container that should deliver to the laboratory along with the 72 h dietary record. Samples should have been delivered within two hours after defecation or, in the case of not being able to do it, they should have been immediately frozen at $-20\ ^\circ$C after deposition and delivery to the laboratory where they were conserved frozen until treated for analysis.

DNA from fecal samples was extracted using the Dneasy Powersoil kit (Qiagen®, Hilden, Germany) following the manufacturer's instructions. Extracted DNA was then quantified using a Qubit™ 4 fluorometer (Invitrogen, Thermo Fisher Scientific, Carlsbad, CA, USA) and the Qubit kit 1X dsDNA High Sensitivity (Thermo Fisher Scientific, Inc., Karlsruhe, Germany). After quantification, DNA samples were frozen and stored at $-20\ ^\circ$C until further analysis.

2.5. 16S rRNA Amplicon Sequencing

For 16S rRNA amplicon sequencing, 2 µL of DNA extracted from each sample was used to construct the libraries, and the Ion GeneStudio™ S5 System (Life Technologies, Carlsbad, CA, USA) was used. For this purpose, the 16S hypervariable regions were amplified with two sets of primers, v2–4–8 and v3–6, 7–9, and the libraries were prepared by using the Ion 16S™ Metagenomics Kit (Life Technologies) and the Ion Xpress™ Plus Fragment Library Kit (Life Technologies). Libraries containing equal amounts of PCR products pooled with a barcode were prepared by using the Ion Xpress™ Barcode Adapters Kit (Life Technologies). Then, these libraries were quantified by using the Ion Universal Library Quantitation Kit (Life Technologies). Next, 10 pM of each library was pooled and loaded on an Ion One-Touch™ 2 System (Life Technologies), which automatically performs template preparation and enrichment. Template-positive ion sphere particles were enriched with Dynabeads™ MyOne™ Streptavidin C1 magnetic beads (Invitrogen, Carlsbad, CA, USA) by using an Ion One Touch ES instrument. Finally, an Ion 520 TM chip (Life Technologies) was loaded with the samples on an Ion GeneStudio™ S5 System sequencer using the Ion 520™ & Ion 530™ Loading Reagents supplied in the OT2-Kit (Life Technologies).

2.6. Statistical and Bioinformatic Analysis

Student's t-test for independent samples was used to compare qualitative variables between different groups (sex or BMI). The X2 test with Yates's correction was used to compare frequencies. In all cases, the obtained differences were considered statistically significant if the p value was less than 0.05.

A two-way ANOVA was used to determine significative differences for time and substrates as the two covariates in the general linear model using Tukey's analysis. For significant differences ($p < 0.05$) a one-way ANOVA was conducted for each substrate comparing 0, 5, 10, and 24 h. Similarly, each substrate was compared using two-way ANOVA; results were significant when $p < 0.05$. The software SPSS® v.27 for Windows (SPSS Inc., Chicago, IL, USA) was used for these analyses.

For the analysis of 16S rRNA amplicon sequencing, the raw sequencing reads were obtained from the Torrent Suite software (v. 5.12.2.) as fastq files. The fastq files were processed with QIIME 2 software v. 2022.11 [25]. To produce amplicon sequence variants (ASVs), the DADA2 method was used for quality filtration (Q score ≥ 30), trimming, denoising, and dereplication. Samples with features (taxa) with a total abundance (summed across all samples) of <10 were removed. Taxonomy was assigned to ASVs by using the q2-feature-classifier classify-sklearn naïve Bayes taxonomy classifier, which was compared to the Greengenes 13_8 99% operational taxonomic unit (OTU) reference sequences.

STAMP software (v 2.1.3) for the "Statistical Analysis of Taxonomic and Functional Profiles" [26] was used to determine statistical differences in the obtained ASVs at the species level. Kruskal–Wallis H test with post hoc Tukey–Kramer test was employed.

The OTUs with taxonomic information, obtained in QIIME2, were used together with a metadata file, in text format, for their analyses in the free platform Microbiome Analyst, "a comprehensive statistical, functional and integrative analysis of microbiome data" [27]. alpha- and beta- diversity, correlation, and LEfSe analysis were carried out.

3. Results

3.1. Nutritional Analysis and Adequation to the Objectives and the Recommended Daily Intakes for the Spanish Population

A total of 108 subjects completed a 72 h dietary recall, and their anthropometric measurements were obtained. Of these, 67 (62%) were women and 41 (38%) were men. The average age of the subjects was 51.0 ± 8.0 years, and the average kilocalorie intake was 2344.0 ± 556.9 kcal/day. Comparing this energy intake by sex, a significantly higher intake ($p = 0.04$) was observed for men (2502.6 ± 538.3) than for women (2247.0 ± 537.0). Data obtained for macronutrients and other parameters are shown in Table 1.

As it can be observed, the average total carbohydrate intake in terms of % of energy is deficient, 88.1% of the individuals do not achieve the recommendations. The same occurs for fiber intake (84.3% of individuals are in deficit). Regarding the lipid profile, 89.6% of the participants are above the objectives, which indicates a diet rich in fat, especially in saturated fat since 88% of the volunteers showed to possess a consumption above the recommendations. For protein, it is necessary to indicate that this macronutrient does not appear in the recommendations for the Spanish population, since its determination is depending on the other two macronutrients. The percent for protein usually recommended is 10–15% of total energy. The data obtained for the participants of this study indicated an adequation of 38.9% and an excess of 61.1%.

For simple sugar, only 13 individuals showed to have a consumption below a 10%, being an average intake of 18.1 ± 7.4%. Regarding fruit and vegetable consumption, the average intake of fruit and vegetables was 1.8 ± 1.5 servings, which is <50% of the recommended five daily servings; only 4.6% of the population surveyed had the recommended intake, while 94.4% did not meet the recommendations. Regarding other parameters such as alcohol consumption, most of the volunteers showed to be below the recommendation of 1 and 2 Standard Drink Units (SDUs) of alcoholic beverages, for women and men, respectively. Regarding water consumption, 45.4% of the participants did not reach the recommendations for water consumption.

Table 1. Participants' diet quality in terms of a caloric lipid profile: adequacy to nutritional objectives for the Spanish population (n = 108). Results are expressed as the average ± standard deviation. Diet adequacy is expressed as the number of individuals meeting the nutritional goals and in brackets is expressed as percent.

CALORIC PROFILE	NUTRITIONAL OBJECTIVES	VALUES OF PARTICIPANTS' DIET	DIET ADEQUACY		
			DÉFICIT	ADEQUATE	EXCESS
Carbohydrates (% Energy)	50–55	38.9 ± 7.8	96 (88.1%)	11 (10.1%)	1 (0.9%)
Fiber (g/1000 kcal)	>14	11.7 ± 7.7	91 (84.3%)	15 (13.9%)	2 (1.9%)
Lipids (% Energy)	30–35	41.8 ± 8.0	7 (6.4%)	15 (13.9%)	86 (79.6%)
LIPID PROFILE					
SFA (% Energy)	≤7–8	12.0 ± 3.2	-	13 (0.0%)	95 (88%)
MUFA (% Energy)	20	20.8 ± 16.1	36 (33.3%)	45 (41.7%)	27 (25.0%)
PUFA (% Energy)	5	5.9 ± 3.6	39 (38.0%)	23 (21.2%)	62 (57.4%)
Cholesterol (mg)	<300	347.0 ± 138.6	0 (0.0%)	46 (42.6%)	62 (57.4%)
OTHERS					
Water (mL)	2000	2063.3 ± 627.9	49 (45.4%)	59 (54.6%)	0 (0.0%)
Fruits and vegetables	5 portions	1.8 ± 1.5	102 (94.4%)	5 (4.6%)	1 (0.9%)
Sugar (% Energy)	6–10	18.1 ± 7.4	-	13 (12.0%)	95 (88.0%)
Alcohol (g)	≤1 SDU women ≤2 SDU men	10.84 ± 44.43	-	100 (92.6%)	8 (7.4%)

SFA: Saturated Fatty Acids; MFA: Monounsaturated Fatty Acids; PUFA: Polyunsaturated Fatty Acids; SDU: Standard Drink Unit.

When the data obtained were compared by sex (Table S1), there were some significant differences in dietary patterns between men and women.

Thus, in general, women accomplish more nutritional objectives than men. On average, men have a higher intake of protein, a lower consumption of carbohydrates, and a higher consumption of fat than women. Regarding the lipid profile, statistical differences were found for SFA, where women, once again, showed to better accomplish the nutritional objectives for the Spanish population.

Comparing intake data according to BMI (Table 2), no statistical differences were found among NW, OW, and OB subjects for all parameters investigated with the exception of total energy, fiber, and MUFAs, for which statistical differences were found. In the case of fiber, a better adequation (32.5%) was observed for NW individuals than for OW/OB (15.2 and 14.3, respectively). For MUFAs, only 14.3% of the OB volunteers accomplish the objectives, whereas for the OW and NW groups, the accomplishment was higher, 36.4 and 25%, respectively. For total energy, 2284.0 ± 658.6 kcal/day were obtained for the NW group, whereas for the OW and OB group, the total energy obtained was 2221.3 ± 497.2 and 2498.4 ± 459.1 kcal/day, respectively. A significantly higher caloric intake was obtained for the OB group (p = 0.0356).

Regarding water, fruit, vegetables, and sugar, no statistical differences were observed according to BMI. However, in general, the NW and the OW groups showed higher adequacy for water and alcohol consumption. For sugar consumption, the worst adequacy was obtained for the NW group, but these values included all the simple sugar consumed, including that provided for fruits and not only the added simple sugar, and this is the group consuming more fruits and vegetables.

Table 2. Macronutrient intake for normal weight (NW), overweight (OW), or obese (OB) subjects, and its adequation to the nutritional objectives for the Spanish population ($n = 108$). Caloric profile, lipidic profile, and others are shown. Results are expressed with mean ± standard deviation. Diet adequacy is expressed as the number of individuals meeting the nutritional goals and in brackets is expressed as percent.

		NW ($n = 40$)		OW ($n = 35$)		OB ($n = 33$)		
CALORIC PROFILE	Nutritional Objectives	Mean ± SD	Intake Adequacy: n (%)	Mean ± SD	Intake Adequacy: n (%)	Mean ± SD	Intake Adequacy: n (%)	p Value
Carbohydrates (% Energy)	50–55%	40.3 ± 7.1	5 (12.5%)	37.4 ± 7.7	1 (3.0%)	38.8 ± 8.6	4 (11.4%)	0.274
Lipids (% Energy)	30–35%	40.6 ± 6.3	6 (15.0%)	43.6 ± 9.6	5 (15.2%)	41.9 ± 7.5	5 (14.3%)	0.280
Fiber (g/1000 Kcal)	>14	14.2 ± 9.5	13 (32.5%)	12.5 ± 10.14	4 (12.0%)	9.1 ± 2.9	5 (14.3%)	0.038
LIPID PROFILE								
SFA (% Energy)	≤7–8	11.8 ± 2.8	3 (7.5%)	11.9 ± 3.0	4 (12.1%)	15.5 ± 8.1	0 (0.0%)	0.559
MUFA (% Energy)	20	20.3 ± 5.7	10 (25.0%)	19.4 ± 5.7	12 (36.4%)	6.5 ± 5.3	5 (14.3%)	<0.001
PUFA (% Energy)	5	5.8 ± 2.1	12 (30.0%)	6.5 ± 5.3	19 (57.6%)	5.4 ± 2.7	6 (17.4%)	0.874
Cholesterol (mg)	<300 mg	340.3 ± 137.7	19 (47.5%)	348.0 ± 129.8	11 (33.0%)	354.1 ± 152.1	10 (28.6%)	0.915
OTHERS								
Water (mL)	2000 mL	2305.36 ± 487.6	23 (57.5%)	2128.0 ± 682.2	20 (57.4%)	2098.1 ± 736.4	16 (48.5%)	0.751
Fruits and vegetables	5 portions	1.9 ± 1.5	3 (7.5%)	1.3 ± 1.4	1 (2.8%)	2.2 ± 1.5	1 (3.0%)	0.785
Sugar	6–10	20.0 ± 9.0	1 (2.5%)	19.0 ± 7.1	5 (14.3%)	16.0 ± 5.1	7 (21.2%)	0.632
Alcohol (g)	≤1 SDU women ≤2 SDU men	3.8 ± 9.8	39 (97.5%)	4.0 ± 8.7	32 (97.0%)	3.9 ± 8.8	31 (88.6%)	0.298

SFA: Saturated Fatty Acids; MFA: Monounsaturated Fatty Acids; PUFA: Polyunsaturated Fatty Acids; SDU: Standard Drink Unit.

Regarding the intake of micronutrients, a comparison between women and men can be seen in Table S2. Significant differences were found between sexes for the intake of thiamine, riboflavin, niacin, vitamin B6, vitamin E, phosphorus, and iron, with the average daily intake being higher in men than in women for all the micronutrients. Regarding adequacy, however, women possess a major percentage of adequacy than men.

When comparing micronutrient intake by BMI (Table 3), it was found that NW subjects consumed higher amounts of some micronutrients such as iron, iodine, and ascorbic acid than OW and OB patients, whereas tocopherol intake was significantly higher for OW subjects and OB patients, and a higher intake of calciferol with respect to both NW and OW subjects was observed. Compliance with intake with current recommendations was higher in NW subjects than in OW subjects for calcium, iron, iodine, zinc, ascorbic acid, and calciferol. Only in the case of magnesium were the highest compliance rates found in OB subjects with respect to NW and OW patients.

Table 3. Micronutrient intake for normal weight (NW), overweight (OW), or obese (OB) subjects, and its adequation to the Dietary Reference Intakes (DRI) for the Spanish population ($n = 108$). Diet adequacy is expressed as the number of individuals meeting the DRI and in brackets is expressed as percent.

	NW ($n = 40$)		OW ($n = 35$)		OB ($n = 33$)		
Vitamins	Average ± SD	Intake Adequacy n (%)	Average ± SD	Intake Adequacy n (%)	Average ± SD	Intake Adequacy n (%)	p Value
Thiamine (mg)	1.5 ± 0.8	32 (80.0%)	1.9 ± 0.9	31 (88.6%)	1.4 ± 0.3	29 (87.9%)	0.009
Riboflavin (mg)	1.7 ± 0.5	30 (75.0%)	2.1 ± 0.6	31 (88.6%)	1.7 ± 0.4	27 (81.9%)	0.007

Table 3. Cont.

Vitamins	NW (n = 40)		OW (n = 35)		OB (n = 33)		p Value
	Average ± SD	Intake Adequacy n (%)	Average ± SD	Intake Adequacy n (%)	Average ± SD	Intake Adequacy n (%)	
Niacin (mg)	30.5 ± 10.7	30 (75.0%)	40.4 ± 14.5	16 (45.7%)	31.6 ± 7.7	25 (75.8%)	0.0005
Vitamin B_6 (µg)	2.0 ± 0.8	35 (87.5%)	2.3 ± 1.1	33 (94.3%)	2.0 ± 0.6	30 (90.9%)	0.159
Folic acid (µg)	281.3 ± 126.3	13 (32.5%)	278.3 ± 105.2	10 (28.6%)	255.3 ± 74.6	8 (24.2%)	0.537
Vitamin B_{12} (µg)	6.1 ± 6.0	40 (100%)	6.4 ± 2.5	35 (100%)	5.6 ± 2.8	33 (100%)	0.697
Vitamin C (mg)	151.2 ± 87.7	35 (87.5%)	166.2 ± 79.6	33 (94.3%)	160.7 ± 68.5	33 (100%)	0.738
Vitamin A (µg)	798.4 ± 603.1	24 (60.0%)	750.5 ± 452.7	19 (54.3%)	745.0 ± 406.8	17 (51.5%)	0.868
Vitamin D (µg)	2.9 ± 3.2	8 (20.0%)	4.6 ± 6.0	11 (31.4%)	4.5 ± 6.5	11 (33.3%)	0.321
Vitamin E (mg)	8.3 ± 8.1	5 (12.5%)	7.8 ± 9.9	4 (11.4%)	5.9 ± 5.6	2 (6.1%)	0.416
Minerals							
Calcium (mg)	719.8 ± 297.1	7 (17.5%)	841.2 ± 415.0	12 (34.3%)	792.9 ± 348.4	10 (30.3%)	0.331
Magnesium (mg)	325.7 ± 134.9	23 (57.5%)	368.9 ± 95.8	23 (65.7%)	308.8 ± 81.0	15 (45.5%)	0.063
Potassium (mg)	3086.7 ± 904.1	22 (55.0%)	4044.5 ± 1135.9	26 (74.3%)	3511.8 ± 745.6	24 (72.7%)	0.0001
Phosporus (mg)	1415.5 ± 500.5	38 (95.0%)	1716.9 ± 472.9	34 (97.1%)	1436.8 ± 380.6	32 (97.0%)	0.009
Iron (mg)	16.7 ± 9.0	23 (57.5%)	18.3 ± 5.8	29 (82.9%)	14.0 ± 2.8	21 (63.6%)	0.035
Iodine (µg)	184.4 ± 150.3	16 (40.0%)	347.5 ± 197.4	25 (71.4%)	292.5 ± 153.6	25 (75.8%)	0.0002
Zinc (mg)	24.4 ± 78.7	29 (72.5%)	14.1 ± 3.5	34 (97.1%)	10.8 ± 2.9	27 (81.8%)	0.0445
Sodium (mg)	2610.9 ± 677.5	6 (15.0%)	5609.5 ± 1219.7	0 (0.0%)	3877.1 ± 346.0	0 (0.0%)	<0.0001

3.2. Analysis of the Gut Microbiota Composition

3.2.1. Alpha- and Beta-Diversity

A total of 95 fecal samples were collected from the volunteers. A first analysis between groups (NW, OW, and OB) was carried out; however, no differences were obtained between the OW and OB groups. Therefore, a second analysis conducted by grouping OW and OB was developed. Although the BMI is the most extended method, in clinical practice, to classify overweight and obesity in adults, it is not the most adequate to determine the amount of body fat. In addition, the nutritional analysis has shown that, in terms of adequacy, the individuals included in the NW group accomplish in higher proportion the nutritional objectives and the DRI for the Spanish population than the OW and OB groups (for example, the % of adequacy for the group of OW and OB is 0, whereas 15% of the individuals in the NW group meet the RDI)

To investigate alpha-diversity, the Chao1 richness and Shannon diversity (richness and abundance) indices were determined. No statistical differences were found between the NW and OW/OB groups for Chao1 (ANOVA, p = 0.1953) nor for Shannon (p = 0.711). For beta-diversity, calculated by Bray-Curtis, no statistical differences were found between groups (F-value: 0.7111; R-squared: 0.0079266; p-value: 0.768) either. See Figure 1.

3.2.2. Relative Abundance of Bacteria

The relative frequency (Figure 2) at the phylum level (a) showed an increase in the Bacteroidetes phlylum in the OW/OB (35.5%) group in comparison with the NW group (33.2%), whereas the Firmicutes phylum decreased in the OW/OB group (53.3% vs. 56.3%) as well as Actinobacteria (3.54 vs. 3.90%). At the genus level (Figure 1b), the main identified bacteria were *Bacteroides* and *Prevotella*, contributing to the Bacteroidetes phylum, while *Blautia* and *Ruminoccocus* formed the Firmicutes phylum, and *Bifidobacterium* contributes to Actinobacteria phylum; in the Proteobacteria phylum, the main genus was *Sutterella* and *Succinivibrio*. Finally, at the species level, 50 species were identified, with the main identified ones being *Prevotella copri*, *Bacteroides uniformis*, *Bifidobacterium adolescentis*, and *Bifidobacterium longum*, among others.

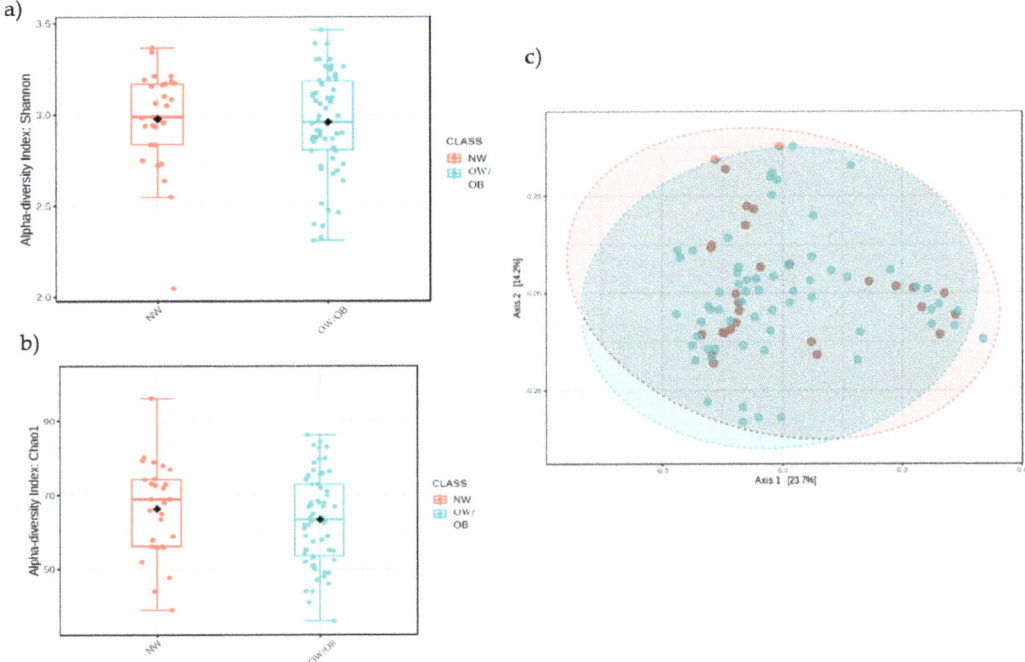

Figure 1. (**a**) Shannon index and (**b**) Chao1 index (alpha-diversity), in red for normal-weight individuals (NW) and, in blue for overweight/obese (OW/OB); (**c**) beta-diversity determined by principal coordinates analysis (PCoA) based on the Bray-Curtis dissimilarity index; red NW group and blue OW/OB group.

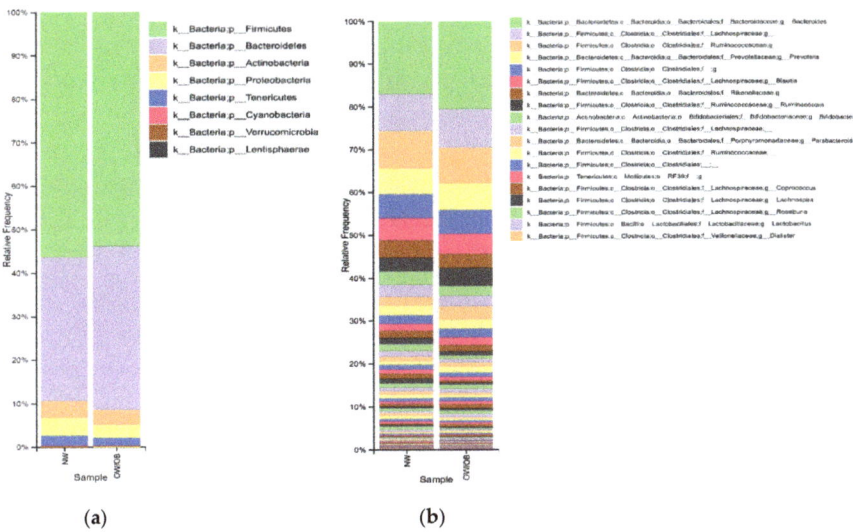

(**a**)   (**b**)

Figure 2. Relative abundance of different bacterial phyla and genera. Bacterial composition (relative abundance, %) was determined using 16S rRNA amplicon sequencing at the phylum (**a**) and genus (**b**) levels. The x-axis shows the different groups evaluated (NW vs. OW/OB). Due to the large number of reported bacteria, only the top 19 most abundant genera were included in the legend. NW: normal weight; OW/OB, overweight/obese individuals.

Regarding the statistical differences, the analysis using the software STAMP showed statistical differences for 18 ASVs (see table in Supplementary Material). In Figure 3, it is possible to see the box plots for three identified bacterial genera and 1 other species. In the graphics, it can be observed as the genera *Anaerostipes* and *Faecalibacterium* decreased in the OW/OB group whereas the genus Oscillospira increased. For the species, *R. faecis*, the proportion of sequence obtained was statistically higher in NW individuals than in OW/OB.

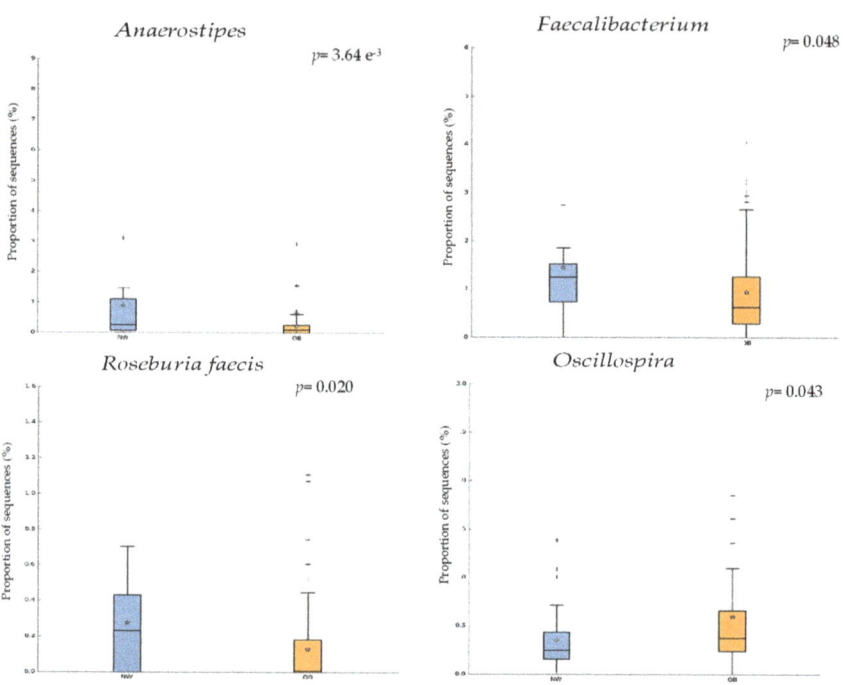

Figure 3. Box plots obtained in the statistical analysis with STAMP for the genera Anaerostipes, *Faecalibacterium, Oscillospira*, and the species *R. faecis*. Blue represents the NW group, and orange is the OW/OB group.

3.2.3. Correlation Analysis: Microbiota-Fiber, Microbiota-MUFAs

Since statistical differences were found for fiber and MUFAs intake in the nutritional analysis, a correlation analysis was carried out with these two factors to establish a linear relationship among the identified species. Individuals were, in this case, classified depending on their adequacy to the recommended intake, reaching or not reaching the recommendation standards for an adequate, lower, or high consumption in the case of MUFAs. Figure 4a,b show the obtained results. As can be seen in Figure 4a, *P. copri* was more abundant in individuals achieving recommendations for fiber, and this species was positively correlated with *F. prausnizii, B. ovatus, B. caccae, B. uniformis*, and *R. faecis*. A negative correlation was found for *B. adolescentis, Collinsella aerofaciens, Dorea formicigenerans, Parabacteroides distasonis, Ruminococcus bromii*, and *B. longum*. The bacteria positively correlated with fiber were those more abundant in NW individuals (see Supplementary Material Figure S1).

Regarding MUFAs (Figure 4b), *P. copri* was more abundant in those individuals with adequate consumption to recommendations, followed by individuals with low consumption, and the lowest abundance was observed for those individuals with high consumption. For this species, a positive correlation was observed with *B. caccae, F. prausnitzii, R. faecis*, and *B. ovatus*.

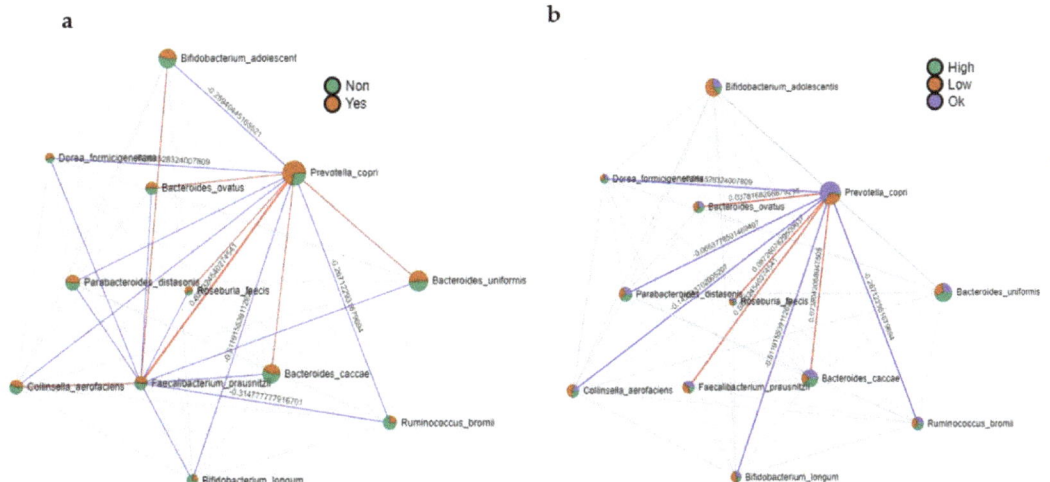

Figure 4. Correlation analysis. Figures show the obtained results for the correlation analysis between identified bacterial species and (**a**) adequation to fiber intake in green, no adequation in red (**b**) MUFAS consumption: above the recommendations(green), below the recommendation(red), and an adequate consumption (purple). Red lines showed a positive correlation among bacterial species, whereas blue lines showed a negative correlation.

3.2.4. LEfSe Analysis

The LEfSE analysis at the feature level for the determination of potential biomarkers shows significant differences for 14 identified bacteria, which are shown in Figure 5. As it can be observed, bacteria such as *R. faecis* or *F. prausnitzii* appear as biomarkers of NW; this bacterium was previously associated with nutritional adequation to fiber and MUFAs intake, whereas the genus *Oscillospira* was associated with OW/OB individuals who showed a lower consumption of fiber.

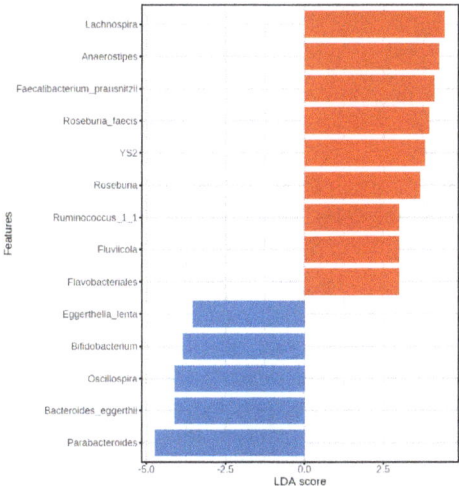

Figure 5. LEfSe analysis at the feature level between the NW group (red) and the OW/OB group (blue) (LDA score > 2). The LDA score (log10) for the most prevalent feature in the OW/OB group is represented on a negative scale, and the LDA score for the most prevalent feature in the NW group is represented on a positive scale.

4. Discussion

4.1. Nutritional Analysis

The results obtained from the nutritional analysis showed that the diet followed by the participants of our study is characterized by an elevated consumption of protein and fat, with a high intake of SFA and simple sugars and reduced carbohydrates and fiber. Regarding energy intake, the European Food Safety Authority (EFSA), for its part, recommends an intake of 2000 kcal/day for women and 2500 kcal/day for men [28]. In the present study, the daily energy intake compared with the EFSA suggestions was higher in women, while men adhered correctly to these recommendations. In 2007, a survey on the eating habits of the Galician adult population was conducted with a sample of 3148 individuals [29]. The average intake in the urban sector (results that can be compared with our population sample) for women was 2227 kcal/day. If a comparison is made with the current data obtained in this work, there is only a difference of 20 kcal per day. The opposite happens with men: subjects in this study consumed 75 kcal/day less than the average obtained in the Galician population survey (2577 kcal/day).

Regarding the values for the intake of protein, the average was $16.6 \pm 3.5\%$, which in grams is equivalent to 97.4 ± 15.71 g, a value that exceeds the recommended dietary allowance of 0.8 g/kg body weight/day [30], which for a person weighing about 70 kg would mean an intake of approximately 56 g of protein. On the opposite side of the spectrum to high protein intake is low carbohydrate intake. In 2010, the EFSA's Technical Commission on Dietetic Products, Nutrition, and Allergies proposed a range of 45–60% as a reference for carbohydrate intake in the European Community [31]. In the case of the Spanish population, the Spanish Society of Community Nutrition (SENC) established nutritional objectives of 50–55% of total energy intake of 50–55% of the total energy [30]. Carbohydrates can be found in five types of food: milk and dairy products, cereals, legumes, fruits, and vegetables [32], and their main function is to provide energy to the body; the human body needs at least 100–150 g/day of this macronutrient to ensure the supply of glucose to glucose-dependent organs and avoid ketosis. From a nutritional point of view, carbohydrates can be divided into two categories. On the one hand, glycemic carbohydrates are considered digested carbohydrates that are absorbed by the small human intestine. On the other hand, dietary fibers are non-digestible carbohydrates that pass into the large intestine [33]. In terms of their influence on the gut microbiome, fiber is considered a key ancestral nutrient that preserves gut ecology, especially by regulating macronutrients and host physiology. Bacterial fermentation of dietary fiber produces key metabolites such as short-chain fatty acids, which are considered beneficial for the host's health. In addition to its already established properties for glycemic control, findings of gut microbiome correlations with glucose homeostasis can be incorporated into clinical nutrition practice. Targeted dietary fiber interventions on microbiome modulation can offer options to improve glucose control and contribute to personalized nutritional practices [34,35].

In the results presented in this work, the average intake of carbohydrates of our volunteers was de $38.9 \pm 7.8\%$ of total energy, which is 11% below the objectives for the Spanish population.

In the case of dietary fiber, the adequacy values are very similar to those for carbohydrates; however, significant statistical differences were observed ($p = 0.038$). It was noted that 84.3% of the volunteers had an intake below the recommendations and only 13.9% were adequate for fiber intake. Dietary fiber has functions such as delaying gastric emptying and maintaining satiety, which may aid in body weight control [35]. It is also associated with a reduction in postprandial peak glucose and insulin, which is a point of interest for people with type 2 diabetes or subjects with glucose intolerance [36]. In terms of BMI, the NW participants in this study had a higher percentage of adequacy (32.5%) than the overweight or obese volunteers (12.0% and 14.3%, respectively). Therefore, this result may indicate the adequacy in fiber intake in participants with NW could be related to a reduction in appetite, which may help the individual to eat less food at subsequent meals, thus balancing daily energy intake [37]. Other studies carried out with the Spanish population, as the ANIBES developed in the year 2019 [38], reported similar results, showing a lower fiber intake of 12.7 ± 5.6 g/day.

Only 2 of the 108 individuals included in the study showed to be fiber intake higher than 50 g/day. High fiber intake can reduce the bioavailability of minerals (iron, calcium, magnesium, and zinc) because phytates, a component present in fiber, can form insoluble compounds with these minerals and affect their absorption at the gastrointestinal level [39]. High fiber consumption is also related to gastrointestinal problems, as fiber can reach the colon intact where it is fermented by the intestinal microbiota of the colon, producing gas that can be accompanied by discomfort with abdominal distension [39]. In terms of the type of bacteria use this fiber, the studies are contradictory. Thus, there are articles reporting an increase in the Bacteroidetes phylum for a diet rich in insoluble fiber, an increase in relative abundance for Proteobacteria for soluble fiber, and for some species of the phylum Firmicutes [40]. Other studies indicate that in humans, it has been reported that Bacteroidetes and Actinobacteria have a positive association with fat but a negative association with fibers, whereas Firmicutes and Proteobacteria show the reverse association [41]. Thus, it seems clear that the metabolism of fiber by the bacteria depends on the type of fiber (soluble and insoluble) and the chemical structure of the fiber (polymerization degree, type of linkages, etc.), as well as the microbiota of the individual. As commented before, the future will allow us to select adequate fiber to develop personalized nutritional practices.

These results, for protein, carbohydrate, and fiber intake, are coincident with previous studies where population diet was analyzed. Thus, a study developed in Buenos Aires (Argentina) [42] evaluated the food intake of 142 adults with an average age of 52 years old, the value for protein intake, in grams, was 97 ± 44 g, 252 ± 117 g of carbohydrates (45% of total energy), and only a 15% of participant achieved the recommendations for fiber. In this study, 49% of the participants showed to be an adequation for refined sugars; however, in the present study, only 13% showed adequacy. In similar studies developed recently in Spain, our results are coincident. Thus, Companys et al. [43] showed, in a study developed with 128 individuals, an elevated protein intake (about 18% of total energy) and a reduced carbohydrate and fiber intake (~38% of energy for carbohydrates and a fiber intake of 25 g/day).

Regarding total lipid intake, 79.6% of the surveyed population exceeded the maximum recommended intake, and only 13.9% accomplished the nutritional objectives of this macronutrient. These data are coincident with the previous studies indicated above [42,43], in which 38.8% and 41% of lipids in terms of total energy, for the two studies, respectively, were reported for the participants.

Fat is one of the macronutrients of greatest interest in the diet, due to its specific nutritional characteristics, as its contribution to the diet is more than twice as many calories per gram (9 kcal/g) as that of carbohydrates or proteins [30]. An adequate intake of total fat provides essential fatty acids and energy to facilitate the absorption of fat-soluble vitamins [44]. A popular belief is that dietary cholesterol is the cause of increased blood cholesterol levels. It is now known that this is not the case, although if consumed in excess, dietary cholesterol can have a detrimental influence on human health [45]. It is worth mentioning that excessive consumption of high-fat foods, accompanied by a sedentary lifestyle, affects body weight and health. In fact, total lipid intake is directly related to BMI and lipid profile; therefore, reducing intake, especially in people with excess body weight, influences weight loss and total and c-LDL cholesterol levels [46].

The SENC recommends a daily intake of three pieces of fruit and two or more pieces of vegetables, adapting to the traditional statement of five portions per day. Of total, 94.4% of the participants surveyed had an intake lower than these recommendations, with an average consumption of 1.8 units. In 2018, through the fruit and vegetable situation report provided by the Spanish Nutrition Foundation, a daily intake of 1.5 pieces of fruit and 1.3 pieces of vegetables was found among the Spanish population [47]. Insufficient fruit and vegetable intake is estimated to be the cause of about 14% of gastrointestinal cancer deaths worldwide, 11% of deaths from ischaemic heart disease, and 90% of deaths from cardiovascular accidents [48]. Scientific research in recent years has focused on the protective role of fruits and vegetables due to their antioxidant potential and their high content of vitamins C, E, and beta-carotene, and other carotenoids, as well as phytochemicals [48].

In general terms, the population studied presented a diet similar to the Western dietary pattern [49]. High intakes of foods rich in fats and sugars reigned supreme, while low intakes of carbohydrates including fiber were conspicuous by their absence. Within these inadequacies, the NW group was those who best met the nutritional targets, compared to the overweight and obese group.

Regarding the data obtained for the nutritional analysis taking into account the BMI, in general, higher adequacy was observed for the NW group. The three groups analyzed presented a similar average intake for nutrients with the exception of fiber ($p < 0.038$) and MUFAs ($p < 0.001$). The OW and OB groups showed to consume lower amounts of fiber with outstanding minor adequacy. For MUFAs, the OB group showed lower intake.

Regarding micronutrients. Data obtained in the function of BMI showed that all groups achieved the DRI for vitamin B_{12} and phosphorus. This can be attributed to the high consumption of meat and fish in the diet of the region of Galicia, where the present study was carried out. In addition, phosphorus is found in many ultra-processed foods, which are abundant in a Western diet. Among the micronutrients for which the DRI was not accomplished, vitamin E, folic acid, and calcium showed the lowest adequation. In Spain, the ANIBES report [37] found that 78% of men and 82% of women do not meet adequate vitamin E intake, which coincides with those found in the present work, i.e., 80.5% of men and 95.5% of women did not reach the minimum intake of vitamin E. Folic acid is a micronutrient found in fruits and vegetables, as well as in legumes and other foods such as nuts. The volunteers in the present study reported inadequate intakes of fruit and vegetables, so the low inadequacy could be due to low intakes of these foods.

The high consumption of sodium for the different BMI groups of the surveyed population is noteworthy. The OW and OB showed a 0% of adequation. In Spain, the DRI established by the Spanish Federation of Nutrition, Food and Dietetic Societies (FESNAD) is 1300 mg/day [25]. EFSA considers that an intake of less than 5 g/day (equivalent to 2000 mg Na) represents a healthy salt intake for the general population [50].

In 2010, the average sodium intake worldwide was 3950 mg/day [51]. The results of the ANIBES study in the Spanish population show that the daily intake was 1846 ± 686 mg/day in women and 2219 ± 876 mg/day in men [37]. The results of the present study reveal a sodium intake that is well above the RDI, similar to the global average consumption mentioned above. In both women and men in the Galician population surveyed, the average consumption is three times the RDI (3855.0 ± 1300.3 mg/day and 4156.8 ± 1779.4 mg/day, respectively).

High salt intake may contribute to increased blood pressure, which is one of the main risk factors for cardiovascular disease [52].

4.2. Analysis of the Gut Microbiota Composition

Results for alpha- and beta- diversity did not show statistical differences among NW and OW/OB groups, which is coincident with previous studies of dietary intake in lean and obese individuals. In the study carried out with Filipino children [53], no statistical differences were found for alpha- and beta- diversity. The study of Companys et al. [43] with Spanish adults, however, found significant differences in the Chao1 index and beta-diversity.

Regarding the profile of intestinal microbiota for both groups, the studies carried out to date have reported that the gut microbiota in obese individuals is different from that of lean people in terms of the dominant phyla Bacteroidetes and Firmicutes [19,54,55]. In this sense, different studies have indicated that when there is an excess of body fat, the relative abundance of the phyla Firmicutes increased [10]. However, our data showed the contrary since this phylum decreased in the OW/OB group. This can be due to the diet since Firmicutes together with the Bacteroidetes phylum are responsible for complex carbohydrate metabolism in the gut [56]. Since our individuals did not achieve the nutritional recommendations for this macronutrient, especially the OW/OB group, the type of carbohydrates could be determinant for the ratio between this phylum and not rely so much on the body fat. In addition, physical activity can also influence the Firmicutes/Bacteroidetes ratio [57]. Since our OW/OB individuals do not achieve the OMS recommendations of at least 75–150 min of vigorous-intensity aerobic physical activity or an equivalent combination of moderate- and vigorous-intensity activity throughout the week [58], the Firmicutes/Bacteroidetes ratio in this population should also be influenced by this situation.

Although most of the studies indicated that the ratio Firmicutes/Bacteroidetes increased in obesity, other studies are constituent with our data [59,60], and there are also a few studies that did not find any correlation between gut microbiota composition and variations in body weight. In addition, some authors indicate that the evidence does not support a pivotal role for the proportion of Bacteroidetes and Firmicutes, at least at the phylum level, in predisposition to increased body weight, but that diet is responsible to decrease or increase this ratio [61].

Among the bacterial analyzed to obtain differences between the NW and the OW/OB group, it should be pointed out that the results indicated a predominance of *Faecalibacterium*, *Anaerostipes*, and *R. faecis* for the NW group and *Oscillospira* for the OW/OB group.

Faecalibacterium is a genus associated with a healthy status, since their species are butyrate producers, taking special relevance to *F. prausnitzii*. Previous studies evaluating intestinal microbiota in OB and NW individuals have reported a decrease in this bacteria in the first one [62], which is one of the most reported lean-associated genera [63]

Anaerostipes, a genus belonging to the family *Lachnospiraceae* of the phylum Firmicutes, was also found in significantly higher abundance in NW individuals. Previous studies have shown that this genus was significantly overrepresented in subjects with low inflammatory index [64] and increased in healthy controls when different pathologies have been evaluated as, for example, major depressive disorder [65]. It has also been reported that *Anaerostipes* may protect against colon cancer in humans as a butyric acid producer. In our study, this genus was indicated more abundant in NW individuals.

R. faecis is also a species belonging to the family *Lachnospiraceae*. The genus *Roseburia* consists of obligate Gram-positive anaerobic bacteria that are slightly curved, rod-shaped, and motile by means of multiple subterminal flagella. It includes five species: *Roseburia intestinalis*, *R. hominis*, *R. inulinivorans*, *R. faecis*, and *R. cecicola*. Gut *Roseburia* spp. metabolize dietary components that stimulate their proliferation and metabolic activities. They are part of commensal bacteria producing short-chain fatty acids, especially butyrate, affecting colonic motility, immunity maintenance, and anti-inflammatory properties. Modification in *Roseburia* spp. representation may affect various metabolic pathways and is associated with several diseases (including irritable bowel syndrome, obesity, Type 2 diabetes, nervous system conditions, and allergies) [66].

Oscillospira was found to increase in OW/OB group. This bacterial genus was associated with constipation in previous studies and predictor of low BMI [67], and it is related in most of the published articles to lean subjects [63,68]; however, our data show the contrary.

For the results obtained from the LefSe analysis, it is remarkable that *Lachnospira*, *Anaerostipes*, *F. prausnitzii*, *R. faecis*, and *Roseburia* together with *YS2* (*Lactobacillus plantarum*), *Ruminococcus_1_1*, *Fluvicola* and *Flavobacteriales* were biomarkers indicative of NW, whereas *Eggerthella lenta*, *Bifidobacterium*, *Oscillospira*, *Bacteroides eggerthii* and *Parabacteroides* were associated with obesity. Some of these bacteria have been discussed above in relation to obesity or lean status. Regarding *L. plantarum*, some studies have reported specific strains that as probiotics can alleviate obesity [69].

B. eggerthii was reported increased in obese children in Mexico [70], but it is true that with *Bacteroides* species, the studies indicated it was associated with a healthy status and other ones with dysbiosis or pathologic one.

Regarding *Bifidobacterium*, it has been reported that the *Lactobacillus* and *Bifidobacterium* genera may have a critical role in weight regulation as an anti-obesity effect in experimental models and humans, or as a growth-promoter effect in agriculture depending on the strains [71]. *B. animalis*, for example, has been associated with normal weight status. Although no significant differences have been found between groups, it was noted, in our OW/OB group, that there was a decrease in *B. animalis*, *B. adolescentis*, and *B. longum* and an increment in *B. breve* and *pseudolongum* (data not shown).

Finally, the study presented showed that *P. copri* was more abundant in individuals achieving recommendations for fiber, and this specie was positively correlated with *F. prausnitzii*, *B. ovatus*, *B. caccae*, *B. uniformis*, and *R. faecis*. A negative correlation was found for *B. adolescentis*. *Collinsella aerofaciens*, *Dorea formicigenerans*, *Parabacteroides distasonis*, *Ruminococcus bromii*, and *B. longum*. The bacteria positively correlated with fiber were those more abundant in NW individuals (see Supplementary Material Figure S1).

These results are consistent with other published studies. For example, Lin et al. [72] found that higher fiber intake can affect the composition of the intestinal microbiota, favouring putative beneficial bacteria such as *F. prausnitzii*. Other authors such as Fritsch et al. [73], in a crossover study of 17 participants, found that the abundance of F. prausnitzii increased after 4 weeks on a low-fat, high-fiber diet compared to a standard American diet enhanced with fiber, while Rosés et al. [74], demonstrated a significantly positive correlation between high-fiber intake within the Mediterranean diet context and *R. faecis* abundance. Similarly, studies have shown that after 14 days on a liquid diet supplemented with fiber-rich foods, the abundance of *F. prausnitzii* and *R. intestinalis* is reduced [75].

Therefore, it seems clear that in our study, fiber is the main component determining intestinal microbiota composition. Regarding MUFAs (Figure 4b), P. copri was more abundant in those individuals with adequate consumption, followed by individuals with low consumption, and the lowest abundance was observed for those individuals with high consumption. The species showing a positive correlation with *B. caccae*, *F. prausnitzii*, *R. faecis*, and *B. ovatus*. *B. caccae*, *F.praunsitzii*, and *R. faecis* were significantly reduced in the OW/OB group (see Supplementary Material Figure S1), indicating that these bacteria in addition to the low consumption of fiber could be affected by MUFAs consumption. Previous scientific studies have shown that diets rich in MUFAs do not affect the number of individual bacterial populations but do reduce the number of total bacteria, serum total cholesterol, and LDL-cholesterol values [76]. Since the chemical structure of the fiber is key for the development of one or other bacteria, more studies focusing on the effect of the type of fiber consumed by individuals and focusing on MUFAs should be carried out to clarify this question.

Thus, for our future studies, it should be interesting to evaluate different types of dietary fiber that could be useful to restore this intestinal microbiota imbalance in these OW/OB individuals, test them in a pre-clinical study using an in vitro colonic model, and then select the most appropriate to develop a clinical study with the volunteers. In this clinical study, different biochemistry and genetic parameters, among others, could be investigated to evaluate the effect of this fiber on intestinal microbiota and the host's health status.

5. Conclusions

In this work, a nutritional analysis of individuals from a Northwest region of Spain, Galicia, was conducted to evaluate their adequacy to the recommendation. When individuals were compared by BMI, significant differences in fiber and monounsaturated fatty acids (MUFAs) intake were observed, showing higher adequacy for the NW group. Additionally, the analysis of the gut microbiota of the volunteers was also evaluated to obtain statistical differences in 18 ASVs. *Anaerostipes* and *Faecalibacterium* decreased in the OW/OB group, whereas the genus *Oscillospira* increased. A genus was also found in the LEFSe analysis as a biomarker for OW/OB. *R. faecis* was found in a significantly higher proportion of NW individuals and identified as a biomarker for the NW group. Correlation analysis showed that adequacy to nutritional recommendation for fiber indicated a higher abundance of *P. copri*, linearly correlated with *F. prautsnitzii*, *Bacteroides caccae*, and *R. faecis*. The same correlation was found for the adequacy of MUFA, with. these bacteria being more abundant when the intake was adjusted to or below the recommendations.

Supplementary Materials: The following supporting information can be downloaded at: https://www.mdpi.com/article/10.3390/nu15153418/s1, Figure S1: Correlation analysis. Figures show the obtained results for the correlation analysis between identified bacterial species and BMI of individual (NW in red and OW/OB in green, groups) Red lines showed a positive correlation among bacterial species whereas blue lines showed a negative correlation; Table S1: Participants' diet quality by sex, in terms of caloric profile and lipid quality: adequacy to nutritional objectives for the Spanish population.; Table S2: Micronutrient intake and adequation to the Dietary Reference Intakes (DRI) for the Spanish population in women and men.

Author Contributions: Conceptualization, A.C. and A.C.-C.; methodology, L.S.-L. and P.A.-L.; software, A.C.-C.; validation, A.C.-C.; formal analysis, J.M.M.; writing—original draft preparation, L.S.-L. and B.I.V.; writing—review and editing, A.C.-C., J.M.M. and A.C.; supervision, A.C.; funding acquisition, A.C. All authors have read and agreed to the published version of the manuscript.

Funding: This research was funded by the Ministry of Economy and Competitiveness through the State Program of I+D+I Oriented to the Challenges of Society 2017–2020 (International Joint Pro-gramming 2018). Project PCI2018-093245.

Institutional Review Board Statement: Ethical approval for this study was obtained from The Regional Ethics Committee for Clinical Research (Galician Health Service, SERGAS, n° 2018/270) in compliance with the Declaration of Helsinki of 1964 regarding privacy, confidentiality, and informed consent. All experiments were carried out in accordance with approved guidelines and regulations.

Informed Consent Statement: Informed consent was obtained from all subjects involved in the study.

Data Availability Statement: The data presented in this study are available on request from the corresponding author.

Acknowledgments: The authors thank the CyTED and each National Organism for Science and Technology for funding the IBEROBDIA project (918PTE0540). In this regard, Spain specifically thanks the Ministry of Economy and Competitiveness for the financial support for this project through the State Program of I+D+I Oriented to the Challenges of Society 2017–2020 (International Joint Programming 2018). Project PCI2018-093245.

Conflicts of Interest: The authors declare no conflict of interest.

References

1. World Health Organization (WHO). *Obesity and Overweight*; World Health Organization: Copenhagen, Denmark, 2021. Available online: https://www.who.int/es/news-room/fact-sheets/detail/obesity-and-overweight (accessed on 9 October 2022).
2. Guyenet, S.J.; Schwartz, M.W. Regulation of food intake, energy balance, and body fat mass: Implications for the pathogenesis and treatment of obesity. *J. Clin. Endocrinol. Metab.* **2012**, *97*, 745–755. [PubMed]
3. Van Dijk, S.J.; Tellam, R.L.; Morrison, J.L.; Muhlhausler, B.S.; Molloy, P.L. Recent developments on the role of epigenetics in obesity and metabolic disease. *Clin. Epigenetics* **2015**, *7*, 66. [CrossRef] [PubMed]
4. Instituto Nacional de Estadística (INE). Encuesta Europea de Salud en España (EESE) 2020. Ministerio de Sanidad. 2020, pp. 1–31. Available online: https://www.mscbs.gob.es/estadEstudios/estadisticas/EncuestaEuropea/EncuestaEuropea2020/EESE2020_inf_evol_princip_result.pdf (accessed on 31 October 2022).
5. Pérez-Rodrigo, C.; Hervás-Bárbara, G.; Gianzo-Citores, M.; Aranceta-Bartrina, J. Prevalencia de obesidad y factores de riesgo cardiovascular asociados en la población general española: Estudio ENPE. *Rev. Esp. Cardiol.* **2021**, *75*, 232–241. [CrossRef]
6. Sinisterra-Loaiza, L.I.; Vazquez, B.I.; Miranda, J.M.; Cepeda, A.; Cardelle-Cobas, A. Food habits in the Galician population during confinement by COVID-19. *Nutr. Hosp.* **2020**, *37*, 1190–1196.
7. Leis-Trabazo, R.; Perez, C.L.; Castro Perez, X.; Solla, P. Atlantic Diet. Nutrion and gastronomy in Galicia. *Nutr. Hosp.* **2019**, *36*, 7–13.
8. Vaz Velho, M.; Pinheiro, R.; Rodriguez, A.S. The Atlantic Diet—Origin and features. *Int. J. Food Stud.* **2016**, *5*, 106–119. [CrossRef]
9. Wolfe, B.; Kvach, E.; Eckel, R. Treatment of obesity: Weight loss and bariatric surgery. *Circ. Res.* **2016**, *118*, 1844–1855.
10. Cheng, S.; Munukka, E.; Wiklund, P.; Pekkala, S.; Völgyi, E.; Xu, L.; Cheng, S.; Lyytikäinen, A.; Marjomäki, V.; Alen, M.; et al. Women with and without metabolic disorder differ in their gut microbiota composition. *Obesity* **2012**, *20*, 1082–1087.
11. Castaner, O.; Goday, A.; Park, Y.M.; Lee, S.H.; Magkos, F.; Shiow, S.A.; Schröder, H. The gut microbiome profile in obesity: A systematic review. *Int. J. Endocrinol.* **2018**, *2018*, 4095789. [CrossRef]
12. Thingholm, L.B.; Rühlemann, M.C.; Koch, M.; Fuqua, B.; Laucke, G.; Boehm, R.; Bang, C.; Franzosa, E.A.; Hübenthal, M.; Rahnavard, G.; et al. Obese individuals with and without type 2 diabetes show different gut microbial functional capacity and composition. *Cell Host Microbe* **2019**, *26*, 252–264e10. [CrossRef]

13. Collado, M.C.; Isolauri, E.; Laitinen, K.Ç.; Salminen, S. Effect of mother's weight on infant's microbiota acquisition, composition, and activity during early infancy: A prospective follow-up study initiated in early pregnancy. *Am. J. Clin. Nutr.* **2010**, *92*, 1023–1030. [CrossRef]
14. Damms-Machado, A.; Mitra, S.; Schollenberger, A.E.; Kramer, K.M.; Meile, T.; Königsrainer, A.; Huson, D.H.; Bischoff, S.C. Effects of surgical and dietary weight loss therapy for obesity on gut microbiota composition and nutrient absorption. *BioMed Res. Int.* **2015**, *2015*, 806248. [CrossRef] [PubMed]
15. Remely, M.; Tesar, I.; Hippe, B.; Gnauer, S.; Rust, P.; Haslberger, A.G. Gut microbiota composition correlates with changes in body fat content due to weight loss. *Benef. Microbes* **2015**, *6*, 431–439. [CrossRef] [PubMed]
16. Santacruz, A.; Collado, M.C.; García-Valdés, L.; Segura, M.T.; Martín-Lagos, J.A.; Anjos, T.; Martí-Romero, M.; Lopez, R.M.; Florido, J.; Campoy, C.; et al. Gut microbiota composition is associated with body weight, weight gain and biochemical parameters in pregnant women. *Br. J. Nutr.* **2010**, *104*, 83–92. [CrossRef]
17. Álvarez, J.; Real, J.M.F.; Guarner, F.; Gueimonde, M.; Rodríguez, J.M.; de Pipaon, M.S.; Sanz, Y. Microbiota intestinal y salud. *Gastroenterol. Hepatol.* **2021**, *44*, 519–535. [CrossRef]
18. Kolodziejczyk, A.A.; Zheng, D.; Elinav, E. Diet–microbiota interactions and personalized nutrition. *Nat. Rev. Microbiol.* **2019**, *17*, 742–753. [CrossRef] [PubMed]
19. Bervoets, L.; Van, H.K.; Kortleven, I.; Van, N.C.; Hens, N.; Vael, C.; Goossens, H.; Desager, K.N.; Vankerckhoven, V. Differences in gut microbiota composition between obese and lean children: A cross-sectional study. *Gut Pathog.* **2013**, *5*, 10. [CrossRef] [PubMed]
20. Reyes, L.M.; Vázquez, R.G.; Arroyo, S.M.C.; Avalos, A.M.; Castillo, P.A.R.; Pérez, D.A.C.; Terrones, I.R.; Ibáñez, N.R.; Magallanes, M.M.R.; Langella, P.; et al. Correlation between diet and gut bacteria in a population of young adults. *Int. J. Food Sci. Nutr.* **2016**, *67*, 470–478. [CrossRef]
21. Fernández-Navarro, T.; Salazar, N.; Gutiérrez-Díaz, I.; De los Reyes-Gavilán, C.G.; Gueimonde, M.; González, S. Different intestinal microbial profile in over-weight and obese subjects consuming a diet with low content of fiber and antioxidants. *Nutrients* **2017**, *9*, 551. [CrossRef]
22. Sociedad Española para el Estudio de la Obesidad [SEEDO]. Consenso SEEDO'2000 para la Evaluación del Sobrepeso y la Obesidad y el Establecimiento de Criterios de Intervención Terapéutica. *Med. Clín.* **2000**, *115*, 587–597.
23. Centro de Investigación de Endocrinología y Nutrición Clínica (IENVA). Calculadora de Dietas-Calibración de Dietas. Available online: https://calcdieta.ienva.org/tu_menu.php (accessed on 14 March 2022).
24. Federación Española de Sociedades de Nutrición, Alimentación, y Dietética (FESNAD). Ingestas dietéticas de referencia (IDR) para la población Española, 2010. *Act. Diet.* **2010**, *14*, 196–197.
25. Bolyen, E.; Rideout, J.R.; Dillon, M.R.; Bokulich, N.A.; Abnet, C.C.; Al-Ghalith, G.A.; Alexander, H.; Alm, E.J.; Arumugam, M.; Asnicar, F.; et al. Reproducible, interactive, scalable and extensible microbiome data science using QIIME 2. *Nat. Biotechnol.* **2019**, *37*, 852–857. [CrossRef]
26. Parks, D.H.; Tyson, G.W.; Hugenholtz, P.; Beiko, R.G. STAMP: Statistical analysis of taxonomic and functional profiles. *Bioinformatics* **2014**, *30*, 3123–3124. [CrossRef]
27. Lu, Y.; Zhou, G.; Ewald, J.; Pang, Z.; Shiri, T.; Xia, J. MicrobiomeAnalyst 2.0: Comprehensive statistical, functional and integrative analysis of microbiome data. *Nucleic Acids Res.* **2023**, *1*, gkad407. [CrossRef] [PubMed]
28. European Food Safety Authority (EFSA). Dietary Reference Values for the EU. DRV Finder. Available online: https://multimedia.efsa.europa.eu/drvs/index.htm (accessed on 28 July 2023).
29. Muñiz Garcia, J.; Pérez Castro, T.; Hervada Vidal, X.; Gómez Amorín, A.; Amigo Quintana, M.; Daporta Padín, P.; Seoane Díaz, B.; Lado Lema, M.E.; Martínez Lorente, A.M.; Blanco Iglesias, O.; et al. Xunta de Galicia, Consellería de Sanidad. 2008; pp. 1–88. Available online: https://www.sergas.es/cas/Publicaciones/Docs/SaludPublica/PDF-2153-es.pdf (accessed on 27 July 2023).
30. Bartrina, J.A.; Majem, L.S. Consenso de la Sociedad Españolade Nutrición Comunitaria 2011. Objetivos nutricionales para la población Española. *Rev. Española Nutr. Comunitaria* **2011**, *17*, 178–199.
31. Agostoni, C.; Bresson, J.L.; Fairweather-Tait, S.; Flynn, A.; Golly, I.; Korhonen, H.; Lagiou, P.; Løvik, M.; Marchelli, R.; Martin, A.; et al. Scientific opinion on dietary reference values for carbohydrates and dietary fibre. *EFSA J.* **2010**, *8*, 1462.
32. Makki, K.; Deehan, E.C.; Walter, J.; Bäckhed, F. The Impact of Dietary Fiber on Gut Microbiota in Host Health and Disease. *Cell Host Microbe* **2018**, *23*, 705–715. [CrossRef]
33. Martínez-Puga, E.; Lendoiro, R. Requerimientos nutricionales de energía y macronutrientes. In *Fisiología y Fisiopatología de la Nutrición: I Curso de Especialización en Nutrición*; Cordido Carballido, F., Ed.; Universidade de A Coruña: A Coruña, Spain, 2005; pp. 53–72.
34. Hoffmann Sarda, F.A.; Giuntini, E.B. Carbohydrates for glycemic control: Functional and microbiome aspects. *Curr. Opin. Clin. Nutr. Metab. Care* **2023**, *26*, 341–346. [CrossRef] [PubMed]
35. Barber, T.M.; Kabisch, S.; Pfeiffer, A.F.H.; Weickert, M.O. The health benefits of dietary fibre. *Nutrients* **2020**, *12*, 3209. [CrossRef] [PubMed]
36. Reynolds, A.N.; Akerman, A.P.; Mann, J. Dietary fibre and whole grains in diabetes management: Systematic review and meta-analyses. *PLoS Med.* **2020**, *17*, e1003053. [CrossRef]
37. Hervik, A.K.; Svihus, B. The Role of Fiber in Energy Balance. *J. Nutr. Metab.* **2019**, *2019*, 4983657. [CrossRef] [PubMed]
38. Partearroyo, T.; Laja, A.; Varela-Moreiras, G. Fortalezas y debilidades de la alimentación en la población española del siglo XXI. *Nutr. Hosp.* **2019**, *36*, 3–6. [PubMed]

39. Álvarez Escudero, E.; Sánchez González, P. La fibra dietética. *Nutr. Hosp.* **2006**, *21*, 61–72.
40. Abreuy Abreu, A.T.; Milke-García, M.P.; Argüello-Arévalo, G.A.; Calderón-de la Barca, A.M.; Carmona-Sánchez, R.I.; Consuelo-Sánchez, A.; Coss-Adame, E.; García-Cedillo, M.F.; Hernández-Rosiles, V.; Icaza-Chávez, M.E.; et al. Dietary fiber and the microbiota: A narrative review by a group of experts from the Asociación Mexicana de Gastroenterología. *Rev. Gastroenterol. México (Engl. Ed.)* **2021**, *86*, 287–304. [CrossRef]
41. Wu, G.D.; Chen, J.; Hoffmann, C.; Bittinger, K.; Chen, Y.Y.; Keilbaugh, S.A.; Bewtra, M.; Knights, D.; Walters, W.A.; Knight, R.; et al. Linking long-term dietary patterns with gut microbial enterotypes. *Science* **2011**, *334*, 105–108. [CrossRef]
42. García, S.M.; Fantuzzi, G.; Angelini, J.M.; Bourgeois, M.J.; Elgart, J.F.; Etchegoyen, G.; Giampieri, C.; González, L.; Kronsbein, P.; Martínez, C.; et al. Ingesta alimentaria en la población adulta de dos ciudades de la provincia de Buenos Aires: Su adecuación a las recomendaciones nutricionales. *Actual. Nutr.* **2018**, *19*, 38–43.
43. Companys, J.; Gosalbes, M.J.; Pla-Pagà, L.; Calderón-Pérez, L.; Llauradó, E.; Pedret, A.; Valls, R.M.; Jiménez-Hernández, N.; Sandoval-Ramirez, B.A.; del Bas, J.M.; et al. Gut microbiota profile and its association with clinical variables and dietary intake in overweight/obese and lean subjects: A cross-sectional study. *Nutrients* **2021**, *13*, 2032. [CrossRef]
44. Carrillo Fernández, L.; Dalmau Serra, J.; Martínez Álvarez, J.R.; Solà Alberich, R.; Pérez Jiménez, F. Grasas de la dieta y salud cardiovascular. *Atención Primaria* **2011**, *43*, 157.e1–157.e16. [CrossRef]
45. Weggemans, R.M.; Zock, P.L.; Tai, E.S.; Ordovas, J.M.; Molhuizen, H.O.F.; Katan, M.B. ATP binding cassette G5 C1950G polymorphism may affect blood cholesterol concentrations in humans. *Clin. Genet.* **2002**, *62*, 226–229. [CrossRef]
46. Brouns, F. Overweight and diabetes prevention: Is a low-carbohydrate-high-fat diet recommendable? *Eur. J. Nutr.* **2018**, *57*, 1301–1312. [CrossRef]
47. Arroyo, P.; Leire, U.; Bergera, M.; Rodríguez, P.; Teresa, A.; Gaspar, V.; Moreno, E.R.; Manuel, J.; Torres, Á.; Moreiras, G.V. Frutas y Hortalizas: Nutrición y Salud en la España del S. XXI. Available online: www.fen.org.es/storage/app/media/imgPublicaciones/INFORME_FRUTAS_Y_HORTALIZAS_FEN_2018-v1.pdf (accessed on 12 June 2023).
48. Afshin, A.; Sur, P.J.; Fay, K.A.; Cornaby, L.; Ferrara, G.; Salama, J.S.; Mullany, E.C.; Abate, K.H.; Abbafati, C.; Abebe, Z.; et al. Health effects of dietary risks in 195 countries, 1990–2017: A systematic analysis for the global burden of disease study 2017. *Lancet* **2019**, *393*, 1958–1972. [CrossRef] [PubMed]
49. Cena, H.; Calder, P.C. Defining a healthy diet: Evidence for the role of contemporary dietary patterns in health and disease. *Nutrients* **2020**, *12*, 334. [CrossRef] [PubMed]
50. Agencia Española de Seguridad Alimentaria y Nutrición (AESAN). Publicación de las Opiniones Científicas de EFSA Sobre Ingestas Diarias de Referencia de Sodio y Cloruro. Ministerio de Consumo. 4 September 2019. Available online: https://www.aesan.gob.es/AECOSAN/web/noticias_y_actualizaciones/noticias/2019/sodio.htm. (accessed on 25 April 2023).
51. Mozaffarian, D.; Fahimi, S.; Singh, G.M.; Micha, R.; Khatibzadeh, S.; Engell, R.E.; Lim, S.; Danaei, G.; Ezzati, M.; Powles, J. Global sodium consumption and death from cardiovascular causes. *N. Engl. J. Med.* **2014**, *371*, 624–634. [CrossRef]
52. Grillo, A.; Salvi, L.; Coruzzi, P.; Salvi, P.; Parati, G. Sodium intake and hypertension. *Nutrients* **2019**, *11*, 1970. [CrossRef]
53. Golloso-Gubat, M.J.; Ducarmon, Q.R.; Tan, R.C.A.; Zwittink, R.D.; Kuijper, E.J.; Nacis, J.S.; Santos, N.L.C. Gut microbiota and dietary intake of normal-weight and overweight Filipino children. *Microorganisms* **2020**, *8*, 1015. [CrossRef] [PubMed]
54. Duca, F.A.; Sakar, Y.; Lepage, P.; Devime, F.; Langelier, B.; Dore, J.; Covasa, M. Replication of obesity and associated signaling pathways through transfer of microbiota from obese-prone rats. *Diabetes* **2014**, *63*, 1624–1636. [CrossRef]
55. Hartstra, A.V.; Bouter, K.E.; Backhed, F.; Nieuwdor, M. Insights into the role of the microbiome in obesity and type 2 diabetes. *Diabetes Care* **2015**, *38*, 159–165. [CrossRef]
56. Devaraj, S.; Hemarajata, P.; Versalovic, J. Metabolismo corporal: Implicaciones con la obesidad y la diabetes. *Acta Bioquim. Clin. Latinoam.* **2013**, *47*, 421–434.
57. Monda, V.; Villano, I.; Messina, A.; Valenzano, A.; Esposito, T.; Moscatelli, F.; Viggiano, A.; Cibelli, G.; Chieffi, S.; Monda, M.; et al. Exercise Modifies the Gut Microbiota with Positive Health Effects. *Oxid. Med. Cell. Longev.* **2017**, *2017*, 3831972. [CrossRef]
58. WHO. Physical Activity. 2022. Available online: https://www.who.int/news-room/fact-sheets/detail/physical-activity (accessed on 27 July 2023).
59. Schwiertz, A.; Taras, D.; Schäfer, K.; Beijer, S.; Bos, N.A.; Donus, C.; Hardt, P.D. Microbiota and SCFA in lean and overweight healthy subjects. *Obesity* **2010**, *18*, 190–195. [CrossRef]
60. Duan, M.; Wang, Y.; Zhang, Q.; Zou, R.; Guo, M.; Zheng, H. Characteristics of gut microbiota in people with obesity. *PLoS ONE* **2021**, *16*, e0255446. [CrossRef] [PubMed]
61. Duncan, S.H.; Lobley, G.E.; Holtrop, G.; Ince, J.; Johnstone, A.M.; Louis, P.; Flint, H.J. Human colonic microbiota associated with diet, obesity and weight loss. *Int. J. Obes.* **2008**, *32*, 1720–1724. [CrossRef] [PubMed]
62. Effendi, R.M.R.A.; Anshory, M.; Kalim, H.; Dwiyana, R.F.; Suwarsa, O.; Pardo, L.M.; Nijsten, T.E.C.; Thio, H.B. *Akkermansia muciniphila* and *Faecalibacterium prausnitzii* in Immune-Related Diseases. *Microorganisms* **2022**, *10*, 2382. [CrossRef]
63. Xu, Z.; Jiang, W.; Huang, W.; Lin, Y.; Chan, F.K.; Ng, S.C. Gut microbiota in patients with obesity and metabolic disorders—A systematic review. *Genes Nutr.* **2022**, *17*, 2. [CrossRef]
64. Aranaz, P.; Ramos-Lopez, O.; Cuevas-Sierra, A. A predictive regression model of the obesity-related inflammatory status based on gut microbiota composition. *Int. J. Obes.* **2021**, *45*, 2261–2268. [CrossRef] [PubMed]
65. Caso, J.R.; MacDowell, K.S.; González-Pinto, A. Gut microbiota, innate immune pathways, and inflammatory control mechanisms in patients with major depressive disorder. *Transl. Psychiatry* **2021**, *11*, 645. [CrossRef] [PubMed]

66. Tamanai-Shacoori, Z.; Smida, I.; Bousarghin, L.; Loreal, O.; Meuric, V.; Fong, S.B.; Bonnaure-Mallet, M.; Jolivet-Gougeon, A. *Roseburia* spp.: A marker of health? *Future Microbiol.* **2017**, *12*, 157–170. [CrossRef]
67. Yang, J.; Li, Y.; Wen, Z.; Liu, W.; Meng, L.; Huang, H. Oscillospira—A candidate for the next-generation probiotics. *Gut Microbes* **2021**, *13*, 1987783. [CrossRef]
68. Chen, Y.R.; Zheng, H.M.; Zhang, G.X.; Chen, F.I.; Yang, Z.C. High Oscillospira abundance indicates constipation and low BMI in the Guangdong Gut Microbiome Project. *Sci. Rep.* **2020**, *10*, 9364. [CrossRef]
69. Cai, H.; Wen, Z.; Zhao, L.; Yu, D.; Meng, K.; Yang, P. *Lactobacillus plantarum* FRT4 alleviated obesity by modulating gut microbiota and liver metabolome in high-fat diet-induced obese mice. *Food Nutr. Res.* **2022**, *9*, 66. [CrossRef]
70. López-Contreras, B.E.; Morán-Ramos, S.; Villarruel-Vázquez, R.; Macías-Kauffer, L.; Villamil-Ramírez, H.; León-Mimila, P.; Vega-Badillo, J.; Sánchez-Muñoz, F.; Llanos-Moreno, L.E.; Canizalez-Román, A.; et al. Composition of gut microbiota in obese and normal-weight Mexican school-age children and its association with metabolic traits. *Pediatr. Obes.* **2018**, *13*, 381–388. [CrossRef]
71. Million, M.; Maraninchi, M.; Henry, M. Obesity-associated gut microbiota is enriched in *Lactobacillus reuteri* and depleted in *Bifidobacterium animalis* and *Methanobrevibacter smithii*. *Int. J. Obes.* **2012**, *36*, 817–825. [CrossRef] [PubMed]
72. Lin, D.; Peters, B.A.; Friedlander, C.; Freiman, H.J.; Goedert, J.J.; Sinha, R.; Miller, G.; Bernstein, M.A.; Hayes, R.B.; Ahn, J. Association of dietary fibre intake and gut microbiota in adults. *Br. J. Nutr.* **2018**, *120*, 1014–1022. [CrossRef] [PubMed]
73. Fritsch, J.; Garces, L.; Quintero, M.A.; Pignac-Kobinger, J.; Santander, A.M.; Fernández, I.; Abreu, M.T. Low-fat, high-fiber diet reduces markers of inflammation and dysbiosis and improves quality of life in patients with ulcerative colitis. *Clin. Gastroenterol. Hepatol.* **2021**, *19*, 1189–1199. [CrossRef] [PubMed]
74. Rosés, C.; Cuevas-Sierra, A.; Quintana, S.; Riezu-Boj, J.I.; Martínez, J.A.; Milagro, F.I.; Barceló, A. Gut microbiota bacterial species associated with Mediterranean Diet-related food groups in a Northern Spanish population. *Nutrients* **2021**, *13*, 636. [CrossRef]
75. Benus, R.F.; van der Werf, T.S.; Welling, G.W.; Judd, P.A.; Taylor, M.A.; Harmsen, H.J.; Whelan, K. Association between *Faecalibacterium prausnitzii* and dietary fibre in colonic fermentation in healthy human subjects. *Br. J. Nutr.* **2010**, *104*, 693–700. [CrossRef]
76. Fava, F.R.; Gitau, R.; Griffin, B.A.; Gibson, G.R.; Tuohy, K.M.; Lovegrove, J.A. The type and quantity of dietary fat and carbohydrate alter faecal microbiome and short-chain fatty acid excretion in a metabolic syndrome 'at-risk' population. *Int. J. Obes.* **2013**, *37*, 216–223. [CrossRef]

Disclaimer/Publisher's Note: The statements, opinions and data contained in all publications are solely those of the individual author(s) and contributor(s) and not of MDPI and/or the editor(s). MDPI and/or the editor(s) disclaim responsibility for any injury to people or property resulting from any ideas, methods, instructions or products referred to in the content.

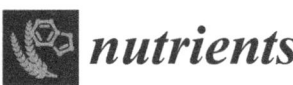

Article

Tartrazine Modifies the Activity of *DNMT* and *HDAC* Genes—Is This a Link between Cancer and Neurological Disorders?

Afshin Zand [1], Sodbuyan Enkhbilguun [1], John M. Macharia [2], Ferenc Budán [3,4], Zoltán Gyöngyi [1,*] and Timea Varjas [1]

[1] Department of Public Health Medicine, Medical School, University of Pécs, H-7624 Pécs, Hungary; af.zand@gmail.com (A.Z.); enkhbiluunsod@gmail.com (S.E.); vtimi_68@yahoo.com (T.V.)
[2] Doctoral School of Health Sciences, Faculty of Health Science, University of Pécs, H-7621 Pécs, Hungary; johnmacharia@rocketmail.com
[3] Institute of Transdisciplinary Discoveries, Medical School, University of Pécs, H-7624 Pécs, Hungary; budfer2@gmail.com
[4] Institute of Physiology, Medical School, University of Pécs, H-7624 Pécs, Hungary
* Correspondence: zoltan.gyongyi@aok.pte.hu

Abstract: In recent years, artificial additives, especially synthetic food colorants, were found to demonstrate wider properties compared to their natural equivalents; however, their health impact is still not totally mapped. Our study aimed to determine the long-term (30 and 90 days) exposure effect of one of the commonly used artificial food colorants, tartrazine, on NMRI mice. The applied dose of tartrazine referred to the human equivalent dose for acceptable daily intake (ADI). Further, we evaluated its impact on the transcription of a range of epigenetic effectors, members of the DNA methyltransferase (*DNMT*) as well as histone deacetylase (*HDAC*) families. Following the exposure, organ biopsies were collected from the lungs, kidneys, liver, and spleen, and the gene expression levels were determined by real-time quantitative reverse transcription PCR (RT-qPCR). Our results demonstrated significant upregulation of genes in the tested organs in various patterns followed by the intake of tartrazine on ADI. Since *DNMT* and *HDAC* genes are involved in different steps of carcinogenesis, have roles in the development of neurological disorders and the effect of dose of everyday exposure is rarely studied, further investigation is warranted to study these possible associations.

Keywords: *DNMT*; *HDAC*; tartrazine; additive; mice; qRT-PCR; gene expression; azo-dye; food colorant; epigenetics

Citation: Zand, A.; Enkhbilguun, S.; Macharia, J.M.; Budán, F.; Gyöngyi, Z.; Varjas, T. Tartrazine Modifies the Activity of *DNMT* and *HDAC* Genes—Is This a Link between Cancer and Neurological Disorders? *Nutrients* **2023**, *15*, 2946. https://doi.org/10.3390/nu15132946

Academic Editor: Jose M. Miranda

Received: 11 June 2023
Revised: 24 June 2023
Accepted: 26 June 2023
Published: 28 June 2023

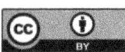

Copyright: © 2023 by the authors. Licensee MDPI, Basel, Switzerland. This article is an open access article distributed under the terms and conditions of the Creative Commons Attribution (CC BY) license (https://creativecommons.org/licenses/by/4.0/).

1. Introduction

Color additives have been widely used since 1500 BC and currently are extensively used by food manufacturers as a vital criterion for food choice. Among them, synthetic food colorants are more favorable due to their stability, low cost, and coloring properties. These artificial food colorants are available in different varieties and colors [1]. Often, we consume them unknowingly. Therefore, it is essential to study the biological consequences of food colorant usage [2].

The consumption of artificial food colorants below the acceptable daily intake (ADI) does not cause any harm, but it may cause for example many disorders among children due to their low body weight [3]. In developing countries, children are the major consumers of artificial food colorants, which is the reason they are at high risk of several illnesses such as asthma [4]. The total world colorant production is estimated to be 80,000,000 tons per year [5].

Azo dyes are a group of vivid synthetic food colorants including tartrazine (TRZ; trisodium-5-hydroxy-1-(4-sulfonatophenyl)-4-(4-sulfonatophenyl-azo)-H-pyrazol-3-carboxylate) and represent about two-thirds of all synthetic dyes, which are undoubtedly the most widely used colorants in our everyday products [6]. Red azo dye TRZ, known as E102 or FD&C Yellow 5, or C.I. 19,140, is a synthetic lemon-yellow colorant used in food, drugs, and cosmetics [7]. Both the FAO/WHO Expert Committee on Food Additives (JECFA) and the European Union Scientific Committee for Food (SCF) determined an acceptable daily intake dose in 1996 [8]. JECFA in 1964 demonstrated TRZ's identity, purity criteria, and toxicological data and defined an ADI of 0–7.5 mg/kg body weight (bw) [9]. TRZ acceptable daily intake was increased in 2016 from 0–7.5 to 0–10 mg/kg bw based on a NOAL of 984 mg/kg bw due to the lack of compelling evidence of harm at the highest tested doses ($\geq$1000 mg/kg bw/day) in both long-term and reproductive and developmental studies [10].

TRZ is synthesized from coal tar, and it is marketed in the form of water-soluble powder. The levels of TRZ and other synthetic colorants in food product samples can exceed the accepted daily consumption limit in adults and children. Among children, the risk of exceeding ADI is usually much higher than adults, because children are the major consumers of colored food. Thus, exposure to excessive colorants may pose a greater health risk such as hyperactivity [11]. The individual response depends on genetic factors as well as on long-term exposure to low doses [12].

TRZ can be metabolized to an aromatic amine such as sulfanilic acid, which is highly sensitizing to allergies such as urticaria and asthma because TRZ is a nitrous derivative [13,14]. In addition, research has focused on its potential to cause genetic mutations and cancer because it can be converted into an aromatic amine, sulfanilic acid, by the microorganisms in the gut [15]. Sufanilic acid has been shown to cause oxidative stress and cellular damage to human pancreatic cells, for instance [16].

TRZ has been demonstrated to exert histopathological effects on the hepatic and renal tissues of rats, indicated by vacuolation, swelling, necrosis, and pyknosis [17]. Red-azo dye such as TRZ can induce DNA damage in vivo and in vitro [18–23]. In one study, the comet assay showed that tartrazine has a genotoxic effect on the white blood cells of rats that were treated [24]. Both TRZ and its metabolites showed genotoxic effects. In addition, TRZ can induce cytotoxicity at high concentrations [24]. The toxic effect of azo dyes has been attributed to the aromatic amines produced from the cleavage of aryl-N=N-aryl [25]. N-hydroxy derivatives, the byproducts of sulfanilic acid, result in neurotoxicity and cause disruptions in redox balance, as evidenced by a significant increase in malondialdehyde (MDA) levels ($p < 0.05$), as well as inhibition of glutathione (GSH) concentration, catalase (CAT), superoxide dismutase (SOD), and glutathione peroxidase (GPx) antioxidant enzyme activities. Additionally, tartrazine-treated rats exhibited elevated levels of acetylcholine (Ach) and gamma-aminobutyric acid (GABA) in the brain, while dopamine (DA) levels were depleted [26].

DNA methyltransferases (DNMTs) and histone deacetylases (HDACs) are groups of enzymes that play a significant role in epigenetics. DNMTs are a family of enzymes that provide a crucial role in genomic stability and integrity. They act on the addition of a methyl group to the 5-position of cytosine residues in DNA. DNA methylation plays a crucial role in regulating gene expression by silencing certain genes by inhibiting their transcription. This can occur through the methylation of promoter regions of genes, preventing the binding of transcriptional factors [27]. There are three active enzymatic members of DNMTs, including DNMT1, DNMT3A, and DNMT3B. Misregulation of them may cause chromosomal instability and carcinogenesis by abnormal DNA methylation. Some studies have shown that DNMT overexpression may lead to the methylation of tumor-suppressor genes, resulting in their silencing and the development of cancer [28]. Hypermethylation of the promoter of DNA repair genes is closely associated with several human tumor types, including colon, breast, and lung cancer [29].

HDACs represent a group of enzymes responsible for the removal of acetyl groups from histones, leading to expressions of several genes. It has been reported that HDACs are responsible for the alteration of acetylation levels, which has been studied in various cancer cells. HDACs could play a significant role in the initiation, progression, and promotion of carcinogenesis [30].

HDAC2, HDAC3, and HDAC8 are all members of the histone deacetylase (HDAC) family of enzymes that play important roles in regulating cell proliferation. They are known to interact with other transcriptional repressors and co-repressors, such as the polycomb group proteins, to silence genes that promote cell proliferation. Studies have shown that *HDAC* genes inhibit cell cycle inhibitors, differentiation, and apoptosis but enhance angiogenesis, invasion, and migration [31,32].

Many food products contain TRZ, which are prepared at different temperatures, such as drinks and juices, cookies, chips, chewing gums, candies, cereals, mustards, dairy products, jellies, ice creams, fillings, liqueurs, powdered juices, soft drinks, yogurts, decoration and coatings, and many other products [33].

This study aimed to evaluate the correlation between TRZ and the expression of *HDAC2*, *HDAC3*, and *HDAC8* as well as *DNMT1*, *DNMT3a*, and *DNMT3b* with the help of qRT-PCR measured in the lungs, kidneys, liver, and spleen of young male and female mice after long-term and short-term exposure, resulting in a detectable enhancing effect of tartrazine on the activity of *DNMT* and *HDAC* genes.

2. Materials and Methods

2.1. Animals

The selected age of the mice was 6–8 weeks. This corresponds to the human infancy and early sedentary age. The duration of treatment was 30 and 90 days for the mice, which corresponds to approximately 3 and 10 years in human life. Thus, our study targets the life stage and duration at which exposure to tartrazine is greatest in the human population. A total number of 48 male and 48 female NMRI mice (Charles River Laboratories International, Budapest, Hungary) were used in the present study, aged between 6 and 8 weeks, and weighing 30–40 g. The study animals were kept at the Experimental Department (University of Pécs, Pécs, Hungary), where they were housed in standard polycarbonate cages (330 × 160 × 137 mm), bedded with shavings under standard conditions (20–22 °C, humidity 40–60%, 12:12 h light–dark cycle photoperiod) and fed with standard rodent pellet (CRLT/n standard rodent pellet, Sindbad Kft., Gödöllő, Hungary); the water was provided ad libitum. The animal experiment was reviewed and approved by the local authorities (Committee on Research of the University of Pécs, permit number: BA02/2000-12/2018) according to Hungarian animal protection laws in accordance with EU guidelines. In line with ethical guidelines, we reduced the number of animals used and refined the experimental conditions and procedures to minimize harm to animals. The cervical dislocation was performed by a properly trained person in full compliance with the regulations of physical euthanasia.

2.2. Treatment of NMRI Mice

NMRI mice were divided into 8 groups of 6 females and 6 males each as described below:

Group I: control group that consumed tap water and rodent chew prepared at room temperature for 30 days.

Group II: control group that consumed tap water and rodent chew prepared at room temperature for 90 days.

Group III: control group that consumed tap water and rodent chew, prepared, and baked after the drying process for 30 min at 160 °C, for the duration of 30 days.

Group IV: control group that consumed tap water and rodent chew, prepared, and baked after the drying process for 30 min at 160 °C, for the duration of 90 days.

Groups V and VI: received special feed consisting of 1×ADI equivalent of human dosage (Human ADI = 7.5 mg/kg/day, which corresponds to 1.845 mg/day of tartrazine, for a mouse with an average body weight of 20 g) [34] of TRZ (Merck-Sigma-Aldrich, Budapest, Hungary), at room temperature for the duration 30 and 90 days, respectively.

Groups VII and VIII: received special feed consisting of 1×ADI equivalent of human dosage of TRZ prepared similar to the control groups and baked at 160 °C for 30 min for the duration of 30 and 90 days, respectively (Table 1)

Table 1. Treatment and sample preparation for the eight groups. The experimental NMRI mice received a daily amount of laboratory rodent chew mixed with an equivalent human dose of TRZ for the duration of the experiment.

Groups	Duration of Consumption	Temperature of Sample Preparation
Group 1 Control	30 days	Room temperature
Group 2 Control	90 days	Room temperature
Group 3 Control	30 days	160 °C
Group 4 Control	90 days	160 °C
Group 5 + TRZ	30 days	Room temperature
Group 6 + TRZ	90 days	Room temperature
Group 7 + TRZ	30 days	160 °C
Group 8 + TRZ	90 days	160 °C

2.3. Sample Collection and mRNA Isolation

After the respective treatment duration, cervical dislocation was performed. The biopsies were collected from various organs such as lungs, liver, kidneys, and spleen, during necropsy. We isolated total RNA from these tissues using TRIzol reagent (MRTR118-20 NucleotestBio Budapest, Hungary) according to the manufacturer's protocol. The tissue samples were homogenized using a Polytron homogenizer with TRIzol reagent (1 mL per 50–100 mg of tissue), and 100 µL of chloroform was added to the TRIzol lysate and thoroughly mixed by shaking. After 5 min at room temperature, the samples were centrifuged for 15 min at 12,000× g at 4 °C, and the upper aqueous phase containing RNA was collected in a fresh Eppendorf tube. Next, 250 µL of isopropanol was added to the sample, mixed, and kept at room temperature for 10 min before being centrifuged for 10 min at 12,000× g at 4 °C. The supernatant was discarded, and the pellet was washed with 70% ethanol and then centrifuged for 5 min at 7500× g at 4 °C. The pellet was air-dried, and either RNase-free water or DEPC-treated water was added to the sample. Finally, RNA was quantified using a Nanodrop spectrophotometer.

2.4. qRT-PCR

Total RNA was evaluated with Roche Lightcycler 480 (Roche, Basel, Switzerland). Assays were run with the Roche 480 instrument, using the KAPA SYBR FAST One-Step qRT-PCR Master Mix kit (Sigma—Budapest, Hungary). Amplifications were carried out in 20 µL of reaction volume, mixing 5 µL of RNA target (50–100 ng) and 15 µL of the master mix containing forward and reverse primers (10 µL KAPA SYBR FASTqPCR Master Mix, 0.4 µL KAPA RT Mix, 0.4 µL dUTP, 0.4 µL primers (200 nM), 3.8 µL sterile double-distilled water). Reactions were performed with the following thermal profile: 42 °C for 5 min, for the reverse transcription step, a hot-start denaturing step of 95 °C for 3 min, followed by 45 cycles of 95 °C for 10 s (denaturation), 60 °C for 20 s (annealing/extension). The fluorogenic signal emitted was read during the annealing–extension step and was analyzed by software. Immediately after amplification, a melting curve protocol was produced by increasing each cycle by 0.5 °C, starting from the set-point temperature (55.0 °C), for 80 cycles, each one at 10 s. The primary sequences of the housekeeping gene used as an internal control, hypoxanthine–guanine phosphoribosyltransferase (*HPRT1*), and the genes of interest, *DNMT1*, *DNMT3A*, *DNMT3B*, *HDAC2*, *HDAC3*, and *HDAC8*, are shown in Table 2. Primers were designed with Primer Express™ Software (Applied Biosystems, Budapest, Hungary) and were synthesized by Integrated DNA Technologies (Bio-Sciences, Budapest, Hungary). The results were analyzed by the relative quantification ($2^{-\Delta\Delta CT}$) method.

Table 2. Sequences of primers used for relative gene expression level measure with qRT-PCR.

Gene name	Forward Primer	Reverse Primer
DNA methyltransferase 1 (*DNMT1*)	AAGAATGGTGTTGTCTACCGAC	CATCCAGGTTGCTCCCCTTG
DNA methyltransferase 3A (*DNMT3a*)	GAGGGAACTGAGACCCCAC	CTGGAAGGTGAGTCTTGGCA
DNA methyltransferase 3B (*DNMT3b*)	AGCGGGTATGAGGAGTGCAT	GGGAGCATCCTTCGTGTCTG
Histone deacetylase 2 (*HDAC2*)	GGAGGAGGCTACACAATCCG	TCTGGAGTGTTCTGGTTTGTCA
Histone deacetylase 3 (*HDAC3*)	GCCAAGACCGTGGCGTATT	GTCCAGCTCCATAGTGGAAGT
Histone deacetylase 8 (*HDAC8*)	ACTATTGCCGGAGATCCAATGT	CCTCCTAAAATCAGAGTTGCCAG
Hypoxanthine phosphoribo-syltransferase 1 (*HPRT1*)	TCAGTCAACGGGGACATAAA	GGGGCTGTACTGCTTAACCAG

2.5. Statistical Analysis

To evaluate our results, we performed an ANOVA test, Levene's F test, and then a post hoc analysis (Scheffe and LSD test). The Kolmogorov–Smirnov test was applied to determine the distribution and standard deviation. Statistical analysis was performed using IBM SPSS statistics for Windows, Version 26.0 (Armonk, NY, USA). Significance was established at $p < 0.05$.

3. Results

3.1. Expression of DNMT Genes

The gene expression of epigenetics-related enzymes was measured in the samples taken from the NMRI mice's spleen, liver, lungs, and kidneys. When *DNMT1* expression (Figure 1) was measured in the spleen, liver, lungs, and kidneys, the 30-day and 90-day room temperature TRZ-treated groups had significantly elevated levels compared to the control groups. When TRZ-containing feed was prepared at high temperatures, significant activation of *DNMT1* was observed in the liver, lungs, and kidneys from the 30-day treatment and the liver and kidneys from the 90-day treatment. Lengthening the treatment from 30 to 90 days significantly activated *DNMT1* expression in the liver and kidneys from the room-temperature TRZ and the spleen, liver, and lungs from the high-temperature TRZ groups. When we examined how the temperature of the chew preparation influenced *DNMT1* expression, the preparation at room temperature had higher gene expression in the spleen, lungs, and kidneys of the 30-day and the liver and kidneys of the 90-day groups.

For the expression of the *DNMT3a* gene (Figure 2), 30- and 90-day room-temperature TRZ-treated samples from the spleen, liver, lungs, and kidneys indicated a significant increase compared to the corresponding control groups. In high-temperature TRZ groups, the spleen and kidneys of 30-day and all tissue samples of the 90-day groups expressed higher *DNMT3a*. Significantly higher *DNMT3a* expressions were observed in the 90-day treatment group than in the 30-day one for spleen, liver, lungs, and kidneys in both unheated and heated TRZ conditions. When the preparation temperatures of the mice chews were analyzed, only lung samples in the 90-day group had significant differences.

DNMT3b gene expression was not statistically different (Figure 3) among all 30- and 90-day room-temperature TRZ treatment groups and their respective control groups, except for the 90 days of tartrazine treatment in the spleen sample. However, during the high-temperature TRZ treatment, the liver sample from 30 days and the spleen and liver from 90 days had increased *DNMT3b* expression compared to their controls. Significant changes were observed in the spleen and liver for 30 days and the spleen and lungs for 90 days when TRZ was prepared at high temperatures.

3.2. Expression of HDAC Genes

Elevated levels of *HDAC2* expression were observed (Figure 4) in the spleen, liver, lungs, and kidneys of the 30- and 90-day room temperature TRZ-treated groups compared to the control groups. When the TRZ was prepared at a high temperature, significant activation of *HDAC2* was found in the liver, lungs, and kidneys of the 30-day group and in the spleen, liver, lungs, and kidneys of the 90-day group. The increase in treatment duration from 30 to 90 days resulted in significant activation of *HDAC2* expression in the spleen of the room-temperature TRZ and the spleen and liver of the high-temperature TRZ group. The gene expression of *HDAC2* was significantly different in the spleen, lungs, and kidneys of the 30-day group and the spleen of the 90-day group when the different chew preparation temperatures were compared.

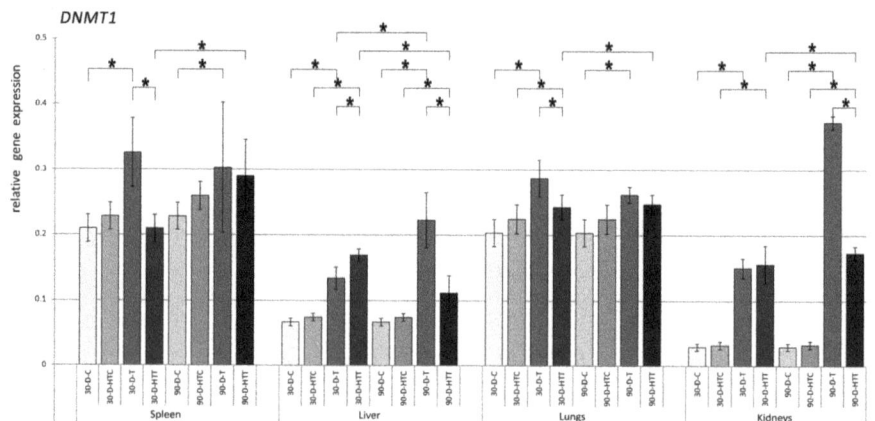

Figure 1. Relative gene expression level of DNMT1 in the spleen, liver, lungs, and kidneys of the animals, $p < 0.05$, after 30- and 90-day consumption of tartrazine prepared at room temperature and treated with high heat (30-D-C: 30-day control, 30-D-HTC: 30-day heat-treated control, 30-D-T: 30-day consumption of TRZ, 30-D-HT: 30-day consumption of heat-treated TRZ, 90-D-C: 90-day control, 90-D-HTC: 90-day heat-treated control, 90-D-T: 90-day consumption of TRZ, 90-D-HT: 90-day consumption of heat-treated TRZ). (* = $p < 0.05$).

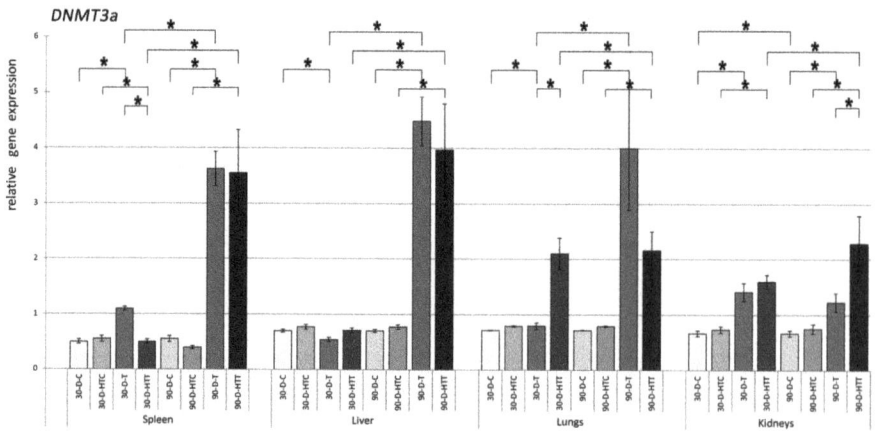

Figure 2. Relative gene expression level of DNMT3a in the spleen, liver, lungs, and kidneys of the animals, $p < 0.05$, after 30- and 90-day consumption of tartrazine prepared at room temperature and treated with high heat (30-D-C: 30-day control, 30-D-HTC: 30-day heat-treated control, 30-D-T: 30-day consumption of TRZ, 30-D-HT: 30-day consumption of heat-treated TRZ, 90-D-C: 90-day control, 90-D-HTC: 90-day heat-treated control, 90-D-T: 90-day consumption of TRZ, 90-D-HT: 90-day consumption of heat-treated TRZ). (* = $p < 0.05$).

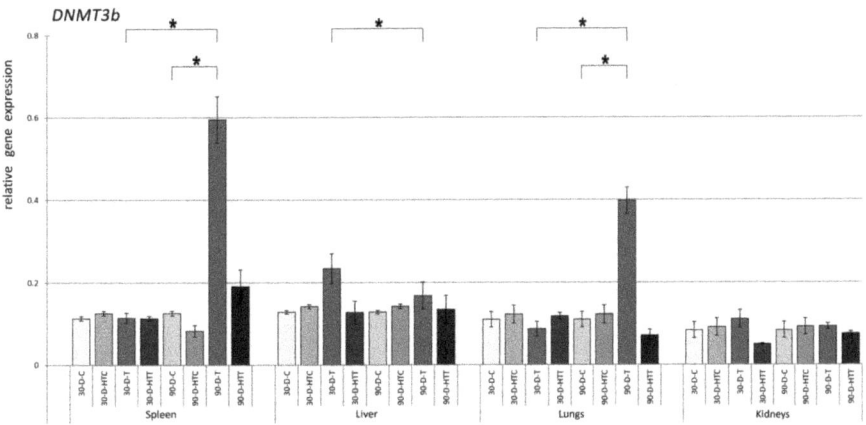

Figure 3. Relative gene expression level of DNMT3b in the spleen, liver, lungs, and kidneys of the animals, $p < 0.05$, after 30- and 90-day consumption of tartrazine prepared at room temperature and treated with high heat (30-D-C: 30-day control, 30-D-HTC: 30-day heat-treated control, 30-D-T: 30-day consumption of TRZ, 30-D-HT: 30-day consumption of heat-treated TRZ, 90-D-C: 90-day control, 90-D-HTC: 90-day heat-treated control, 90-D-T: 90-day consumption of TRZ, 90-D-HT: 90-day consumption of heat-treated TRZ). (* = $p < 0.05$).

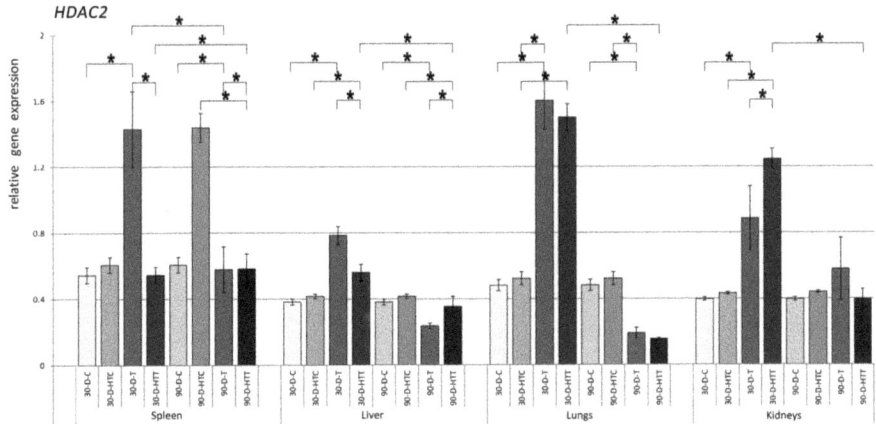

Figure 4. Relative gene expression level of HDAC2 in the spleen, liver, lungs, and kidneys of the animals, $p < 0.05$, after 30- and 90-day consumption of tartrazine prepared at room temperature and treated with high heat (30-D-C: 30-day control, 30-D-HTC: 30-day heat-treated control, 30-D-T: 30-day consumption of TRZ, 30-D-HT: 30-day consumption of heat-treated TRZ, 90-D-C: 90-day control, 90-D-HTC: 90-day heat-treated control, 90-D-T: 90-day consumption of TRZ, 90-D-HT: 90-day consumption of heat-treated TRZ). (* = $p < 0.05$).

The expression pattern of the *HDAC3* gene was very similar to that of *HDAC2*, but there were some differences (Figure 5). It was also found that, in general, *HDAC3* expression was lower than that of *HDAC2*. Nevertheless, there was a clearly significant increase in *HDAC3* expression caused by TRZ. The greatest difference was observed in the liver and lungs, where TRZ diets prepared at room temperature after 90 days of administration resulted in a relatively higher significant increase in *HDAC3* expression compared to *HDAC2*. The expression levels of the *HDAC8* gene were significantly increased (Figure 6) in the spleen, liver, and lungs of both 30- and 90-day room-temperature TRZ-treated groups compared to the control groups that did not receive TRZ treatment. However, in the kidneys, only the

90-day TRZ treatment group showed a significant increase in expression compared to the control. When TRZ was prepared at a high temperature, none of the samples tested caused significant changes in *HDAC8* expression. When the treatment duration was increased from 30 to 90 days, there was a significant rise in *HDAC8* expression in the spleen, liver, and kidneys of room-temperature TRZ and the spleen of the high-temperature TRZ group. In addition, the gene expression of *HDAC8* was found to be substantially different in the spleen, liver, and lungs of both the 30- and 90-day groups, depending on the temperature at which the chew preparation was made.

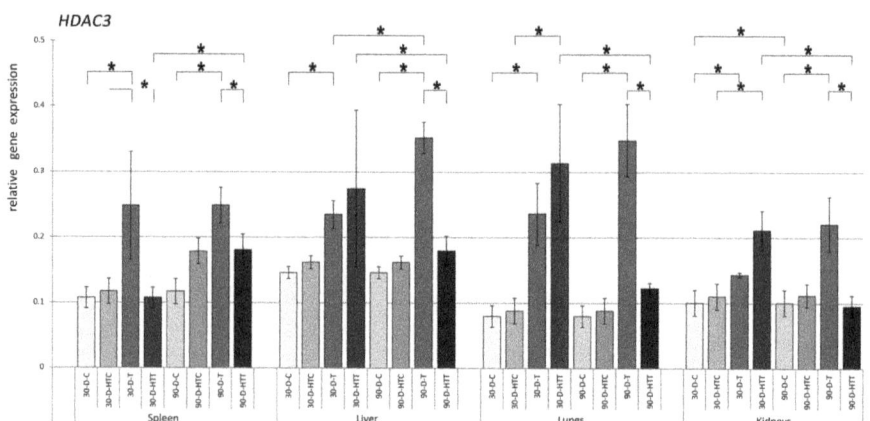

Figure 5. Relative gene expression level of HDAC3 in the spleen, liver, lungs, and kidneys of the animals, $p < 0.05$, after 30- and 90-day consumption of tartrazine prepared at room temperature and treated with high heat (30-D-C: 30-day control, 30-D-HTC: 30-day heat-treated control, 30-D-T: 30-day consumption of TRZ, 30-D-HT: 30-day consumption of heat-treated TRZ, 90-D-C: 90-day control, 90-D-HTC: 90-day heat-treated control, 90-D-T: 90-day consumption of TRZ, 90-D-HT: 90-day consumption of heat-treated TRZ). (* = $p < 0.05$).

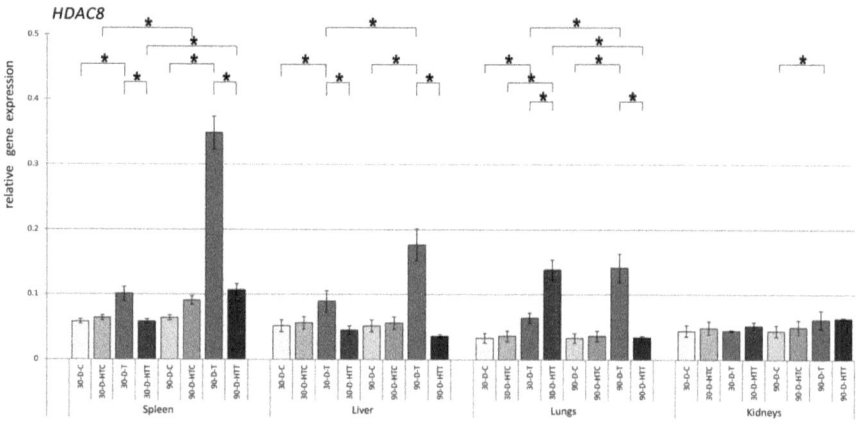

Figure 6. Relative gene expression level of HDAC8 in the spleen, liver, lungs, and kidneys of the animals, $p < 0.05$, after 30- and 90-day consumption of tartrazine prepared at room temperature and treated with high heat (30-D-C: 30-day control, 30-D-HTC: 30-day heat-treated control, 30-D-T: 30-day consumption of TRZ, 30-D-HT: 30-day consumption of heat-treated TRZ, 90-D-C: 90-day control, 90-D-HTC: 90-day heat-treated control, 90-D-T: 90-day consumption of TRZ, 90-D-HT: 90-day consumption of heat-treated TRZ). (* = $p < 0.05$).

In summary, the results show that tartrazine affected the activity of all the genes tested in the *HDAC* and *DNMT* families. In addition, all organs were affected. However, the strongest response varied depending on which time point, which organ, and which gene.

4. Discussion

Our study examined the impact of the acceptable daily intake of tartrazine, a food azo dye, on a set of genes of DNA epigenetic modifiers, *DNMTs*, and *HDACs*.

The widespread use of dye in the food industry has raised significant concerns regarding its excessive utilization in food products. Although the literature is available on the toxicity of food azo dyes at both high and low doses, little information is available on the ADI of these dyes. A range of azo dye products display genotoxic properties only when they are reduced by enteral bacteria such as *Enterococcus faecalis*. This mechanism appears to be linked to the formation of superoxide and oxygen radicals [35]. Azo compounds comprise an aromatic ring that is connected via an azo bond to a second naphthalene or benzene ring [12]. After oral consumption, azo compounds are reduced by azo reductases present in intestinal bacteria and the liver's cytosolic and microsomal enzyme fraction. This process results in the formation of aromatic amines, which have been detected in the urine of experimental animals and paint industry workers following the administration of food azo dyes [36].

It has been reported that gastrointestinal microflora can metabolize tartrazine and produce aromatic amine sulfanilic acid [15]. Consequently, there is a possibility that these aromatic amines may produce reactive oxygen species, including hydrogen peroxide, superoxide anion, and hydroxyl radical, during their metabolism. This could potentially lead to oxidative stress [37]. Based on oxidative stress, TRZ induced dose-related DNA damage in rat colons, which may lead to the formation of tumor cells [38]. Peroxynitrite, a potent RNA formed by the reaction of nitric oxide and ROS, may also play a role in DNA damage [39].

To study the long-term effects, Himri and colleagues (2011) found that ADI doses of TRZ and its consequent metabolic byproducts, namely, sulfanilic acid, have the ability to produce reactive oxygen species (ROS), which leads to oxidative stress and potentially impacts the hepatic and renal structures as well as their respective biochemical profiles [40]. Administration of tartrazine led to a significant increase in plasma aspartate transaminase (AST), alanine transaminase (ALT), and alkaline phosphatase (AlP) levels compared to the control group ($p < 0.05$). Additionally, there was a significant reduction in the total antioxidant capacity observed following tartrazine treatment [41]. The increased levels of malondialdehyde (MDA), which is a product of lipid peroxidation, and nitric oxide (NO) in the rats treated with tartrazine strongly suggest the occurrence of oxidative stress [42]. Related to our study, reactive oxygen species (ROS) can trigger the overexpression of *DNMTs*, which can result in DNA hypermethylation [43]. In the present study, tartrazine significantly increased *DNMT1*, *DNMT3a*, *HDAC2*, and *HDAC3* in both liver and kidneys along with *HDAC8* in the kidney tissues, but the level of *DNMT3b* did not change noticeably in the kidney.

There is limited research on the specific molecular pathways in the lungs that may be affected by tartrazine. However, some studies have suggested that tartrazine may induce oxidative stress and inflammation [44]; however, it may contribute to lung damage and exacerbation of respiratory conditions such as asthma. Ram Prasad's research group discovered that elevated levels of prostaglandin E2 and cyclooxygenase-2 (Cox-2) are associated with increased *DNMT* activity in the epithelial cells [45]. In current research, tartrazine has elevated the relative expression of *DNMTs* and *HDACs*, which suggests that tartrazine may have a negative effect on lung health by inducing oxidative stress, inflammation, and upregulation of pro-inflammatory cytokines. However, further research is needed to fully understand the mechanisms underlying these effects.

Recently, there have been several studies published regarding the effect of epigenetic mechanisms such as *HDACs* and *DMNTs* overexpression in the brain. One study conducted by Valera et al. suggested that modulating the *DNMT* and *HDAC* enzymes could potentially contribute to the manifestation of anti-manic effects. This was concluded because effectively regulating these enzymes has been observed to reverse the effects of Ouabain (OUA), an inhibitor of Na+/K+ATPase. OUA is known to extend the depolarized state of neurons and to induce hyperactivity [46]. Another study by Dash et al. found that the occurrence of traumatic brain injury (TBI) triggers a multifaceted cascade of neurochemical and signaling transformations that give rise to a range of pathological consequences. These include heightened neuronal activity, an excessive release of glutamate, inflammation, increased permeability of the blood–brain barrier (BBB), cerebral edema, modified gene expression, and impaired neuronal function. The administration of valproate shortly after a traumatic brain injury has the potential to provide neuroprotection. This medication can exert its protective effects by inhibiting the activity of *GSK-3* and *HDACs* [47]. Wang et al. demonstrated that a brief treatment with the class I HDAC inhibitors MS-275 or romidepsin improved social and cognitive impairments in transgenic mice carrying the 16p11.2 deletion (16p11del/+). These findings strongly indicate that inhibiting HDACs can serve as an immensely effective therapeutic approach for addressing behavioral deficits in 16p11del/+ mice [48]. The mentioned research has concluded that *HDAC* and *DNMT* genes can alleviate conditions such as mania, hyperactivity, bipolar disorders, neurological disorders, and behavior deficits, which can be reversed with medications that act as HDAC inhibitors, such as valproate. In the current study, we witnessed an overexpression of these genes in several organs due to the exposure of the experimental animals to tartrazine; meanwhile, tartrazine and its metabolites can pass the blood–brain barrier and induce neurotoxicity. Although we gained data from different organs other than the brain, we hypothesize that tartrazine may play a role in behavior and neurological disorders from consuming a food product that meets the current regulations regarding ADI. We believe that further investigations of everyday doses of tartrazine are needed to study the long-term impact on brain function.

5. Conclusions

This is the first study to investigate the effects of oral administration of tartrazine on *DNMT* and *HDAC* genes over a long treatment period while keeping the recommended dose of intake. The present study shows that tartrazine can cause a change in the gene expressions of *DNMT1*, *DNMT3a*, *DNMT3b*, *HDAC2*, *HDAC3*, and *HDAC8* over a long period even at a dose at the ADI level in different organs. Based on the data, compared with the literature, we hypothesize that tartrazine consumption may contribute to cell proliferation and may even increase the likelihood of carcinogenesis. Furthermore, the observed effect in various organs highlights the possibility that the genes under investigation may also be activated in the brain, with proven consequences for brain function.

In view of these findings, it is of great importance to investigate the direct effect of tartrazine on brain function, and replacing the artificial mono-azo dyes with natural food dyes in the food industry, where it is necessary to color food and beverages, should be considered.

Author Contributions: Conceptualization, A.Z. and T.V.; data curation, T.V.; formal analysis, A.Z. and T.V.; investigation, A.Z. and T.V.; methodology, A.Z. and T.V.; project administration, Z.G.; resources, T.V.; supervision, T.V.; validation, S.E., J.M.M. and F.B.; visualization, A.Z., J.M.M., F.B. and T.V.; writing—original draft, A.Z., S.E. and T.V.; writing—review and editing, F.B. and Z.G. All authors have read and agreed to the published version of the manuscript.

Funding: The APC was funded by University of Pécs, Medical School.

Institutional Review Board Statement: The animal study protocol was approved by the Ethics Committee of University of Pécs (BA02/2000-12/2018, 14 March 2018).

Informed Consent Statement: Not applicable.

Data Availability Statement: Data will be made available on request.

Conflicts of Interest: The authors declare no conflict of interest.

References

1. Mpountoukas, P.; Pantazaki, A.; Kostareli, E.; Christodoulou, P.; Kareli, D.; Poliliou, S.; Mourelatos, C.; Lambropoulou, V.; Lialiaris, T. Cytogenetic Evaluation and DNA Interaction Studies of the Food Colorants Amaranth, Erythrosine and Tartrazine. *Food Chem. Toxicol.* **2010**, *48*, 2934–2944. [CrossRef]
2. Merinas-Amo, R.; Martínez-Jurado, M.; Jurado-Güeto, S.; Alonso-Moraga, Á.; Merinas-Amo, T. Biological Effects of Food Coloring in In Vivo and In Vitro Model Systems. *Foods* **2019**, *8*, 176. [CrossRef]
3. Dixit, S.; Purshottam, S.K.; Khanna, S.K.; Das, M. Usage Pattern of Synthetic Food Colours in Different States of India and Exposure Assessment through Commodities Preferentially Consumed by Children. *Food Addit. Contam. Part A Chem. Anal. Control Expo. Risk Assess.* **2011**, *28*, 996–1005. [CrossRef]
4. Husain, A.; Sawaya, W.; Al-Omair, A.; Al-Zenki, S.; Al-Amiri, H.; Ahmed, N.; Al-Sinan, M. Estimates of Dietary Exposure of Children to Artificial Food Colours in Kuwait. *Food Addit. Contam.* **2006**, *23*, 245–251. [CrossRef] [PubMed]
5. Revankar, M.S.; Lele, S.S. Synthetic Dye Decolorization by White Rot Fungus, Ganoderma Sp. WR-1. *Bioresour. Technol.* **2007**, *98*, 775–780. [CrossRef] [PubMed]
6. Chung, K.T. Azo Dyes and Human Health: A Review. *J. Environ. Sci. Health C Environ. Carcinog. Ecotoxicol. Rev.* **2016**, *34*, 233–261. [CrossRef]
7. Mittal, A.; Kurup, L.; Mittal, J. Freundlich and Langmuir Adsorption Isotherms and Kinetics for the Removal of Tartrazine from Aqueous Solutions Using Hen Feathers. *J. Hazard. Mater.* **2007**, *146*, 243–248. [CrossRef] [PubMed]
8. Joint FAO/WHO Expert Committee on Food Additives. 44th Meeting, Rome, Ialy, 1995; International Program on Chemical Safety. In *Toxicological Evaluation of Certain Food Additives and Contaminants in Food*; Joint FAO/WHO Expert Committee on Food Additives: Geneva, Switzerland, 1996; p. 465.
9. Specifications for the Identity and Purity of Food Additives and Their Toxicological Evaluation: Food Colours and Some Antimicrobials and Antioxidants, Eighth Report of the Joint FAO/WHO Expert Committee on Food Additives, Geneva, Switzerland, 8–17 December 1964. Available online: https://apps.who.int/iris/handle/10665/40627 (accessed on 10 June 2023).
10. Joint FAO World Health Organization, & WHO Expert Committee on Food Additives. Evaluation of Certain Food Additives: Eighty-Second Report of the Joint FAO. World Health Organization. 2016. Available online: http://apps.who.int/iris/bitstream/handle/10665/250277/9789241210003-eng.pdf?sequence=1#page=75%22%3E (accessed on 10 June 2023).
11. McCann, D.; Barrett, A.; Cooper, A.; Crumpler, D.; Dalen, L.; Grimshaw, K.; Kitchin, E.; Lok, K.; Porteous, L.; Prince, E.; et al. Food Additives and Hyperactive Behaviour in 3-Year-Old and 8/9-Year-Old Children in the Community: A Randomised, Double-Blinded, Placebo-Controlled Trial. *Lancet* **2007**, *370*, 1560–1567. [CrossRef]
12. Amin, K.A.; Abdel Hameid, H.; Abd Elsttar, A.H. Effect of Food Azo Dyes Tartrazine and Carmoisine on Biochemical Parameters Related to Renal, Hepatic Function and Oxidative Stress Biomarkers in Young Male Rats. *Food Chem. Toxicol.* **2010**, *48*, 2994–2999. [CrossRef]
13. Maekawa, A.; Matsuoka, C.; Onodera, H.; Tanigawa, H.; Furuta, K.; Kanno, J.; Jang, J.J.; Hayashi, Y.; Ogiu, T. Lack of Carcinogenicity of Tartrazine (FD & C Yellow No. 5) in the F344 Rat. *Food Chem. Toxicol.* **1987**, *25*, 891–896. [CrossRef]
14. Chung, K.T.; Stevens, S.E.; Cerniglia, C.E. The Reduction of Azo Dyes by the Intestinal Microflora. *Crit. Rev. Microbiol.* **1992**, *18*, 175–190. [CrossRef]
15. Moutinho, I.L.D.; Bertges, L.C.; Assis, R.V.C. Prolonged Use of the Food Dye Tartrazine (FD&C Yellow N° 5) and Its Effects on the Gastric Mucosa of Wistar Rats. *Braz. J. Biol.* **2007**, *67*, 141–145. [CrossRef] [PubMed]
16. Ameur, F.Z.; Mehedi, N.; Kheroua, O.; Saïdi, D.; Salido, G.M.; Gonzalez, A. Sulfanilic Acid Increases Intracellular Free-Calcium Concentration, Induces Reactive Oxygen Species Production and Impairs Trypsin Secretion in Pancreatic AR42J Cells. *Food Chem. Toxicol.* **2018**, *120*, 71–80. [CrossRef] [PubMed]
17. Mekkawy, H.A.; Ali, M.O.; El-Zawahry, A.M. Toxic Effect of Synthetic and Natural Food Dyes on Renal and Hepatic Functions in Rats. *Toxicol. Lett.* **1998**, *95*, 155. [CrossRef]
18. Sarikaya, R.; Selvi, M.; Erkoç, F. Evaluation of Potential Genotoxicity of Five Food Dyes Using the Somatic Mutation and Recombination Test. *Chemosphere* **2012**, *88*, 974–979. [CrossRef] [PubMed]
19. Sarikaya, R.; Çakir, Ş. Genotoxicity Testing of Four Food Preservatives and Their Combinations in the Drosophila Wing Spot Test. *Environ. Toxicol. Pharmacol.* **2005**, *20*, 424–430. [CrossRef]
20. Poul, M.; Jarry, G.; Elhkim, M.O.; Poul, J.M. Lack of Genotoxic Effect of Food Dyes Amaranth, Sunset Yellow and Tartrazine and Their Metabolites in the Gut Micronucleus Assay in Mice. *Food Chem. Toxicol.* **2009**, *47*, 443–448. [CrossRef]
21. Hassan, G.M. Effects of Some Synthetic Coloring Additives on DNA Damage and Chromosomal Aberrations of Rats. *Arab. J. Biotechnol.* **2010**, *13*, 13–24.
22. Yurchenko, V.V.; Ingel, F.I.; Akhaltseva, L.V.; Konyashkina, M.A.; Yurtseva, N.A.; Nikitina, T.A.; Krivtsova, E.K. Genotoxic Safety of Synthetic Food Colours. Review. *Ecol. Genet.* **2021**, *19*, 323–341. [CrossRef]
23. An, Y.; Jiang, L.; Cao, J.; Geng, C.; Zhong, L. Sudan I Induces Genotoxic Effects and Oxidative DNA Damage in HepG2 Cells. *Mutat. Res.* **2007**, *627*, 164–170. [CrossRef]
24. Atlı Şekeroğlu, Z.; Güneş, B.; Kontaş Yedier, S.; Şekeroğlu, V.; Aydın, B. Effects of Tartrazine on Proliferation and Genetic Damage in Human Lymphocytes. *Toxicol. Mech. Method.* **2017**, *27*, 370–375. [CrossRef] [PubMed]
25. Albasher, G.; Maashi, N.; Alfarraj, S.; Almeer, R.; Albrahim, T.; Alotibi, F.; Bin-Jumah, M.; Mahmoud, A.M. Perinatal Exposure to Tartrazine Triggers Oxidative Stress and Neurobehavioral Alterations in Mice Offspring. *Antioxidants* **2020**, *9*, 53. [CrossRef]

26. Essawy, A.E.; Mohamed, A.I.; Ali, R.G.; Ali, A.M.; Abdou, H.M. Analysis of Melatonin-Modulating Effects Against Tartrazine-Induced Neurotoxicity in Male Rats: Biochemical, Pathological and Immunohistochemical Markers. *Neurochem. Res.* **2023**, *48*, 131–141. [CrossRef] [PubMed]
27. Taylor, R.W.; Turnbull, D.M. Mitochondrial DNA Mutations in Human Disease. *Nat. Rev. Genet.* **2005**, *6*, 389–402. [CrossRef] [PubMed]
28. Esteller, M. Epigenetics in Cancer. *N. Engl. J. Med.* **2008**, *358*, 1148–1159. [CrossRef] [PubMed]
29. Poh, W.J.; Wee, C.P.P.; Gao, Z. DNA Methyltransferase Activity Assays: Advances and Challenges. *Theranostics* **2016**, *6*, 369–391. [CrossRef]
30. de Ruijter, A.J.M.; van Gennip, A.H.; Caron, H.N.; Kemp, S.; van Kuilenburg, A.B.P. Histone Deacetylases (HDACs): Characterization of the Classical HDAC Family. *Biochem. J.* **2003**, *370*, 737. [CrossRef]
31. Park, S.Y.; Kim, J.S. A Short Guide to Histone Deacetylases Including Recent Progress on Class II Enzymes. *Exp. Mol. Med.* **2020**, *52*, 204–212. [CrossRef]
32. Glozak, M.A.; Seto, E. Histone Deacetylases and Cancer. *Oncogene* **2007**, *26*, 5420–5432. [CrossRef]
33. Shrestha, S.; Bharat, R.B.; Lee, K.H.; Cho, H. Some of the Food Color Additives Are Potent Inhibitors of Human Protein Tyrosine Phosphatases. *Bull. Korean Chem. Soc.* **2006**, *27*, 1567–1571. [CrossRef]
34. Reagan-Shaw, S.; Nihal, M.; Ahmad, N. Dose Translation from Animal to Human Studies Revisited. *FASEB J.* **2008**, *22*, 659–661. [CrossRef]
35. Sweeney, E.A.; Chipman, J.K.; Forsythe, S.J. Evidence for Direct-Acting Oxidative Genotoxicity by Reduction Products of Azo Dyes. *Environ. Health Perspect.* **1994**, *102* (Suppl. S6), 119–122. [CrossRef]
36. Cerniglia, C.E.; Zhuo, Z.; Manning, B.W.; Federle, T.W.; Heflich, R.H. Mutagenic Activation of the Benzidine-Based Dye Direct Black 38 by Human Intestinal Microflora. *Mutat. Res. Lett.* **1986**, *175*, 11–16. [CrossRef] [PubMed]
37. Bansal, A.K.; Bansal, M.; Soni, G.; Bhatnagar, D. Modulation of N-Nitrosodiethylamine (NDEA) Induced Oxidative Stress by Vitamin E in Rat Erythrocytes. *Hum. Exp. Toxicol.* **2016**, *24*, 297–302. [CrossRef] [PubMed]
38. Abo-EL-Sooud, K.; Hashem, M.M.; Badr, Y.A.; Eleiwa, M.M.E.; Gab-Allaha, A.Q.; Abd-Elhakim, Y.M.; Bahy-EL-Dien, A. Assessment of Hepato-Renal Damage and Genotoxicity Induced by Long-Term Exposure to Five Permitted Food Additives in Rats. *Environ. Sci. Pollut. Res. Int.* **2018**, *25*, 26341–26350. [CrossRef]
39. Islam, B.U.; Habib, S.; Ahmad, P.; Allarakha, S.; Moinuddin; Ali, A. Pathophysiological role of peroxynitrite induced DNA damage in human diseases: A special focus on poly (ADP-ribose) polymerase (PARP). *Ind. J. Clin. Biochem.* **2015**, *30*, 368–385. [CrossRef]
40. Himri, I.; Souna, F.; Belmekki, F.; Aziz, M.; Bnouham, M.; Zoheir, J.; Berkia, Z.; Mekhfi, H.; Saalaoui, E. A 90-day oral toxicity study of tartrazine, a synthetic food dye, in Wistar rats. *Int. J. Pharm. Pharm. Sci.* **2011**, *3*, 159–169.
41. Khayyat, L.; Essawy, A.; Sorour, J.; Soffar, A. Tartrazine Induces Structural and Functional Aberrations and Genotoxic Effects in Vivo. *PeerJ* **2017**, *5*, e3041. [CrossRef]
42. Demirkol, O.; Zhang, X.; Ercal, N. Oxidative Effects of Tartrazine (CAS No. 1934-21-0) and New Coccin (CAS No. 2611-82-7) Azo Dyes on CHO Cells. *J. Verbrauch. Lebensm.* **2012**, *7*, 229–236. [CrossRef]
43. Kietzmann, T.; Petry, A.; Shvetsova, A.; Gerhold, J.M.; Görlach, A. The epigenetic landscape related to reactive oxygen species formation in the cardiovascular system. *Brit. J. Pharmacol.* **2017**, *174*, 1533–1554. [CrossRef] [PubMed]
44. Shakoor, S.; Ismail, A.; Redzwan Sabran, M.; Mohtarrudin, N. Effect of Food Colorants Supplementation on Reactive Oxygen Species, Antioxidant Vitamins Level and DNA Damage (Kesan Tambahan Pewarna Makanan Pada Spesies Oksigen Reaktif, Tahap Antioksidan Vitamin Dan Kerosakan DNA). *Sains. Malays.* **2021**, *50*, 1343–1356. [CrossRef]
45. Prasad, R.; Katiyar, S.K. Prostaglandin E2 Promotes UV Radiation-Induced Immune Suppression through DNA Hypermethylation. *Neoplasia* **2013**, *15*, 795–804. [CrossRef] [PubMed]
46. Varela, R.B.; Resende, W.R.; Dal-Pont, G.C.; Gava, F.F.; Tye, S.J.; Quevedo, J.; Valvassori, S.S. HDAC Inhibitors Reverse Mania-like Behavior and Modulate Epigenetic Regulatory Enzymes in an Animal Model of Mania Induced by Ouabain. *Pharmacol. Biochem. Behav.* **2020**, *193*, 172917. [CrossRef]
47. Dash, P.K.; Orsi, S.A.; Zhang, M.; Grill, R.J.; Pati, S.; Zhao, J.; Moore, A.N. Valproate Administered after Traumatic Brain Injury Provides Neuroprotection and Improves Cognitive Function in Rats. *PLoS ONE* **2010**, *5*, e11383. [CrossRef] [PubMed]
48. Wang, W.; Tan, T.; Cao, Q.; Zhang, F.; Rein, B.; Duan, W.M.; Yan, Z. Histone Deacetylase Inhibition Restores Behavioral and Synaptic Function in a Mouse Model of 16p11.2 Deletion. *Int. J. Neuropsychopharmacol.* **2022**, *25*, 877–889. [CrossRef] [PubMed]

Disclaimer/Publisher's Note: The statements, opinions and data contained in all publications are solely those of the individual author(s) and contributor(s) and not of MDPI and/or the editor(s). MDPI and/or the editor(s) disclaim responsibility for any injury to people or property resulting from any ideas, methods, instructions or products referred to in the content.

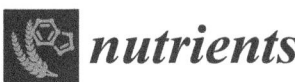

Article

A Positive Causal Relationship between Noodle Intake and Metabolic Syndrome: A Two-Sample Mendelian Randomization Study

Sunmin Park [1,*] and Meiling Liu [1,2]

1 Obesity/Diabetes Research Center, Department of Food and Nutrition, Hoseo University, Asan 31499, Republic of Korea; meiling1125@naver.com
2 Shanxi Institute of Science and Technology, College of Chemical Engineering, Jincheng 048011, China
* Correspondence: smpark@hoseo.edu; Tel.: +82-41-540-5633; Fax: +82-41-540-5638

Abstract: The controversy over the link between noodle consumption and metabolic syndrome (MetS) persists. Using a two-sample Mendelian randomization (MR) approach, we aimed to examine the potential causal relationship between noodle consumption and the risk of MetS and its components in adult populations of city hospital-based (n = 58,701) and Ansan/Ansung plus rural (AAR; n = 13,598) cohorts. The instrumental variables were assigned with genetic variants associated with low- and high-noodle intake (cutoff: 130 g/day) by a genome-wide association study (GWAS) with $p < 5 \times 10^{-5}$ and linkage disequilibrium (r^2 = 0.001), following adjustment for covariates related to MetS, in the city cohort. MR-Egger, inverse-variance weighted (IVW), and weighted median were applied to investigate the causal association of noodle intake with MetS risk in the AAR. The quality of the MR results was checked with leave-one-out sensitivity and heterogeneity analyses. A higher energy intake with lower carbohydrates and higher fats, proteins, and higher sodium and a lower intake of calcium, vitamin D, vitamin C, and flavonoids were shown in the high-noodle group, indicating poor diet quality. The glycemic index and glycemic load of daily meals were much higher in the high-noodle intake group than in the low-noodle intake group. In the observational studies, not only the total noodle intake but also the different types of noodle intake were also positively associated with MetS risk. In the MR analysis, high-noodle intake elevated MetS, hypertension, dyslipidemia, hyperglycemia, hypertriglyceridemia, and abdominal obesity in an IVW model ($p < 0.05$) but not the MR-Egger model. No single genetic variant among the instrumental variables changed their relationship in the leave-one-out sensitivity analysis. No likelihood of horizontal pleiotropy and heterogeneity was exhibited in the association between noodle intake and MetS. In conclusion, noddle intake had a positive causal association with MetS and its components in Asian adults.

Keywords: Mendelian randomization; noodle intake; diet quality; metabolic syndrome

Citation: Park, S.; Liu, M. A Positive Causal Relationship between Noodle Intake and Metabolic Syndrome: A Two-Sample Mendelian Randomization Study. Nutrients 2023, 15, 2091. https://doi.org/10.3390/nu15092091

Academic Editor: Santiago Navas-Carretero

Received: 7 April 2023
Revised: 24 April 2023
Accepted: 25 April 2023
Published: 26 April 2023

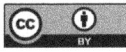

Copyright: © 2023 by the authors. Licensee MDPI, Basel, Switzerland. This article is an open access article distributed under the terms and conditions of the Creative Commons Attribution (CC BY) license (https://creativecommons.org/licenses/by/4.0/).

1. Introduction

Metabolic syndrome (MetS) is a group of disease conditions that raise the risk of type 2 diabetes (T2DM), coronary heart disease, and stroke. A diagnosis of MetS is made when an individual has three or more of the following components: abdominal obesity, hypertension, hyperglycemia, hypo-HDL-cholesterolemia, and hypertriglyceridemia. MetS is a significant global public health issue, affecting approximately one-quarter of the world's population [1]. The prevalence of MetS is higher in developed countries, with rates ranging from 20 to 30% in Europe and North America to over 40% in India and China among the Asian countries and in Mexico in South America. Indeed, the incidence of MetS is rising rapidly in developing countries. In Korea, MetS increased among men from 24.5% to 28.1% during the decade 2008–2017. However, it was 20.5% among women in 2008 and 18.7% in 2017 [2].

The incidence of MetS differs between locations depending on environmental factors, although genetics can interact with environmental factors to affect the probability of developing MetS. The rapid increase in MetS incidence in developing countries has been linked to a shift toward more sedentary lifestyles and the higher consumption of high-calorie and fat-rich diets that increase insulin resistance [3]. A healthy diet full of fruits, vegetables, whole grains, nuts, legumes, and fish, and with low levels of saturated fats, trans fats, and added sugars, has been linked to a reduced risk of MetS. These healthy dietary patterns include the Mediterranean diet, Dietary Approaches to Stop Hypertension (DASH), and Korean-balanced diets [4]. These dietary patterns have been reported to have an inverse relationship with MetS risk [5]. The shift from a Korean-balanced diet to a Western-style diet (WSD) increases MetS incidence, and a WSD is positively associated with MetS risk [5]. However, Koreans have not consumed meat as much as people in Western countries (men: 96 g/day and women: 76 g/day), and meat intake does not differ between non-MetS and MetS groups in Korea [6,7]. Interestingly, the WSD among Koreans is characterized by a high intake of noodles consumed with meat and processed meats. However, since the intake of meats and processed meats remains lower in Korea than in Western countries, a high carbohydrate diet (about 70 percent energy) and not a high-fat diet strongly correlates with MetS risk in Korea [8]. Therefore, a higher intake of noodles rich in carbohydrates may be linked to MetS risk.

The association of noodle (or pasta) intake on MetS risk has been evaluated in previous studies. Noodles are made not only of refined flour but also rice and buckwheat. However, noodle dishes are high carbohydrate and calorie-rich foods. In an earlier study conducted on the data from the Korean National Health and Nutrition Examination Survey (KNHANES) IV 2007–2009, increased intake of instant noodles (≥ 2 times/week) was positively associated with MetS risk by 1.68-fold in women [7]. In addition, the higher intake of instant noodles (≥ 3 times/week) was positively linked to a 2.6-fold higher risk of dyslipidemia among Korean college students [9]. However, the effects of other types of noodles or pasta on MetS risk in Korea remain unknown. In a systematic review and meta-analysis of thirteen randomized clinical trials conducted in Western countries, the intake of pasta was found to have significantly lower standard mean differences in postprandial glucose responses compared to bread (seven studies) or potatoes (six studies) [10]. However, the intake of pasta made from whole grains has not shown beneficial effects on glucose metabolism compared to that made from refined grains [10]. Furthermore, pasta meals substituted for bread or potatoes were inversely associated with stroke and cardiovascular disease in the Women's Health Initiative (WHI), a series of clinical studies initiated by the US National Institutes of Health (NIH). However, pasta intake did not show a significant association with T2DM risk [10]. Moreover, pasta consumption had an inverse relationship with the risk of being overweight and obese in an Italian Nutrition & Health Survey (INHES) [11]. Therefore, the effects of pasta consumption on MetS risk remain controversial.

The present study aimed to determine the effects of consuming different types of noodles on MetS risk and its components. Their causal relationship was studied by carrying out a two-sample Mendelian randomization (MR) analysis on adults aged over 40 in the Korean Genomic Epidemiology Study (KoGES), a long-term population-based cohort study. It is novel to demonstrate that different types of noodle intake were similarly associated with the risk of MetS and its components and to show the causal association of overall noodle consumption with the risk of MetS and its components by randomizing participants with genetic variants related to the noodle consumption.

2. Methods

2.1. Participants

Between 2004 and 2013, the Korea Centers for Disease Control and Prevention (KCDC) established the KoGES, which contained three cohorts—rural (n = 8105), Ansan/Ansung (n = 5493), and hospital-based urban (n = 58,701). The KoGES obtained approval from the KoGES Institutional Review Board (KBP-2019-055), and this study was approved by Hoseo University Institutional Review Board (1041231-150811-HR-034-01) to comply with the Declaration of Helsinki. All the participants agreed to the terms after providing written informed consent.

2.2. Demographic, Anthropometric, Biochemical, and Clinical Parameter Assessment

At the first visit, the participants completed the survey questionnaire providing data such as their gender, age, monthly income (<$2000, $2000–4000, or >$4000), education (<high school, high school, or college plus above), type, amount, and frequency of alcohol consumption, smoking status, and physical activity [12,13]. The daily alcohol intake (g/day) was calculated by multiplying the alcohol percentage according to alcohol drink types and amount on a single occasion by the frequency of consumption. It was categorized into low (0–19 g) and high drinkers ($\geq$20 g) [14]. Current and past smokers were divided based on smoking over 100 cigarettes during the six months prior to the survey in their lifetimes [13].

According to a standardized procedure, anthropometric measurements were taken, with the participants wearing light clothes and barefoot [15]. Blood was drawn from the participants after they had fasted for over 12 h, with and without anticoagulants. The plasma and serum were separated from the blood after it was centrifuged at $500\times g$. Plasma glucose, serum lipid profiles, serum alanine transaminase (ALT), serum aspartate transaminase (AST), and serum creatinine concentrations were analyzed using an automatic analyzer (Hitachi 7600, Hitachi, Tokyo, Japan) [12]. The glycated hemoglobin (hemoglobin A1c; HbA1c) levels were measured using ethylenediaminetetraacetic acid (EDTA)-treated blood, and serum high-sensitive C-reactive protein (hs-CRP) concentrations were assessed with an enzyme-linked immunosorbent assay (ELISA) kit (R&D system, Minneapolis, MN, USA). The estimated glomerular filtration rate (eGFR) was calculated using MDRD Study Equation [16]. Blood pressure was taken three times from the right arm in a sitting position while the participant was sitting, and the averages of SBP and DBP were used.

2.3. MetS Definition

MetS is a cluster of conditions that includes a minimum of three of the following criteria, according to the International Diabetes Federation (IDF) and the criteria for MetS of the Korean Society for the Study of Obesity (KSSO): abdominal obesity (90 cm for men and 85 cm for women), hypertension (average systolic blood pressure $\geq$ 130 mmHg or diastolic blood pressure $\geq$ 85 mmHg or currently on antihypertensive medication), hyperglycemia ($\geq$100 mg/dL or currently on the hypoglycemic agent), hypertriglyceridemia ($\geq$150 mg/dL or currently on anti-dyslipidemic medication), and hypo-HDL-cholesterolemia (<40 mg/dL for men, and <50 mg/dL for women or currently on anti-dyslipidemic medication) [17]. MetS can be considered a borderline or a "pre"-condition between healthy and disturbed metabolisms, which could progress to specific metabolic diseases such as T2DM.

2.4. Food and Nutrient Intake Measurement

The semi-quantitative food frequency questionnaire (SQFFQ), fitted to the eating habits of Koreans, has been developed and validated for the KoGES [18] and was completed based on the food consumed within the 6-month period prior to the survey. According to the SQFFQ results, the daily intake of 106 foods was assessed from the frequencies and amounts of each food. The intake of noodles was divided into five categories, namely, instant noodles, Chinese noodles (Chajangmyon/Jambbong), buckwheat noodles, wheat noodles, and starch noodles. The total noodle intake was calculated by summing the noodle intake of the five categories. The nutrients present in the results were calculated based on the food intake from the SQFFQ using the computer-aided nutrition analysis program (CAN-Pro) 3.0, a nutrient database program developed by the Korean Nutrition Society (Seoul, Republic of Korea) [18].

2.5. Dietary Patterns, Dietary Inflammatory Index (DII), Glycemic Index (GI), and Glycemic Load (GL)

Foods in the SQFFQ were categorized into 29 food groups according to nutrient similarity. Dietary patterns were chosen according to an eigenvalue >1.5 by performing the principal component analysis (PCA) [18]. The predominant food groups in each pattern were selected with ≥0.40 factor-loading values after applying the orthogonal rotation procedure [15]. The names of each dietary pattern were based on the primary food group chosen (Supplementary Table S1).

The dietary inflammatory index (DII) of each participant was determined by multiplying the inflammatory weights of the following four groups: energy sources, thirty-two nutrients, caffeine, and four spices by the intake of each participant and divided by 100 [19].

The GI and GL were calculated with the corresponding equations. The GI of the same food can vary due to differences in the types of the food and its nutritional composition. Hence the GI values commonly listed for Korean foods were used [20,21]. The GI and GL of daily food intake in the form of meals were calculated by following equations [22]:

GI of daily food intake = $\sum_{i=1}^{i=n}$(GI of a food X carbohydrate in the food)i/total carbohydrate intake for a day.

GL of daily food intake = $\sum_{i=1}^{i=n}$(GI of a food X carbohydrate in the food)i/100

n: the number of foods consumed in a day.

2.6. Genotyping and Quality Control

The participants' genotypes were assessed at the Center for Genome Science of the Korea National Institute of Health (Osong, Republic of Korea). The resulting data were then provided to the researchers. Genomic DNA extracted from the whole blood was used to perform genotyping using a Korean chip (Affymetrix, Santa Clara, CA, USA) that was specifically designed to look for genetic variants linked to chronic metabolic diseases (dyslipidemia, diabetes, hypertension, osteoporosis, kidney disease, and autoimmune diseases) and cancers in Korean adults [15,23]. The genotyping accuracy was verified by the Bayesian Robust Linear Model (BRLMM) genotyping algorithm [24]. The quality of the genotyping was further checked with the following criteria: absence of gender bias, low heterozygosity (<30%), genotyping accuracy (≥98%), missing genotype call rates (<4%), minor alleles frequency (MAF, >1%), and Hardy–Weinberg Equilibrium (HWE; $p > 0.05$) [23]. After genotype imputation, the genotype quality was then verified with additional inclusion criteria of a posterior probability score > 0.90 and low informative content of genotype informative > 0.5.

2.7. Identification of Instrumental Variables in a Two-Sample MR Analysis

A genome-wide association study (GWAS) was conducted to investigate the genetic variants in relation to the daily total noodle intake. The daily total noodle intake was divided into two categories with a cutoff of 130 g cooked noodles per day (3 times/week): low-noodle (<130 g/d) and high-noodle (≥130 g/d) [14,25]. This study was performed utilizing PLINK v.2.0 (http://pngu.mgh.harvard.edu/~purcell/plink accessed on 12 May 2022) in a city hospital-based cohort (n = 58,701). The following factors were considered as covariates: participants' age, residential area, gender, body mass index (BMI), education, daily physical activity, energy intake, carbohydrate intake, alcohol consumption, and smoking status. The p-values of the genetic variants from the association between the low- and high-noodle groups were plotted with the GWAS. The p-values of the genetic variants were then plotted in a Manhattan plot to distinguish significant genetic variants on chromosome 12 (Supplementary Figure S1A). The quantile–quantile (Q-Q) plot of the observed and expected p-values revealed only a few sources of spurious associations (Supplementary Figure S1B). The genome inflation factor (λGC) value in the Q-Q plot was estimated to be 1.016, indicating that the genetic variants from the GWAS did not have large inflation and an excessive false positive rate. The gene name of the SNP was identified by searching the g: profiler database website (https://biit.cs.ut.ee/gprofiler/snpense, accessed on 3 June 2022).

The linkage disequilibrium (LD) of all selected genetic variants within a 10,000 kb distance was checked: the variants were considered for inclusion if their r2 value was less than 0.001 (or D′ < 0.2) in the R program. The significance of the genetic variants influencing noodle intake was liberally set to $p < 5 \times 10^{-5}$ as the majority of the variants (over 50%) showed linkage disequilibrium and a large number of participants (n = 58,701) were included in the study. Previous studies also used a liberal significance level, especially where lifestyles were instrumental variables [26]. Supplementary Table S2 presents potential instrumental variables related to noodle intake, with the respective gene names sourced from the g:profiler database website (https://biit.cs.ut.ee/gprofiler/snpense, accessed on 18 June 2022).

2.8. A Two-Sample MR Analysis Design

In the noodle intake (exposure) and MetS and its components (outcomes), the genetic variants (instrumental variables) that affect noodle intake were used to randomize the participants to evaluate the association between noodle intake and MetS and its components. Figure 1 displays the diagram of the two-sample MR design. The results of the two-sample MR analysis can show the causal relationship between the noodle intake and MetS and its components when the assumptions are fulfilled. The assumptions were as follows: (1) The genetic variants should be connected to the noodle intake and serve as instrumental variables; (2) The instrumental variables must not be associated with confounders; (3) The instrumental variables should have no effect on the risk of MetS and its components [25]. The confounders included categorical variables (gender, residential area, education, income, exercise, and smoking) and continuous variables (age, BMI, and energy, carbohydrates, and alcohol intake). The assumptions were tested at a statistical significance level at $p < 5 \times 10^{-5}$, the same as the significance level for the instrumental variables. The assumptions in this study achieved the required statistical significance.

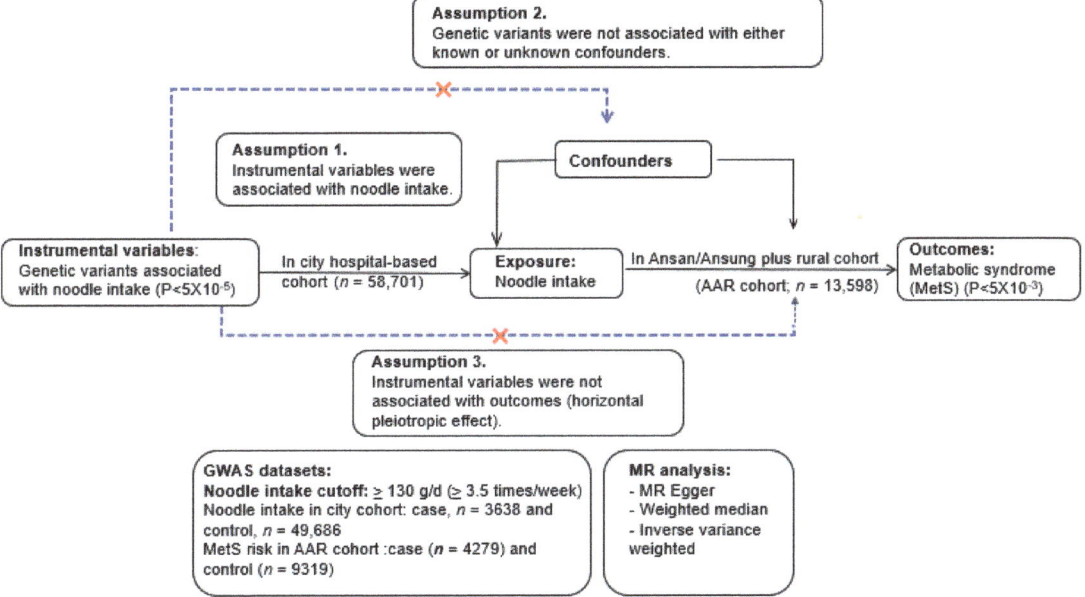

Figure 1. Experimental flow and assumptions for a two-sample Mendelian randomization (MR) of the causal association of daily total noodle intake with the risk of metabolic syndrome and its components.

A two-sample MR analysis was conducted with the Mendelian Randomization package (v.0.5.1) and Two-Sample MR (v.0.4.26) in the R program. The scheme of a two-sample MR analysis is depicted in Figure 1. The KoGES cohorts were separated into two cohorts in order to satisfy the two-sample MR assumptions: (1) A city hospital-based cohort (n = 58,701) and (2) Ansan/Ansung plus rural cohorts (n = 13,598). Instrumental variables were created from the GWAS between individuals with low- and high-noodle consumption in the city hospital-based cohort (low-noodle: n = 52,408; high-noodle: n = 4493), as mentioned above. The association of instrumental variables with MetS and its components was conducted by logistic regression analysis in the Ansan/Ansung plus rural cohorts (n = 13,598). If the genetic variants selected for instrumental variables were linked to T2DM at $p < 5 \times 10^{-5}$ in the Ansan/Ansung plus rural cohorts, they were taken out of the instrumental variables. The number of participants in MetS and its metabolic traits in the Ansan/Ansung plus rural cohorts (n = 13,598) were (1) MetS (n = 4279); (2) abdominal obesity determined by waist circumferences (n = 4144); (3) hyperglycemia (n = 999); (4) hypo-HDL-cholesterolemia (n = 6277); (5) hypertriglyceridemia (n = 2306); and (6) hypertension (n = 4355).

The correlation between the amount of noodles consumed daily and the risk of metabolic syndrome and its components was calculated using a two-sample MR. The figure outlines the criteria of the instrumental variables as well as the assumptions for the MR analysis. All three assumptions of the MR analysis were fulfilled in this study.

The causal relationship between noodle intake and MetS incidence was determined with the two-sample MR analysis using the Mendelian Randomization package (v.0.5.1) and Two-Sample MR (v.0.4.26) in the R program. The MR package included the inverse-variance weighted (IVW) method, MR-Egger, weighted median, and weighted mode. IVW is the primary causal effect estimate with a robust ability to assume that all genetic variants are effective instrumental variables [27,28]. However, it requires exposure to the genetic variants (instrumental variables) that affect the target outcome only. Furthermore, other unknown confounding factors may contribute to horizontal pleiotropy and bias in effect size estimates, although the confounding factors that affect exposure were mostly excluded [27,28]. MR-Egger, IVW, and weighted median approaches were used to analyze the causal relationship of noodle intake to MetS and its components in the Ansan/Ansung plus rural cohorts (n = 13,598).

The heterogeneity test was used mainly to examine the differences between the selected IVs. The selected IVs were inappropriate if there was a strong heterogeneity between IVs with a small p value. The heterogeneity should not exist in IVs to use for MR study. The leave-one-out sensitivity test was used to conduct the MR with the remaining IVs after excluding IVs one by one. When the MR results estimated by removing one IV were very different from those with all IVs, the MR result was sensitive to excluding one IV. If one IV occupies a big portion of the MR results, the MR model is not robust. No matter which SNP is removed, the results are similar, indicating the MR result is robust. The analysis was included in the two-sample MR analysis.

2.9. Statistical Analysis

It was conducted using SAS v.9.3 (SAS Institute, Cary, NC, USA). The descriptive summaries for the categorical variables (e.g., gender, education, income, and smoking) were computed with frequency distribution according to the low- and high-noodle intake groups. The Chi-square test was utilized to determine the considerable variations in frequency distributions between the low- and high-noodle intake groups. After adjusting for the covariates, the adjusted means and standard deviations of the continuous variables were studied in the low- and high-noodle intake groups. Analysis of covariance (ANCOVA) was employed to assess the statistical discrepancies between the low- and high-noodle intake groups.

3. Results

3.1. Demographic Characteristics and Lifestyles of the Participants

The participants in the high-noodle group were, on average, younger than those in the low-noodle group (Table 1). A higher proportion of males was found within the high-noodle group than females (Table 1). Additionally, women with a higher education level and income were more likely to be in the high-noodle group than the low-noodle group (Table 1). Furthermore, the high-noodle group had a greater rate of alcohol consumption, less physical activity, and more smoking than the low-noodle group (Table 1).

Table 1. Demographic characteristics and lifestyles according to gender and noodle intake status.

	Men (n = 20,293)		Women (n = 38,408)	
	Low Intake of Noodles (n = 17,799)	High Intake of Noodle (n = 2494)	Low Intake of Noodles (n = 36,409)	High Intake of Noodle (n = 1999)
Age (years)	56.7 ± 0.06 [a]	54.3 ± 0.16 [b]	52.5 ± 0.04 [c]	50.3 ± 0.179 [d***+++]
Education (Yes, %)				
≤Middle school	1554 (14.2)	199 (13.2) [‡]	6529 (22.6)	209 (14.1) [‡‡‡]
High school	8314 (75.8)	1120 (74.4)	20,711 (71.7)	1160 (78.1)
≥College	1105 (10.1)	186 (12.4)	1665 (5.76)	117 (7.87)
Income (Yes, %)				
≤$2000	1449 (8.57)	157 (6.55) [‡‡]	4038 (11.8)	134 (7.07) [‡‡‡]
$2000–4000	7179 (42.4)	1028 (42.9)	15,144 (44.2)	841 (44.4)
>$4000	8287 (49.0)	1213 (50.6)	15,049 (44.0)	921 (48.6)
Past smoker	7795 (43.9)	1000 (40.1)	418 (1.15)	42 (2.11)
Smoker (Yes, %)	4740 (26.7)	924 (37.1) [‡‡‡]	663 (1.83)	86 (4.31) [‡‡‡]
Alcohol intake (g/day)	6.5 ± 0.11 [b]	10.3 ± 0.28 [a]	1.7 ± 0.08 [c]	2.2 ± 0.31 [c***+++##]
Physical activity (Yes, %)	10,547 (59.5)	1405 (56.4) [‡‡]	19,091 (52.6)	933 (46.7) [‡‡‡]
Energy (EER percent)	86.9 ± 0.24 [d]	110.5 ± 0.61 [b]	97.7 ± 0.16 [c]	131.5 ± 0.66 [a***+++###]
Carbohydrates (En%)	72.0 ± 0.06 [a]	68.8 ± 0.14 [b]	72.0 ± 0.04 [a]	68.5 ± 0.15 [b+++]
Protein (En%)	13.0 ± 0.02 [d]	13.7 ± 0.05 [b]	13.5 ± 0.01 [c]	14.1 ± 0.06 [a***+++]
Fat (En%)	13.7 ± 0.04 [b]	16.5 ± 0.11 [a]	13.6 ± 0.03 [b]	16.5 ± 0.12 [a+++]
Saturated fat (En%)	4.27 ± 0.01 [c]	5.37 ± 0.03 [a]	4.35 ± 0.01 [b]	5.22 ± 0.03 [a+++###]
Monounsaturated fat (En%)	5.46 ± 0.01 [c]	6.86 ± 0.02 [a]	5.35 ± 0.01 [d]	6.72 ± 0.03 [b***+++]
Polyunsaturated fat (En%)	3.10 ± 0.02 [b]	3.80 ± 0.04 [a]	3.08 ± 0.01 [b]	3.78 ± 0.05 [a+++]
Cholesterol (mg/day)	162.7 ± 0.79 [d]	193.3 ± 1.99 [b]	168.0 ± 0.53 [c]	210.1 ± 2.16 [a***+++##]
Fiber (g/day)	16.1 ± 0.07 [a]	16.4 ± 0.16 [a]	14.0 ± 0.04 [b]	13.1 ± 0.18 [c**]
Calcium (mg/day)	453 ± 1.50 [a]	373 ± 3.73 [c]	449 ± 0.99 [a]	390 ± 5.1 [b***+++###]
Sodium (g/day)	2.67 ± 0.01 [b]	2.82 ± 0.02 [a]	2.29 ± 0.01 [c]	2.30 ± 0.03 [c***+++##]
Potassium (g/day)	2.34 ± 0.01 [a]	2.13 ± 0.01 [c]	2.20 ± 0.003 [b]	1.81 ± 0.02 [d***+++###]
Vitamin C (mg/day)	105 ± 0.47 [b]	87.3 ± 1.18 [d]	109 ± 0.32 [a]	77.3 ± 1.31 [c***+++##]
Vitamin D (ug/day)	6.2 ± 0.04 [b]	4.2 ± 0.09 [c]	6.8 ± 0.02 [a]	4.0 ± 0.10 [c***+++###]
DII (scores)	−20.6 ± 0.12 [a]	−18.6 ± 0.29 [b]	−19.1 ± 0.08 [b]	−15.0 ± 0.32 [c***+++###]
Flavonoids (mg/day)	36.3 ± 0.25 [b]	27.8 ± 0.62 [c]	40.9 ± 0.16 [a]	26.3 ± 0.68 [c***+++###]

The values represent adjusted means ± standard deviations or the number of participants (percentage of each group). Covariates included age, residence areas, gender, body mass index, education, income, energy intake, carbohydrate intake, daily activity, and smoking status. EER, estimated energy requirement; CHO, carbohydrates; DII, dietary inflammatory index. A total noodle intake was the sum of instant noodles, wheat noodle soup, Chinese noodles (Chajangmyon/Jambbong), buckwheat noodles, and starch noodles daily. The cutoff of total noodle intake was 130 g/day, equivalent to three times a week. * Significant differences by gender at $p < 0.05$, ** at $p < 0.01$, *** $p < 0.001$. ++ Significant differences by noodle intake at $p < 0.01$, +++ $p < 0.001$ ## Significant effect of the interaction between gender and the noodle intake groups at $p < 0.01$, ### $p < 0.001$. a,b,c,d Different superscript letters indicated significant differences among the groups in Tukey's test at $p < 0.05$. ‡ Significant differences from the low-noodle intake in each gender at $p < 0.05$, ‡‡ at $p < 0.01$, and ‡‡‡ at $p < 0.001$.

3.2. Food and Nutrient Intake

The participants in the high-noodle group had a much higher energy intake than those in the low-noodle group, with the former consuming more energy than the estimated requirement (Table 1). Carbohydrates intake was lower in the high-noodle group, while fat and protein intake were higher (as shown in Table 1). Moreover, the former had a lower calcium, potassium, vitamin C, vitamin D, flavonoids, and cholesterol intake than the latter. However, sodium intake and DII were higher in the high-noodle group compared to the low-noodle group (Table 1).

The consumption of noodles among males in the high-noodle group was 4.6 times more than in the low-noodle group. The intake of noodles among females in the high-noodle group was 7.6 times more than among those in the low-noodle group (Table 2). The varieties of noodles were divided into instant noodles, wheat noodle soup, Chinese noodles, buckwheat noodles, and starch noodles, with intakes of all types except starch noodles significantly greater in the high-noodle group than in the low-noodle group (Table 2). The most regularly consumed noodles were wheat noodle soup and Chinese noodles.

Table 2. Usual food intake according to gender and noodle intake (unit: g/day).

	Men (n = 20,293)		Women (n = 38,408)	
	Low Intake of Noodles (n = 17,799)	High Intake of Noodle (n = 2494)	Low Intake of Noodles (n = 36,409)	High Intake of Noodle (n = 1999)
Total noodle	47.6 ± 0.49 [c]	213.1 ± 1.22 [b]	30.6 ± 0.32 [d]	221.2 ± 1.35 [a***+++###]
Instant noodles	10.8 ± 0.13 [c]	30.9 ± 0.32 [a]	5.21 ± 0.09 [d]	22.7 ± 0.35 [b***+++##]
Wheat noodle soup	18.3 ± 0.28 [c]	85.3 ± 0.70 [b]	15.6 ± 0.18 [d]	108.5 ± 0.77 [a***+++###]
Chinese noodle	14.7 ± 0.29 [c]	84.3 ± 0.73 [a]	7.1 ± 0.20 [d]	74.7 ± 0.81 [b***+++]
Buckwheat noodle	3.23 ± 0.08 [c]	12.1 ± 0.20 [b]	2.23 ± 0.05 [d]	14.7 ± 0.22 [a***+++###]
Starch noodle	0.56 ± 0.02 [a]	0.57 ± 0.05 [a]	0.43 ± 0.01 [b]	0.54 ± 0.05 [ab*]
White rice	147 ± 2.0 [b]	179 ± 5.03 [a]	82.6 ± 1.34 [d]	113 ± 5.58 [c***+++]
Whole grains	523 ± 2.04 [a]	431 ± 5.07 [c]	457 ± 1.35 [b]	329 ± 5.62 [d***+++###]
Bread	12.5 ± 0.19 [c]	13.9 ± 0.46 [b]	12.7 ± 0.12 [c]	21.2 ± 0.51 [a***+++###]
Cookie	3.07 ± 0.06 [a]	2.44 ± 0.16 [c]	2.72 ± 0.04 [b]	2.53 ± 0.18 [bc+++]
Potato	17.4 ± 0.21 [b]	13.9 ± 0.52 [c]	20.7 ± 0.14 [a]	16.0 ± 0.57 [b***+++]
Green vegetables	70.8 ± 0.52 [a]	54.4 ± 1.30 [c]	75.0 ± 0.35 [b]	54.0 ± 1.47 [c+++#]
White vegetables	45.9 ± 0.33 [a]	39.6 ± 0.83 [b]	41.0 ± 0.22 [b]	30.6 ± 0.92 [c***+++##]
Kimchi	158 ± 0.91 [a]	143 ± 2.26 [b]	131 ± 0.60 [c]	103 ± 2.51 [d***+++###]
Fruits	199 ± 1.68 [b]	147 ± 4.19 [c]	237 ± 1.11 [a]	144 ± 4.64 [c***+++###]
Beans	30.3 ± 0.20 [a]	27.0 ± 0.50 [c]	29.2 ± 0.13 [b]	24.3 ± 0.55 [d***+++#]
Seaweeds	1.81 ± 0.02 [b]	1.40 ± 0.04 [c]	2.12 ± 0.01 [a]	1.55 ± 0.05 [c***+++##]
Meats	47.7 ± 0.28 [a]	44.3 ± 0.69 [b]	33.8 ± 0.18 [c]	25.8 ± 0.76 [d***+++###]
Fish	35.5 ± 0.24 [a]	26.3 ± 0.60 [c]	33.5 ± 0.16 [b]	20.5 ± 0.67 [d***+++###]
Process meats	48.7 ± 0.72 [a]	41.7 ± 1.79 [b]	44.8 ± 0.48 [b]	38.0 ± 1.99 [bc***+++]
Milk and milk products	109.2 ± 1.04 [b]	69.6 ± 2.60 [c]	128.7 ± 0.69 [a]	75.4 ± 2.88 [c***+++##]
Nuts	1.6 ± 0.03 [b]	1.1 ± 0.08 [c]	1.9 ± 0.02 [a]	1.3 ± 0.09 [c***+++]
Coffee	4.2 ± 0.03 [a]	4.2 ± 0.06 [a]	3.3 ± 0.02 [c]	3.5 ± 0.07 [b***#]
Glycemic index	49.4 ± 0.10 [c]	59.8 ± 0.28 [a]	45.6 ± 0.08 [d]	58.2 ± 0.32 [b***+++###]
Glycemic load	154 ± 0.35 [b]	193 ± 0.97 [a]	142 ± 0.25 [d]	186 ± 1.1576 [b***+++###]
KBD (N, %)	6909 (38.8)	1278 (51.2) ‡‡‡	10,678 (29.3)	750 (37.5) ‡‡‡
PBD (N, %)	3719 (20.9)	563 (22.6) ‡	14,499 (39.8)	999 (50.0) ‡‡‡
WSD (N, %)	8044 (45.2)	2379 (95.4) ‡‡‡	11,389 (31.3)	1822 (91.2) ‡‡‡
RMD (N, %)	5577 (31.3)	947 (38.0) ‡‡‡	12,235 (33.9)	749 (37.5) ‡‡

The values are expressed as adjusted means ± standard deviations or the number of participants (percentage of each group). The covariates covered age, place of residence, gender, BMI, education, income, daily activity, energy consumption, carbohydrate consumption, and smoking status. A total noodle intake was the sum of instant noodles, wheat noodle soup, Chinese noodles (Chajangmyon/Jambbong), buckwheat noodles, and starch noodles daily. The cutoff of total noodle intake was 130 g/day, equivalent to three times a week. KBD, Korean-style balanced diet; PBD, plant-based diet; WSD, Western-style diet; RMD, rice-main diet. * Significant differences by gender at $p < 0.05$, ** $p < 0.01$, and *** $p < 0.001$. +++ $p < 0.001$ # Significant effect of the interaction between gender and the noodle intake groups at $p < 0.05$, ## $p < 0.01$, and ### $p < 0.001$. [a,b,c,d] Different superscript letters indicated significant differences among the groups in Tukey's test at $p < 0.05$. ‡ Significant differences from the low-noodle intake in each gender at $p < 0.05$, ‡‡ at $p < 0.01$, and ‡‡‡ at $p < 0.001$.

GI and GL values of the daily meal were substantially higher for the high-noodle group than the low-noodle group for both genders, with men having higher values than women (Table 2). The high-noodle group participants had a higher intake of white rice but lower consumption of other foods such as whole grains, potatoes, vegetables, kimchi, fruits, beans, seaweed, meats, processed meats, fish, and nuts (Table 2).

The four dietary patterns were the Korean-balanced diet (KBD) for factor 1, the plant-based diet (PBD) for factor 2, the Western-style diet (WSD) for factor 3, and the rice-main diet (RMD) for factor 4. Regardless of dietary patterns, the proportion of noodle intake was higher in the high-noodle intake groups than in the low-noodle intake groups (Table 2). Interestingly, the proportion of noodle intake was 95.4% in men and 91.2% in women in WSD (Table 2), indicating that adults having WSD highly consumed noodles.

3.3. Observational Association of Noodle Intake, MetS, and Its Components

After adjusting for two different sets of covariates, the total intake of noodles was positively associated with MetS risk in a dose-dependent manner (Figure 2A). The 130 g/day total noodle intake showed the highest adjusted ORs for MetS risk, and it was used as the cutoff. The association of each type of noodle with MetS is presented in Figure 2B, where the cutoff of 25 g, 55 g, 40 g, 9 g, and 0.8 g per day was assigned for instant noodles, noodle soup, Chinese noodles, buckwheat noodles, and starch noodles, respectively. Among the types of noodles, the intake of instant noodles, noodle soup, Chinese noodles, and buckwheat noodles was associated with MetS, but the intake of starch noodles was not. Participants with high total noodle intake ($\geq$130 g/day) had a higher risk of MetS and its components compared with those with low-noodle intake in both genders after adjusting for the covariates related to MetS (Table 3).

Among the MetS components, total noodle intake showed a positive relationship with abdominal obesity, hyperglycemia, hypertension, and hypertriglyceridemia in total participants. However, noodle intake had no association with hypo-HDL-cholesterolemia (Figure 2C). Table 3 also showed that the total noodle intake was positively linked to abdominal obesity, hyperglycemia, hypertension, hypertriglyceridemia in both genders. There were no specific gender differences. The total noodle intake had a higher association with insulin resistance in both genders, but significant differences were shown only in men. However, the total noodle intake was not significantly associated with serum hs-CRP, AST and ALT concentrations, and eGFR (Table 4).

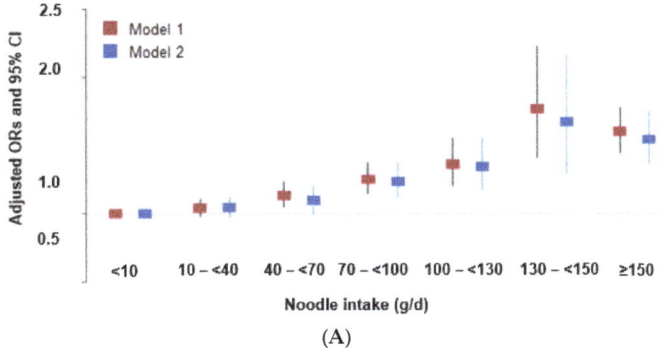

(A)

Figure 2. *Cont.*

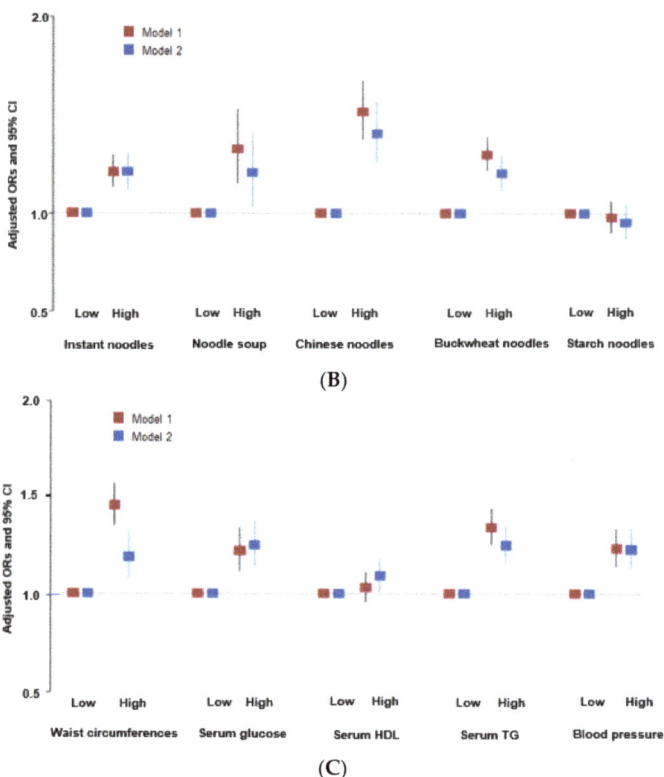

Figure 2. Association of noodle intake and its components with the risk of metabolic syndrome and its components in observational estimates in a city hospital-based cohort. (**A**) Association of the total noodle intakes by six groups (<10 g, 10–40 g, 40–70 g, 100–130 g, 130–150 g, ≥150 g total noodle intake/day) with metabolic syndrome and its components. Daily total noodle intake was calculated by summing up the daily intakes of instant noodles, noodle soup, Chinese noodles, buckwheat noodles, and starch noodles. (**B**) Association of the individual noodle intakes by two groups (cutoff of 130 g/day) with metabolic syndrome. The cutoffs of instant noodles, noodle soup, Chinese noodles, buckwheat noodles, and starch noodles were 25, 55, 40, 9, and 0.8 g/day, respectively. (**C**) Association of the daily total noodle intake by two groups (cutoff of 130 g/day) with metabolic syndrome components. Daily total noodle intake was calculated by summing the daily intakes of instant noodles, noodle soup, Chinese noodles, buckwheat noodles, and starch noodles.

Table 3. Metabolic parameters related to metabolic syndrome (MetS) according to gender and noodle intake status.

	Men (n = 20,293)			Women (n = 38,408)		
	Low Intake of Noodles (n = 17,799)	High Intake of Noodles (n = 2494)	Adjusted OR	Low Intake of Noodles (n = 36,409)	High Intake of Noodle (n = 1999)	Adjusted OR
MetS (Yes, %) [1]	3052 (17.2)	546 (21.9) ‡‡	1.341 (1.182–1.523)	4438 (12.2)	264 (13.2)	1.345 (1.144–1.580)
BMI (mg/kg²) [2]	24.4 ± 0.02 [b]	24.7 ± 0.07 [a]	1.147 (1.045–1.260)	23.6 ± 0.02 [c]	23.7 ± 0.08 [c]*** +++	1.165 (1.047–1.296)
Waist C. (cm) [3]	84.3 ± 0.04 [b]	84.7 ± 0.11 [a]	1.263 (1.141–1.398)	78.8 ± 0.03 [c]	79 ± 0.13 [c]*** +#	1.257 (1.111–1.423)
SMI (kg/m²) [4]	7.2 ± 0.01 [a]	7.3 ± 0.02 [a]	1.047 (0.951–1.153)	6.1 ± 0 [b]	6.1 ± 0.02 [b]	1.068 (0.946–1.206)
Fat mass (%) [5]	22.6 ± 0.01 [c]	22.6 ± 0.02 [b]	1.232 (1.115–1.361)	31.4 ± 0.01 [a]	31.5 ± 0.03 [a]*** +++	1.169 (1.055–1.295)
Plasma glucose (mg/dL) [6]	98 ± 0.17 [b]	100.1 ± 0.47 [a]	1.210 (1.074–1.363)	93.5 ± 0.12 [c]	94.5 ± 0.52 [c]*** +++	1.248 (1.053–1.479)
Blood HbA1c (%) [7]	5.67 ± 0.01 [b]	5.73 ± 0.02 [a]	1.297 (1.068–1.575)	5.73 ± 0.01 [b]	5.73 ± 0.02 [b]#	1.578 (1.226–2.031)
Insulin resistance (%) [8]	1910 (11.1)	299 (14.5) ‡‡	1.288 (1.118–1.484)	1961 (6.04)	105 (6.65)	1.196 (0.970–1.475)
Serum total cholesterol (mg/dL) [9]	190.6 ± 0.31 [c]	193.2 ± 0.85 [b]	1.202 (1.071–1.350)	201.3 ± 0.22 [a]	200.3 ± 0.95 [a]+##	1.028 (0.915–1.155)
Serum HDL (mg/dL) [10]	49.4 ± 0.11 [b]	49.7 ± 0.3 [b]	1.063 (0.945–1.195)	56.1 ± 0.08 [a]	56.3 ± 0.33 [a]***	1.071 (0.963–1.191)
Serum LDL (mg/dL) [11]	113 ± 0.28 [b]	112.8 ± 0.78 [b]	1.137 (0.990–1.306)	122.1 ± 0.2 [a]	119.9 ± 0.87 [a]***	1.142 (1.001–1.302)
Serum TG (mg/dL) [12]	140.9 ± 0.72 [b]	153.4 ± 2 [a]	1.199 (1.087–1.321)	116 ± 0.51 [c]	120.8 ± 2.23 [c]*** +++#	1.284 (1.144–1.441)
SBP (mmHg) [13]	124.6 ± 0.12 [a]	125.1 ± 0.33 [a]	1.097 (0.997–1.208)	121.3 ± 0.09 [b]	121.2 ± 0.37 [b]***	1.099 (0.981–1.230)
DBP (mmHg) [14]	77.8 ± 0.08 [a]	78.3 ± 0.22 [a]	1.233 (1.079–1.409)	74.7 ± 0.06 [b]	74.6 ± 0.25 [b]***	0.971 (0.798–1.182)
Serum hs-CRP (mg/L) [15]	0.142 ± 0.004	0.154 ± 0.01	1.013 (0.708–1.449)	0.136 ± 0.003	0.148 ± 0.011	1.093 (0.696–1.716)
Serum urate (mg/dL) [16]	5.54 ± 0.01	5.62 ± 0.02	1.126 (1.023–1.240)	4.22 ± 0.01	4.25 ± 0.02	1.360 (1.065–1.736)
eGFR (ml/min) [17]	84.7 ± 0.13 [b]	84.6 ± 0.33 [b]	1.273 (0.996–1.628)	86.5 ± 0.09 [a]	86.7 ± 0.36 [a]***	1.288 (0.962–1.724)
Serum AST (U/L) [18]	24.7 ± 0.24 [a]	26 ± 0.59 [a]	1.169 (0.972–1.407)	23.1 ± 0.16 [b]	23.1 ± 0.64 [b]***	1.025 (0.790–1.329)
Serum ALT (U/L) [19]	25.5 ± 0.23 [b]	27.2 ± 0.56 [a]	1.065 (0.945–1.201)	20.7 ± 0.16 [c]	20.4 ± 0.61 [a]*** +#	0.905 (0.751–1.092)

Values represent adjusted mean ± standard errors and adjusted odds ratio (OR) with 95% confidence intervals (CI). Adjusted OR was calculated with low-noodle intake as the reference using logistic regression with the adjustment of covariates and the cutoff points of each variable as following: [1] MetS criteria; [2] <25 kg/m² for body mass index (BMI); [3] <90 cm for men and 85 cm for women waist circumferences (C.); [4] <7.4 kg/m² for men, 6.2 kg/m² for women skeletal mass index (SMI) calculated with dividing skeletal muscle mass by squares of height; [5] <25% for men and 30% for women fat mass; [6] <126 mL/dL fasting serum glucose plus diabetic drug intake; [7] <6.5% hemoglobin A1c (HbA1c) plus diabetic drug intake; [8] <HOMA-IR for insulin resistance; [9] <230 mg/dL serum total cholesterol (chol) concentrations; [10] >40 mg/dL for men and 50 mg/dL for women serum high density lipoprotein (HDL) cholesterol; [11] <160 mg/dL low-density lipoprotein (LDL) concentrations; [12] <150 mg/dL plasma triglyceride (TG) concentrations; [13] <140 mmHg systolic blood pressure (SBP); [14] <90 mmHg diastolic blood pressure (DBP) plus hypertension medication; [15] <0.5 mg/dL serum high-sensitive C-reactive protein (hs-CRP) concentrations; [16] <6 mg/dL Uric acid; [17] Estimated glomerular filtration rate (eGFR) <60; [18] Aspartate aminotransferase (AST) <40 U/L; [19] Alanine aminotransferase (ALT) <35 U/L. CI, 95% confidence intervals. A total noodle intake was the sum of instant noodles, wheat noodle soup, Chinese noodles (Chajangmyon/Jambbong), buckwheat noodles, and starch noodles daily. The cutoff of total noodle intake was 130 g/day, equivalent to three times a week. *** Significant differences by gender at $p < 0.001$. ++ Significant differences by noodle intake at $p < 0.01$ and +++ $p < 0.001$. [a,b,c,d] Different superscript letters indicated significant differences among the groups in Tukey's test at $p < 0.05$. ‡‡ Significant differences from the low-noodle intake groups at $p < 0.05$ and ## $p < 0.01$. # Significant the interaction of gender and the noodle intake groups at ‡‡ at $p < 0.001$.

Table 4. Association of noodle intake with metabolic syndrome and its components using genetic variant randomization in different MR methods.

9	Method	MR OR (95% CI)	p	Method	Heterogeneity Q	p-Value	Intercept	Pleiotropy SE	p-Value
Metabolic syndrome	MR-Egger	1.204(0.811~1.787)	0.362	MR-Egger	5.214	1	−0.0005	0.014	0.973
	WMD [a]	1.137(0.957~1.352)	0.145						
	IVW	1.196(1.045~1.368)	0.0009	IVW	5.215	1			
	WMO [b]	1.061(0.740~1.521)	0.748						
Hypertension	MR-Egger	1.089(0.858~1.383)	0.486	MR-Egger	4.436	1	0.002	0.008	0.787
	WMD [a]	1.097(0.984~1.222)	0.095						
	IVW	1.124(1.036~1.218)	0.005	IVW	4.510	1			
	WMO [b]	1.095(0.872~1.375)	0.437						
Dyslipidemia	MR-Egger	1.236(0.833~1.835)	0.298	MR-Egger	3.878	1	−0.002	0.014	0.899
	WMD [a]	1.151(0.966~1.373)	0.116						
	IVW	1.206(1.055~1.379)	0.006	IVW	3.894	1			
	WMO [b]	1.105(0.743~1.644)	0.624						
Exposures	Method	β (95% CI)	p	Method	Q	p-value	Intercept	SE	p-value
Serum triglyceride concentrations (mg/dL)	MR-Egger	0.145(−0.181~0.471)	0.387	MR-Egger	2.285	1	−0.000089	0.011	0.994
	WMD [a]	0.117(−0.022~0.257)	0.100						
	IVW	0.144(0.033~0.255)	0.011	IVW	2.285	1			
	WMO [b]	0.103(−0.185~0.392)	0.486						
Serum LDL concentrations (mg/dL)	MR-Egger	0.119(−0.210~0.447)	0.482	MR-Egger	3.301	1	0.0007	0.011	0.949
	WMD [a]	0.107(−0.034~0.248)	0.138						
	IVW	0.129(0.017~0.240)	0.024	IVW	3.306	1			
	WMO [b]	0.049(−0.249~0.346)	0.750						
Serum HDL concentrations (mg/dL)	MR-Egger	0.121(−0.105~0.346)	0.300	MR-Egger	3.081	1	−0.002	0.008	0.788
	WMD [a]	0.080(−0.013~0.173)	0.091						
	IVW	0.091(0.015~0.168)	0.020	IVW	3.154	1			
	WMO [b]	0.061(−0.147~0.269)	0.569						
Serum glucose concentrations (mg/dL)	MR-Egger	0.282(−0.084~0.648)	0.138	MR-Egger	5.709	1	−0.007	0.013	0.580
	WMD [a]	0.141(−0.020~0.303)	0.086						
	IVW	0.184(0.060~0.308)	0.004	IVW	6.019	1			
	WMO [b]	0.074(−0.237~0.386)	0.642						
BMI	MR-Egger	0.097(−0.119~0.313)	0.384	MR-Egger	3.729	1	0.0007	0.007	0.922
	WMD [a]	0.087(−0.005~0.180)	0.064						
	IVW	0.107(0.034~0.180)	0.004	IVW	3.739	1			
	WMO [b]	0.068(−0.133~0.269)	0.511						
Waist circumferences (cm)	MR-Egger	0.208(−0.243~0.659)	0.370	MR-Egger	2.479	1	−0.001	0.016	0.945
	WMD [a]	0.179(−0.012~0.370)	0.066						
	IVW	0.193(0.039~0.347)	0.014	IVW	2.484	1			
	WMO [b]	0.136(−0.240~0.513)	0.481						
Body fat	MR-Egger	0.218(−0.222~0.658)	0.337	MR-Egger	4.117	1	−0.002	0.015	0.889
	WMD [a]	0.151(−0.047~0.349)	0.134						
	IVW	0.188(0.038~0.338)	0.014	IVW	4.136	1			
	WMO [b]	0.100(−0.303~0.502)	0.630						

MR, Mendelian randomization; WMD [a], Weighted median; IVW, inverse-variance weighted mode. WMO [b], Weighted mode.

3.4. A Causal Relationship between Total Noodle Intake with MetS and Its Components by a Two-Sample MR Analysis

Genetic variants linked to noodle intake were explored by conducting GWAS between low- and high-noodle intake groups according to the cutoff of 130 g/day noodle intake. The Q-Q plot in Supplementary Figure S1A showed the logarithm of the observed and expected p-values on the y-axis and x-axis, respectively. The inflation factor was 1.036, which suggested no inflation (Figure S1A). The Q-Q plot revealed that there were no biased genetic variants between the groups with low and high-noodle intake.

The p-values of genetic variants in the GWAS results are presented as a Manhattan plot in the Supplementary Figure S1B. Their associations were marginal since the intake of noodles is a lifestyle-related parameter. Furthermore, potential LD in the genetic variants was eliminated using an r^2 threshold of < 0.001 within a distance of 10,000 kb using the R package. Therefore, the p-value cutoff for the GWAS between the categories of noodle intake was assigned as $p < 5 \times 10^{-5}$. The selected genetic variants from the GWAS that had a significant relationship with MetS and its components ($p < 5 \times 10^{-5}$) were removed. It resulted in 53 genetic variants that met the requirements for use as instrumental variables, the features of which are displayed in Supplementary Table S2.

Noodle intake with the cutoff of ≥130 g/day was only causally linked to a heightened risk of MetS in the IVW approach (OR = 1.196, 95% CI = 1.045~1.368, p = 0.0009) and not in the MR-Egger, weighted median, and weighted mode methods (p > 0.05; Table 3). Figure 2A revealed a positive correlation between a predicted MetS incidence from genetics and noodle intake, and the line passed zero in the IVW, MR-Egger, and weighted median methods. The slope of the lines, which represented the effect size of the connection between noodle intake and MetS risk, was equivalent in the IVW and MR-Egger methods (Figure 2A). Figure 2B showed the MR effect size for noodle intake on MetS in each instrumental variable. MetS was significantly associated with noodle intake in the overall instrumental variables in the IVW but not in the MR-Egger method (Figure 2B). Thus, the association in MR-Egger is similar to IVW, although MR-Egger was not significant. Since the MR-Egger method is known to be a reference for the direction of a causal and positive association in the two-sample MR analysis [28], the positive direction of the association was correctly represented. The slope in the weighted median was smaller than that in the IVW and MR-Egger.

Among the MetS components, the intake of noodles showed a positive association with hypertension and dyslipidemia only in the logistic regression analysis in the IVW method (p = 0.005 and p = 0.006, respectively; Table 3). In linear association, noodle intake was positively associated with serum triglycerides, LDL, hypo-HDL, and glucose concentrations only in the IVW method (p = 0.01, 0.02, 0.02, and 0.004, respectively) but not in the MR-Egger, weighted median, and weighted mode methods (p > 0.05; Table 3 and Figure 3A). Furthermore, body composition, BMI, waist circumferences, and fat mass exhibited a positive relationship with noodle intake only in the IVW method (p = 0.004, 0.01, and 0.01, respectively, Table 3). However, serum glucose concentrations, BMI, and waist circumferences were close to statistical significance in the weighted median method (p = 0.086, 0.064, 0.066, respectively). Since the weighted median estimator retained greater precision than the MR-Egger analysis, serum glucose concentrations, BMI, and waist circumferences were causally positively associated with noodle intake.

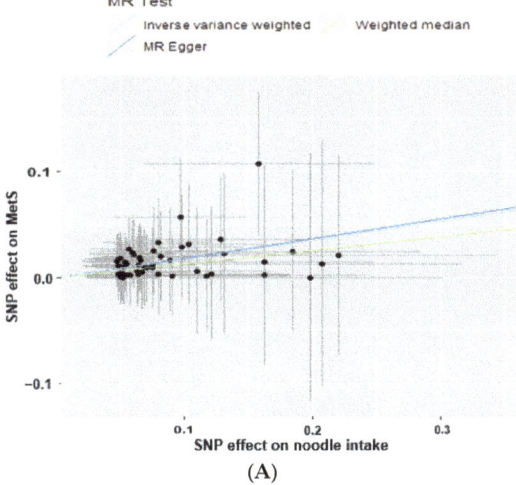

Figure 3. Cont.

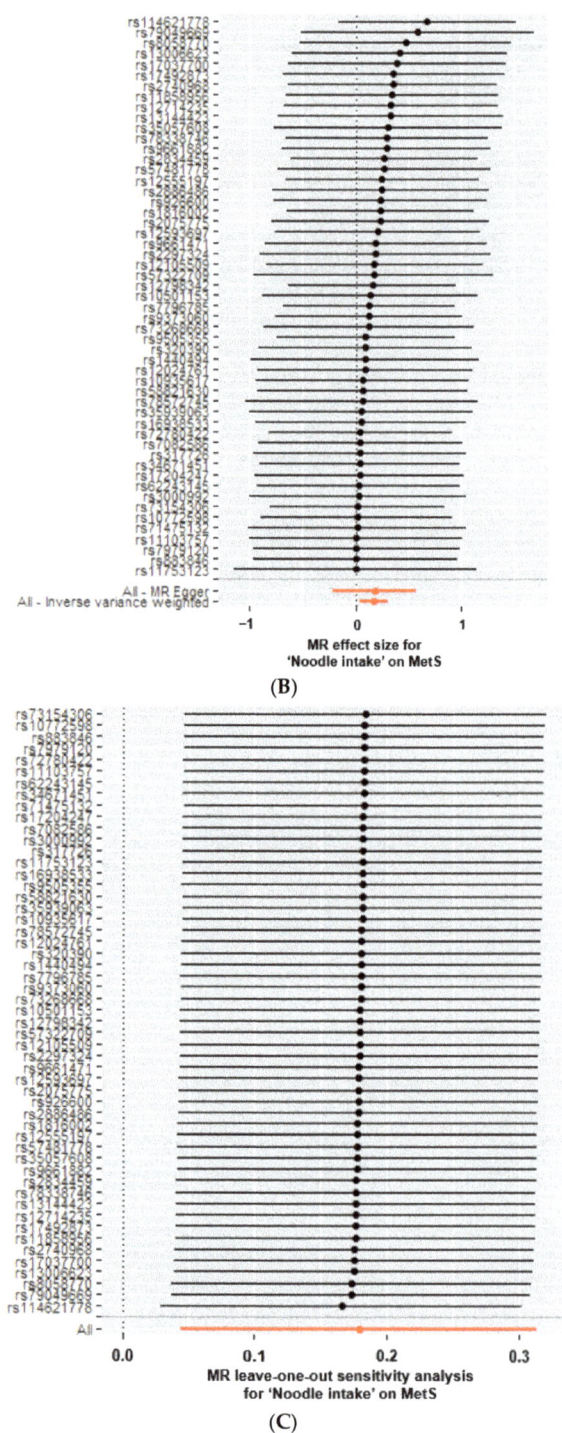

Figure 3. Cont.

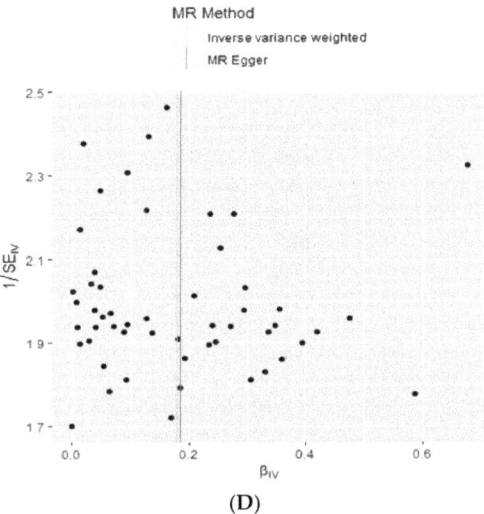

(D)

Figure 3. Two-sample Mendelian randomization (MR) analysis of the association between daily total noodle intake (cutoff: 130 g/day) and metabolic syndrome (MetS) risk. (**A**) Correlation between the effect size of the single nucleotide polymorphism (SNP)-total noodle intake (x-axis, standard deviation (SD) units) and SNP-MetS association (y-axis, log OR) to the SD bars. (**B**) Forest plot between daily total noodle intake and MetS. Each black dot represents an increase in the log OR of each SD in MetS, using each SNP of daily total noodle intake as a separate instrumental tool in the MR-Egger method. All–Egger and all-inverse-variance weighted (IVW) indicated a combined causal estimate using all SNPs in a single instrumental variable, using each MR-Egger and IVW random effects. The horizontal lines in each SNP represented the 95% confidence intervals. (**C**) Leave-one-out sensitivity analysis of MR for the effect of daily total noodle intake on the MetS. Each black dot indicated an IVW method for estimating the causal effect of daily total noodle intake on MetS, from which the single SNP was excluded. All described the IVW estimate using eight SNPs in the leave-one-out sensitivity analysis. (**D**) IVW and MR-Egger regression funnel plot for the effect of the daily total noodle intake on MetS. The vertical line represented a causal estimate using all SNPs combined into a single instrumental variable for each IVW and MR-Egger method. SNP, single nucleotide polymorphism; IVW, inverse-variance weighted.

No heterogeneity was observed between noodle intake and MetS and its components in the MR-Egger and IVW analysis ($p = 1$; Table 3 and Figure 3B). The intercept of the association between noodle intake and the risk of MetS and its components was not significantly different from zero in the MR-Egger and IVW tests, demonstrating no significant horizontal pleiotropy of the association between them ($p > 0.05$; Table 3). Cochran's Q test further indicated no heterogeneities in MetS and its components (all p-values of Cochran's Q = 1). The exclusion of individual genetic variants in the leave-one-out analysis did not affect the association between total noodle intake and MetS and its components without removing one genetic variant by one (Figure 3C). Moreover, the lines for IVW and MR-Egger in the funnel plot for MetS were closely placed together. The distribution of genetic variants was close to symmetrical in the IVW and MR-Egger tests (Figure 3D). It indicates that the association between noodle intake and MetS did not manifest any signs of bias of the instrumental variables in the IVW and MR-Egger methods. The MR estimate of each SNP was plotted as a function of its MAF-corrected association with MetS. A MAF correction was used in proportion to the standard error of the SNP-MetS since a low MAF is likely to be measured with low accuracy. The plot revealed symmetry in the IVW and asymmetry in the MR-Egger method. Thus, noodle intake was causally and positively associated with MetS in the IVW method.

4. Discussion

Asians have a high grain intake from boiled grains or noodles. Noodles vary according to noodle sources, thickness, length, and shape. Noodles are mainly made of wheat and durum wheat, but rice, buckwheat, and potato starch are also used as raw materials to make noodles. Previous studies have demonstrated that noodle and pasta intake exhibit controversial results in MetS risk, possibly due to the differences in the sources and types of noodles [7,10]. Intake of instant noodles is shown to increase MetS risk in adults in the data from KNHANES IV 2007–2009 [7]. However, WHI in 84,555 postmenopausal women has shown that substituting pasta meals for other starchy foods could improve cardiometabolic outcomes [29]. In the INHES, pasta consumption was found to be inversely associated with the incidence of being overweight and obese [11]. However, few observational studies have been conducted on the relationship between the intake of noodles and MetS and its components. No study to date has been performed to identify their causal association. The present study revealed that not only the intake of instant noodles but also the intake of noodles overall was positively linked to MetS and waist circumference, hypo-HDL-cholesterolemia, hypertriglyceridemia, and hypertension. Furthermore, to our knowledge, overall noodle intake increased MetS incidence in a two-sample MR.

The association between noodle intake and MetS risk remains controversial. The differences in the relationship between noodle intake and MetS risk between Western countries and Asia are attributed to the differences in the dietary patterns between the two geographical regions. Consistent with the results of the present study, Asians having a high intake of noodles were also observed to consume a small amount of rice and a high amount of meat intake, including processed meats, as seen in two studies, one based on a Nutrition and Diet Investigation Project in Jiangsu Province, China [30] and the other from the China Health and Nutrition Survey (CHNS) [31]. Two studies have indicated that adults with WSD consume more wheat flour and meat and less rice, associated with an increased risk of MetS [31]. This present study confirmed the same results as the CHNS and revealed that WSD had a slight link with the risk of MetS. Additionally, when the consumption of noodles and meats was separated, it was apparent that noodles had a bigger influence on MetS than WSD. As a result, Koreans who often eat noodles are more vulnerable to MetS and its related components. More research needs to be conducted to understand the correlation between noodle consumption and the development of MetS in various populations in order to develop efficient interventions to reduce the MetS risk.

The relationship between noodle intake and MetS risk may be related to both GI and GL. Both parameters determine the postprandial glucose levels in insulin-sensitive and insulin-resistant individuals. GI is a measure of the quality of carbohydrates, and GL is the amount of glucose released based on the carbohydrate consumed [31–33]. GI is estimated based on increased serum glucose concentrations when a given amount of carbohydrates is consumed. Dietary GI, but not GL, was positively linked to MetS risk in a meta-analysis of observational studies, but the results remain inconsistent [31,34]. In a randomized clinical trial, serum glucose variability during 24 h decreased in the low-GI group compared to the high-GI group in people on a Mediterranean-style healthy eating pattern [32]. Noodles are reported to have a lower GI than rice, although this may vary according to the type of noodle or rice (GI: 48–52 for noodles and 50–93 for rice). The GI values of noodles (about 44–60), rice (70), and grains (41–60) are different depending on their gluten and amylose contents. We, therefore, used the GI values commonly listed in Korea [33]. The intake of noodles alone has lower GI and GL values than rice intake. However, the GI of mixed foods in a meal may affect MetS risk differently. The present study revealed that the daily food consumption of people in the high-noodle group had much higher total GI and GL values than those in the low-noodle group. This result could be due to more noodles being consumed in the meals of the former, with fewer vegetables, as opposed to a meal with rice, which includes soup, meat or a fish dish, two vegetable dishes, and kimchi. As such, this could explain the positive correlation between noodle intake and the risk of MetS, as the GI of the mixed food in a meal may affect the risk differently. In Korea, people who often consume meals composed mainly of noodles also consume a high-GI meal.

The current study was the first to demonstrate a causal connection between consuming noodles (at least three times a week and at least 130 g a day) and MetS and its components by utilizing a two-sample Mendelian randomization and a study of observation in people from Asia. In the present study, instrumental variables were generated with the GWAS between low- and high-noodle intake at a p-value of 5×10^{-5} after adjusting for covariates including age, gender, education, income, energy, carbohydrates, and alcohol consumption, smoking, and physical exercise. Those variables associated with MetS and its components were excluded from the instrumental variables. Finally, 53 genetic variants were selected as instrumental variables, and only six were at p-values of 5×10^{-7}–5×10^{-6}, and most were between 5×10^{-5} and 5×10^{-6}. No study to date has explored the genetic variants related to noodle intake. However, the noodle-rich dietary pattern was observed to interact with the 22q13 loci, including patatin-like phospholipase domain-containing protein 3 (PNPLA3), which has been shown to influence non-alcoholic fatty liver risk in KoGES [34]. The genetic association of meat intake has been studied, but the genetic variants do not meet the Bonferroni statistical significance. However, rs7166776 in 15q26.1 is marginally significantly associated with total meat intake per 1000 kcal energy ($p = 5.54 \times 10^{-8}$). Furthermore, they are not genetically linked, and many genetic variants show LD relationships [35,36]. Therefore, loose statistical significance should be applied for selecting the instrumental variables associated with lifestyle-related parameters.

The instrumental variables selected for the MR were 53 genetic variants. IVW, weighted median, and MR-Egger are all methods used in two-sample MR studies that assess the causal relationship between exposures (noodle intake) and outcomes (MetS). The main difference between these three methods is their causal effect estimate. IVW uses a weighted average of all available genetic instruments to estimate the causal effect, while MR-Egger uses a linear regression model to assess the relationship between the genetic instrument and the outcome [28,37]. A weighted median of the available genetic instruments is also used to estimate the causal effect. IVW is often considered the gold standard in two-sample MR studies, as it has been shown to be more robust and reliable than MR-Egger in small sample sizes but to have more bias [38]. The present study showed a positive association of noodle intake with MetS and its components, including hypertension, dyslipidemia, hypertriglyceridemia, hypo-HDL concentrations, hyperglycemia, and abdominal obesity in the IVW but not the MR-Egger method. The results suggest that noodles may have a link to MetS and its components. Nonetheless, the MR-Egger and weighted median tests did not detect a significant association between noodle intake and MetS, implying that a larger sample size may be necessary to strengthen the statistical analysis. Further research would also be necessary to understand the relationship between them better.

The current study was novel as it demonstrated that noodle intake ($\geq$130 g/day, $\geq$3 times/week) has a causal relationship with MetS and its components in Asians. The other advantage was using the large cohort data, which were conducted in a well-controlled manner, such as anthropometric, biochemical, and genotyping measurements. Usual food intake was determined with SQFFQ designed for Korean dietary patterns, and nutrient intake was calculated from the food intake using a computer-aided nutrition analysis program containing nutrient composition for Korean foods. However, this study has some limitations: First, the instrumental variables to explain the causal association between noodles and MetS risk included some bias since a loose statistical significance was applied [39]. Second, the two cohorts included 58,701 and 13,598 participants, which may not be sufficient to show statistical power in a two-sample MR study, although the participants were ethnically homogeneous. Third, SQFFQ can under- or overestimate the participants' food intake since it contained only 106 food items and the portion size was 0.5, 1, or 1.5 of the one portion size. Finally, MetS-related environmental parameters were used as confounding factors. These included age, gender, education, income, smoking, physical exercise, energy, carbohydrates, and alcohol consumption. However, some factors could have been missed out, leading to bias. Therefore, the causal relationship between the intake of noodles and MetS may include a bias and requires further confirmation with a large randomized clinical trial.

5. Conclusions

Adults with a high intake of noodles ($\geq$130 g/day, $\geq$3 times/week), regardless of the type of noodle, namely, wheat noodles, instant noodles, Chinese noodles, and buckwheat noodles, had a higher energy intake with poorer diet quality than those with a low-noodle intake in the KoGES. The intake of noodles, related to high GI, was positively associated with a 1.34-fold MetS risk. Furthermore, in a two-sample MR, the noodle intake exhibited a positive causal relationship with MetS and its components, including hypertension, dyslipidemia, hypertriglyceridemia, hypo-HDL concentration, hyperglycemia, and abdominal obesity in Asians who consume a high carbohydrate diet. Therefore, it is essential to recognize the potential health risks associated with the high consumption of noodles. Public health intervention strategies should be implemented to reduce the prevalence of MetS and its components by decreasing noodle consumption and/or consuming it with various quality foods, especially for Asians.

Supplementary Materials: The following supporting information can be downloaded at: https://www.mdpi.com/article/10.3390/nu15092091/s1. Table S1: The factor-loading values of the predefined 29 food groups in each dietary pattern. Table S2: Instrumental variables for metabolic syndrome according to total noodle intake. Figure S1: Manhattan and quantile-quantile (QQ) plots for single nucleotide polymorphism (SNP) association with noodle intake.

Author Contributions: S.P. formulated the research question, interpreted the data, and wrote the first draft of the manuscript. M.L. analyzed the data. All authors have read and agreed to the published version of the manuscript.

Funding: This study was supported by a grant from the National Research Foundation of Korea (NRF) funded by the Ministry of Science and ICT (RS-2023-00208567).

Institutional Review Board Statement: The KoGES obtained approval from the KoGES Institutional Review Board (KBP-2019-055), and this study was approved by Hoseo University Institutional Review Board (1041231-150811-HR-034-01) to comply with the Declaration of Helsinki. All the partici-pants agreed to the terms after providing written informed consent.

Data Availability Statement: Data can be obtained from Korea Biobank.

Conflicts of Interest: The authors declare no conflict of interest.

References

1. Park, S.; Zhang, T. A Positive Association of Overactivated Immunity with Metabolic Syndrome Risk and Mitigation of Its Association by a Plant-Based Diet and Physical Activity in a Large Cohort Study. *Nutrients* **2021**, *13*, 2308. [CrossRef]
2. Kim, M.; Lee, S.; Shin, K.; Son, D.; Kim, S.; Joe, H.; Yoo, B.; Hong, S.; Cho, C.; Shin, H.; et al. The Change of Metabolic Syndrome Prevalence and Its Risk Factors in Korean Adults for Decade: Korea National Health and Nutrition Examination Survey for 2008–2017. *Korean J. Fam. Pr.* **2020**, *10*, 44–52. [CrossRef]
3. Saklayen, M.G. The Global Epidemic of the Metabolic Syndrome. *Curr. Hypertens. Rep.* **2018**, *20*, 12. [CrossRef] [PubMed]
4. Yang, H.J.; Kim, M.J.; Hur, H.J.; Lee, B.K.; Kim, M.S.; Park, S. Association Between Korean-Style Balanced Diet and Risk of Abdominal Obesity in Korean Adults: An Analysis Using KNHANES-VI (2013–2016). *Front. Nutr.* **2021**, *8*, 772347. [CrossRef] [PubMed]
5. Kim, M.J.; Hur, H.J.; Jang, D.J.; Kim, M.S.; Park, S.; Yang, H.J. Inverse association of a traditional Korean diet composed of a multigrain rice-containing meal with fruits and nuts with metabolic syndrome risk: The KoGES. *Front. Nutr.* **2022**, *9*, 1051637. [CrossRef] [PubMed]
6. Cho, Y.A.; Kim, J.; Cho, E.R.; Shin, A. Dietary patterns and the prevalence of metabolic syndrome in Korean women. *Nutr. Metab. Cardiovasc. Dis.* **2011**, *21*, 893–900. [CrossRef] [PubMed]
7. Shin, H.J.; Cho, E.; Lee, H.-J.; Fung, T.T.; Rimm, E.; Rosner, B.; Manson, J.E.; Wheelan, K.; Hu, F.B. Instant Noodle Intake and Dietary Patterns Are Associated with Distinct Cardiometabolic Risk Factors in Korea. *J. Nutr.* **2014**, *144*, 1247–1255. [CrossRef] [PubMed]

8. Ha, K.; Kim, K.; Chun, O.K.; Joung, H.; Song, Y. Differential association of dietary carbohydrate intake with metabolic syndrome in the US and Korean adults: Data from the 2007–2012 NHANES and KNHANES. *Eur. J. Clin. Nutr.* **2018**, *72*, 848–860. [CrossRef]
9. Huh, I.S.; Kim, H.; Jo, H.K.; Lim, C.S.; Kim, J.S.; Kim, S.J.; Kwon, O.; Oh, B.; Chang, N. Instant noodle consumption is associated with cardiometabolic risk factors among college students in Seoul. *Nutr. Res. Pract.* **2017**, *11*, 232–239. [CrossRef]
10. Huang, M.; Li, J.; Ha, M.A.; Riccardi, G.; Liu, S. A systematic review on the relations between pasta consumption and cardiometabolic risk factors. *Nutr. Metab. Cardiovasc. Dis.* **2017**, *27*, 939–948. [CrossRef]
11. Pounis, G.; Castelnuovo, A.D.; Costanzo, S.; Persichillo, M.; Bonaccio, M.; Bonanni, A.; Cerletti, C.; Donati, M.B.; de Gaetano, G.; Iacoviello, L.; et al. Association of pasta consumption with body mass index and waist-to-hip ratio: Results from Moli-sani and INHES studies. *Nutr. Diabetes* **2016**, *6*, e218. [CrossRef] [PubMed]
12. Park, S. Association between polygenetic risk scores related to sarcopenia risk and their interactions with regular exercise in a large cohort of Korean adults. *Clin. Nutr.* **2021**, *40*, 5355–5364. [CrossRef] [PubMed]
13. Park, S.; Ahn, J.; Lee, B.-K. Self-rated subjective health status is strongly associated with sociodemographic factors, lifestyle, nutrient intakes, and biochemical indices, but not smoking status: KNHANES 2007–2012. *J. Korean Med. Sci.* **2015**, *30*, 1279–1287. [CrossRef]
14. Park, S.; Liu, M.; Kang, S. Alcohol intake interacts with CDKAL1, HHEX, and OAS3 genetic variants, associated with the risk of type 2 diabetes by lowering insulin secretion in Korean adults. *Alcohol. Clin. Exp. Res.* **2018**, *42*, 2326–2336. [CrossRef] [PubMed]
15. Kim, Y.; Han, B.-G.; Group, K. Cohort profile: The Korean genome and epidemiology study (KoGES) consortium. *Int. J. Epidemiol.* **2017**, *46*, e20. [CrossRef] [PubMed]
16. Levey, A.S.; Bosch, J.P.; Lewis, J.B.; Greene, T.; Rogers, N.; Roth, D. A more accurate method to estimate glomerular filtration rate from serum creatinine: A new prediction equation. Modification of Diet in Renal Disease Study Group. *Ann. Intern. Med.* **1999**, *130*, 461–470. [CrossRef]
17. Liu, J.; Grundy, S.M.; Wang, W.; Smith, S.C., Jr.; Vega, G.L.; Wu, Z.; Zeng, Z.; Wang, W.; Zhao, D. Ethnic-Specific Criteria for the Metabolic Syndrome: Evidence from China. *Diabetes Care* **2006**, *29*, 1414–1416. [CrossRef] [PubMed]
18. Ahn, Y.; Kwon, E.; Shim, J.; Park, M.; Joo, Y.; Kimm, K.; Park, C.; Kim, D. Validation and reproducibility of food frequency questionnaire for Korean genome epidemiologic study. *Eur. J. Clin. Nutr.* **2007**, *61*, 1435–1441. [CrossRef]
19. Park, S.; Kang, S. A Western-style diet interacts with genetic variants of the LDL receptor to hyper-LDL cholesterolemia in Korean adults. *Public Health Nutr.* **2021**, *24*, 2964–2974. [CrossRef]
20. Kim, D.-Y.; Kim, Y.; Lim, H. Glycaemic indices and glycaemic loads of common Korean carbohydrate-rich foods. *Br. J. Nutr.* **2019**, *121*, 416–425. [CrossRef]
21. Foster-Powell, K.; Holt, S.H.; Brand-Miller, J.C. International table of glycemic index and glycemic load values: 2002. *Am. J. Clin. Nutr.* **2002**, *76*, 5–56. [CrossRef] [PubMed]
22. Wolever, T.M.S.; Jenkins, D.J.A. The use of the glycemic index in predicting the blood glucose response to mixed meals. *Am. J. Clin. Nutr.* **1986**, *43*, 167–172. [CrossRef] [PubMed]
23. Hong, K.W.; Kim, S.H.; Zhang, X.; Park, S. Interactions among the variants of insulin-related genes and nutrients increase the risk of type 2 diabetes. *Nutr. Res.* **2018**, *51*, 82–92. [CrossRef] [PubMed]
24. Rabbee, N.; Speed, T.P. A genotype calling algorithm for affymetrix SNP arrays. *Bioinformatics* **2006**, *22*, 7–12. [CrossRef]
25. Park, S.; Zhang, X.; Lee, N.R.; Jin, H.-S. TRPV1 gene polymorphisms are associated with type 2 diabetes by their interaction with fat consumption in the Korean genome epidemiology study. *J. Nutr. Nutr.* **2016**, *9*, 47–61. [CrossRef]
26. Storey, J.D.; Tibshirani, R. Statistical significance for genome wide studies. *Proc. Natl. Acad. Sci. USA* **2003**, *100*, 9440–9445. [CrossRef]
27. De Leeuw, C.; Savage, J.; Bucur, I.G.; Heskes, T.; Posthuma, D. Understanding the assumptions underlying Mendelian randomization. *Eur. J. Hum. Genet.* **2022**, *30*, 653–660. [CrossRef]
28. Burgess, S.; Thompson, S.G. Interpreting findings from Mendelian randomization using the MR-Egger method. *Eur. J. Epidemiol.* **2017**, *32*, 377–389. [CrossRef]
29. Huang, M.; Lo, K.; Li, J.; Allison, M.; Wu, W.-C.; Liu, S. Pasta meal intake in relation to risks of type 2 diabetes and atherosclerotic cardiovascular disease in postmenopausal women: Findings from the Women's Health Initiative. *BMJ Nutr. Prev. Health* **2021**, *4*, 195–205. [CrossRef]
30. Wang, Y.; Dai, Y.; Tian, T.; Zhang, J.; Xie, W.; Pan, D.; Xu, D.; Lu, Y.; Wang, S.; Xia, H.; et al. The Effects of Dietary Pattern on Metabolic Syndrome in Jiangsu Province of China: Based on a Nutrition and Diet Investigation Project in Jiangsu Province. *Nutrients* **2021**, *13*, 4451. [CrossRef]
31. Chen, Y.; Kang, M.; Kim, H.; Xu, W.; Lee, J.E. Associations of dietary patterns with obesity and weight change for adults aged 18–65 years: Evidence from the China Health and Nutrition Survey (CHNS). *PLoS ONE* **2023**, *18*, e0279625. [CrossRef] [PubMed]
32. Bergia, R.E.; Giacco, R.; Hjorth, T.; Biskup, I.; Zhu, W.; Costabile, G.; Vitale, M.; Campbell, W.W.; Landberg, R.; Riccardi, G. Differential Glycemic Effects of Low- versus High-Glycemic Index Mediterranean-Style Eating Patterns in Adults at Risk for Type 2 Diabetes: The MEDGI-Carb Randomized Controlled Trial. *Nutrients* **2022**, *14*, 706. [CrossRef] [PubMed]
33. Kim, M.J.; Park, S.; Yang, H.J.; Shin, P.K.; Hur, H.J.; Park, S.J.; Lee, K.H.; Hong, M.; Kim, J.H.; Choi, S.W.; et al. Alleviation of Dyslipidemia via a Traditional Balanced Korean Diet Represented by a Low Glycemic and Low Cholesterol Diet in Obese Women in a Randomized Controlled Trial. *Nutrients* **2022**, *14*, 235. [CrossRef] [PubMed]

34. Park, S.; Kang, S. High carbohydrate and noodle/meat-rich dietary patterns interact with the minor haplotype in the 22q13 loci to increase its association with non-alcoholic fatty liver disease risk in Koreans. *Nutr. Res.* **2020**, *82*, 88–98. [CrossRef]
35. Burgess, S.; Small, D.S.; Thompson, S.G. A review of instrumental variable estimators for Mendelian randomization. *Stat. Methods Med. Res.* **2017**, *26*, 2333–2355. [CrossRef]
36. Bowden, J.; Davey Smith, G.; Burgess, S. Mendelian randomization with invalid instruments: Effect estimation and bias detection through Egger regression. *Int. J. Epidemiol.* **2015**, *44*, 512–525. [CrossRef]
37. Park, S. A Causal and Inverse Relationship between Plant-Based Diet Intake and in a Two-Sample Mendelian Randomization Study. *Foods* **2023**, *12*, 545. [CrossRef]
38. Bowden, J. Misconceptions on the use of MR-Egger regression and the evaluation of the InSIDE assumption. *Int. J. Epidemiol.* **2017**, *46*, 2097–2099. [CrossRef] [PubMed]
39. Lee, Y.H. Overview of Mendelian Randomization Analysis. *J. Rheum. Dis.* **2020**, *27*, 241–246. [CrossRef]

Disclaimer/Publisher's Note: The statements, opinions and data contained in all publications are solely those of the individual author(s) and contributor(s) and not of MDPI and/or the editor(s). MDPI and/or the editor(s) disclaim responsibility for any injury to people or property resulting from any ideas, methods, instructions or products referred to in the content.

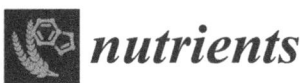

Article

Dietary Supplementation of *Caulerpa racemosa* Ameliorates Cardiometabolic Syndrome via Regulation of PRMT-1/DDAH/ADMA Pathway and Gut Microbiome in Mice

Fahrul Nurkolis [1], Nurpudji Astuti Taslim [2,*], Dionysius Subali [3], Rudy Kurniawan [4], Hardinsyah Hardinsyah [5], William Ben Gunawan [6], Rio Jati Kusuma [7,8], Vincentius Mario Yusuf [9], Adriyan Pramono [6], Sojin Kang [10], Nelly Mayulu [11], Andi Yasmin Syauki [2], Trina Ekawati Tallei [12], Apollinaire Tsopmo [13,14] and Bonglee Kim [10]

[1] Department of Biological Sciences, Faculty of Sciences and Technology, State Islamic University of Sunan Kalijaga (UIN Sunan Kalijaga), Yogyakarta 55281, Indonesia
[2] Division of Clinical Nutrition, Department of Nutrition, Faculty of Medicine, Hasanuddin University, Makassar 90245, Indonesia
[3] Department of Biotechnology, Faculty of Biotechnology, Atma Jaya Catholic University of Indonesia, Jakarta 12930, Indonesia
[4] Department of Internal Medicine, Faculty of Medicine, University of Indonesia—Cipto Mangunkusumo Hospital, Jakarta 10430, Indonesia
[5] Division of Applied Nutrition, Department of Community Nutrition, Faculty of Human Ecology, IPB University, Bogor 16680, Indonesia
[6] Department of Nutrition Science, Faculty of Medicine, Diponegoro University, Semarang 50275, Indonesia
[7] Department of Nutrition and Health, Faculty of Medicine, Public Health, and Nursing, Gadjah Mada University, Yogyakarta 55223, Indonesia
[8] Center for Herbal Medicine, Faculty of Medicine, Public Health, and Nursing, Universitas Gadjah Mada, Yogyakarta 55223, Indonesia
[9] Medical Study Programme, Faculty of Medicine, Brawijaya University, Malang 65145, Indonesia
[10] Department of Pathology, College of Korean Medicine, Kyung Hee University, Kyungheedae-ro 26, Dongdaemun-gu, Seoul 05254, Republic of Korea
[11] Department of Nutrition, Faculty of Medicine, Sam Ratulangi University, Manado 95115, Indonesia
[12] Department of Biology, Faculty of Mathematics and Natural Sciences, Universitas Sam Ratulangi, Manado 95115, Indonesia
[13] Food Science and Nutrition Program, Department of Chemistry, Carleton University, 1125 Colonel by Drive, Ottawa, ON K1S 5B6, Canada
[14] Institute of Biochemistry, Carleton University, Ottawa, ON K1S 5B6, Canada
* Correspondence: pudji_taslim@yahoo.com

Abstract: This study evaluated the effects of an aqueous extract of *Caulerpa racemosa* (AEC) on cardiometabolic syndrome markers, and the modulation of the gut microbiome in mice administered a cholesterol- and fat-enriched diet (CFED). Four groups of mice received different treatments: normal diet, CFED, and CFED added with AEC extract at 65 and 130 mg/kg body weight (BW). The effective concentration (EC_{50}) values of AEC for 2,2-diphenyl-1-picrylhydrazyl (DPPH), 2,2′-azino-bis(3-ethylbenzothiazoline-6-sulfonic acid) (ABTS), and lipase inhibition were lower than those of the controls in vitro. In the mice model, the administration of high-dose AEC showed improved lipid and blood glucose profiles and a reduction in endothelial dysfunction markers (PRMT-1 and ADMA). Furthermore, a correlation between specific gut microbiomes and biomarkers associated with cardiometabolic diseases was also observed. In vitro studies highlighted the antioxidant properties of AEC, while in vivo data demonstrated that AEC plays a role in the management of cardiometabolic syndrome via regulation of oxidative stress, inflammation, endothelial function (PRMT-1/DDAH/ADMA pathway), and gut microbiota.

Keywords: cardiometabolic syndrome; *Caulerpa racemosa*; PRMT-1/DDAH/ADMA pathway; gut microbiota; cardioprotective; sea grapes; nutraceuticals; seaweed; green algae

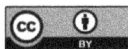

1. Introduction

Cardiometabolic syndrome is a group of metabolic disorders that increase the risk of developing cardiovascular diseases. Metabolic dysfunctions associated with the syndrome include insulin resistance, glucose intolerance, atherogenic dyslipidemia, hypertension, and intra-abdominal adiposity. The prevalence of cardiometabolic syndrome ranges from 7% to 45% [1]. The discovery of a novel cardiometabolic syndrome therapy is challenging due to a multitude of etiopathogenesis factors, including the diabetes triumvirate (insulin resistance in muscles, liver, and pancreatic beta cell failure), omnibus octet, egregious eleven, dirty dozen, treacherous thirteen, formative fifteen, microbiota dysbiosis, and intestinal barrier dysfunction [2–4]. The complexity of the syndrome makes the available therapy costly and also limits its availability [5]. Hence, countries with higher per capita incomes tend to get therapy more easily [6]. Therapeutic innovations based on bioresources can offer an alternative approach that is easily accessible and relatively inexpensive to help control metabolic syndrome. As a tropical and archipelagic country, Indonesia has a wealth of natural products that can be used as health agents, such as nutraceuticals. Some of these products are algae and seaweed [7].

Indonesia has more than 30,000 species of plants and marine resources [7], of which many have been only partially investigated or not studied at all [7]. Our group has directed its attention to seaweed as a potential source of functional ingredients with health benefits. Unlike terrestrial plants, marine algae have not been widely used as an alternative medicine or adjuvant to medicines [7]. *Caulerpa racemosa* (green seaweed, known as "sea grapes") is widely distributed in tropical regions, notably Indo-Pacific Asia, and is a member of the *Caulerpaceae* family [8]. This species contains peptides, fibers (polysaccharides), polyphenols, and flavonoids, which are known to possess diverse biological activities [9,10]. Consumption of food rich in polyphenols and other antioxidant molecules may attenuate cardiometabolic syndrome [11]. Previous studies on *C. racemosa* have reported anti-obesity and antiaging effects through the modulation of blood glucose and lipid profiles [12–14]. However, to date, no studies have successfully reported the effects of dietary supplementation of *Caulerpa racemosa* on the markers of cardiometabolic syndrome. Therefore, the aim of this study was to determine the effect of *C. racemosa* on balancing the markers of the cardiometabolic syndrome in a mice model. The markers investigated are related to oxidative stress, inflammation, endothelial function, digestion of sugars and lipids, and modulation of the gut microbiome.

2. Materials and Methods

2.1. Collection and Preparation of Caulerpa Racemosa

Green sea grapes (*Caulerpa racemosa*) were obtained from the *C. racemosa* Aquaculture Pond Waters in Jepara Regency, Central Java Province, Indonesia (6°35′12.5″ S latitude; 110°38′36.0″ E longitude). Once obtained, *C. racemosa* samples were washed immediately to remove dirt. The authentication and identification of the botanical species were carried out in the laboratory of Biological Sciences, Faculty of Science and Technology, State Islamic University of Sunan Kalijaga (UIN Sunan Kalijaga), Yogyakarta, Indonesia, and complied with the National Center for Biotechnology Information (NCBI) Taxonomy ID 76,317 (Eukaryota/Viridiplantae/Chlorophyta/Ulvophyceae/Bryopsidales/Caulerpaceae/Caulerpa). The whole body of the collected specimen was thoroughly rinsed with distilled water, dried in a hybrid hot water Goodle dryer, and lyophilized (Lyovapor™ L-200 by BÜCHI Labortechnik AG, Flawil, Switzerland). The obtained dehydrated coarse powder was then ground, as reported in previous studies [12,13,15]. The fine powder was packed in aluminum foil and deep-frozen at −20 °C before use for subsequent experiments.

2.2. Preparation of the Aqueous Extract of Caulerpa Racemosa (AEC)

The procedure for aqueous extraction was adapted from previous studies [16,17]. *C. racemosa* fine powder samples were mixed with distilled water at a solid-liquid ratio of 1:19 and sonicated (60 min, 40 °C) using an ultrasound sonicator (400 W, Branson

2510 model; Danbury, CT, USA). After filtration, the AEC powder was stored airtight in aluminum foil at −20 °C until use for in vitro and in vivo tests. The concentration of caulerpin, the major bioactive secondary metabolite (e.g., antioxidant and anti-inflammatory effects) of *Caulerpa sp.*, was quantified by high-performance liquid chromatography-mass spectrometry (HPLC-MS), as shown in Supplementary Table S1 [12].

2.3. In Vitro Studies

2.3.1. Antioxidant Activity by ABTS and DPPH Radical Scavenging Activity Assays (ABTS and DPPH Inhibition, %)

The scavenging of 2,2′-azino-bis(3-ethylbenzothiazoline-6-sulfonic acid) or its diammonium salt radical cation (ABTS+; Sigma-Aldrich, Saint Louis, MO, USA) was determined based on a published procedure [18,19]. Potassium persulfate (2.4 mM) and 7 mM ABTS (7 mM) were mixed at a ratio of 1:1, protected from light with aluminum foil, and allowed to react for 14 h at 22 °C. The mixture was further diluted (e.g., 1 mL of the stock solution plus 60 mL of ethanol) to obtain a working solution with an absorbance of 0.706 at 734 nm. A fresh working solution was prepared for each test. The AEC extracts (50, 100, 150, 200, and 250 µg/mL) were diluted with ABTS working solution (1 mL), and the absorbance was measured at 734 nm after 7 min. Trolox, a known antioxidant molecule, was used as a positive control.

The antioxidant activity in the 2,2-diphenyl-1-picrylhydrazyl radical-scavenging activity (DPPH) test was assayed according to [12,18,19]. In the testing vial, a concentration of 50, 100, 150, 200, and 250 µg/mL of AEC was added to the DPPH reagent (3 mL). The DPPH-AEC mixture was then cooled at room temperature for 30 min. A change in the concentration of DPPH was observed based on 517 nm absorbance. Glutathione (GSH; Sigma-Aldrich, 354102) was used as a positive control.

To ensure the validity of the data results (ABTS and DPPH tests), each sample was analyzed in triplicate ($n = 3$).

Inhibition of DPPH and ABTS was expressed as a percentage and determined according to the formula below:

$$Inhibition\ Activity\ (\%) = \frac{A0 - A1}{A0} \times 100\% \quad (1)$$

$A0$ = absorbance of the blank; $A1$ = absorbance of the standard or sample.

The half-maximal effective concentration ratio (EC_{50}) was used to express the radical-scavenging capability of AEC and Trolox for ABTS and AEC and glutathione for the DPPH assay. EC_{50} was defined as the concentration of a sample that caused a 50% decrease in the initial radical concentration.

2.3.2. α-Glucosidase Inhibition Assay

The inhibitory activity was evaluated according to the literature [19]. The enzyme (1 mg, 76 UI) was mixed with 50 mL of phosphate buffer (pH 6.9) to obtain a concentration of 1.52 UI/mL. In the reaction tube, 0.35 mL of sucrose (65 mM), maltose solution (65 mM), and AEC extract (0.1 mL of 50, 100, 150, 200, and 250 µg/mL) were added, one at a time. After homogenization, α-glucosidase solution (1.52 UI/mL, 0.2 mL) was added to each tube, which was then maintained at 37 °C for 20 min. The enzyme was heat-inactivated in a water bath for 2 min at 100 °C. Acarbose served as the positive control. To develop the color, 0.2 mL of testing solution and color reagent (3 mL) were reacted. Next, the system was heated (37 °C) for 5 min, and the absorbance of the solution was examined at 505 nm. The amount of glucose released during the reaction served as a sign of inhibitory activity.

2.3.3. α-Amylase Inhibition Assay (%)

The α-amylase inhibition activity of the AEC extract was measured based on a published method [12]. Diluted AEC at five different concentrations (50, 100, 150, 200, and 250 µg/mL) was incubated for 10 min at 25 °C with sodium phosphate buffer (0.02 M, pH 6.9), 0.006 M NaCl, and 0.5 mg/mL of porcine pancreatic amylase. Then, 500 µL of a 1% starch solution in assay buffer was added to each mixture. After 10 min of incubation at 25 °C, 3,5-dinitrosalicylic acid was added to complete the process and incubated in a water bath at 100 °C for 5 min. The test tube was then allowed to cool down to 22 °C. To obtain the values in the permissible range for recording the absorbance at 540 nm, a dilution with distilled water (10 mL) was performed. Acarbose was used as the positive control.

2.3.4. Lipase Inhibition Assay (%)

Crude pig pancreatic lipase (PPL, 1 mg/mL) was first dissolved in phosphate buffer (50 mM, pH 7) before centrifugation at 12,000× g to remove insoluble components. Preparing an enzyme stock (0.1 mg/mL) required a 10-fold dilution of the supernatant with buffer. The lipase inhibition potential was assessed based on prior research [20]. A transparent 96-well microplate containing 100 µL of AEC was combined with 20 µL of p-nitrophenyl butyrate (pNPB, 10 mM in buffer) and incubated for 10 min at 37 °C. The outcome was compared to the reference drug orlistat, a well-known PPL inhibitor. Measurements were taken at 405 nm using a microplate reader. The unit of activity was calculated using the yield from the reaction rate of 1 mol of p-nitrophenol/min at 37 °C. To measure the lipase inhibition activity, PPL activity was reduced in the test mixture by a specific amount. To ensure the validity of the study results, each sample was verified in triplicate. The inhibitory data were obtained using the equation below.

$$Inhibition\ of\ Lipase\ Activity\ (\%) = 100 - \frac{B - Bc}{A - Ac} \times 100\% \qquad (2)$$

A = activity without inhibitor; Ac = negative control without inhibitor; B = activity with inhibitor; Bc = negative control with inhibitor.

2.4. In Vivo Study Design

2.4.1. Animal Handling and Ethical Approval

Forty male albino Swiss mice (*Mus musculus*), each weighing 21.53 ± 1.92 g (3–5 weeks old), were provided by Animal Model Farm Yogyakarta, Indonesia, and then shipped to the research site. Mice were housed in cages and kept in a climate-controlled environment (27 °C, 50–60% relative humidity) with a balanced light-dark cycle. All mice were acclimated in the lab for 10 days before the experiment. During the research, mice had unrestricted access to conventional animal feed or pellets from PT Citra Ina Feedmill as well as drinking water. The mice were randomly divided into four treatment groups after the 10-day acclimatization period. The animal research protocol used mentions the Declaration of Helsinki and the Council of International Organizations of Medical Sciences (CIOMS). In addition, all procedures involving animals adhered to the Guidelines for Reporting In Vivo Experiments (ARRIVE) and obtained approval from the ethics board of the International Register of Preclinical Trial Animal Studies Protocols (preclinicaltrials.eu) with registration number PCTE0000329.

2.4.2. Study Design of Treatments

Throughout the study, skilled veterinarians looked out for any signs of animal welfare problems, such as lack of food, ruffling, lethargy, indifference, hiding, or curling up. Moreover, mice got weekly examinations for specific health and weight loss markers. Forty mice were randomly divided into four treatment groups. Based on Federer's equation, a minimum sample of six is required for an animal experiment consisting of four groups. Ten mice were used in this study as backup and for further sample harvest. Group A was given a normal diet and water ad libitum. Group B was given a cholesterol- and fat-enriched (CFED) diet with ad libitum water. Groups C and D were given a CFED diet and water ad libitum with daily supplementation of 65 and 130 mg/kg of body-weight (BW) AEC, respectively. An expert administered the AEC dosages orally. The daily consumption of animal feed and drinking water was tracked during the entire experiment; therefore, there was no difference between the control and experimental groups.

2.4.3. Feed or Pellet Composition and CFED Production

Normal pellets contained 12% moisture, 20% protein, 4% fat, 14% calcium, 1% fiber, 0.7% phosphorus, 11.5% total ash, 0.3% vitamin C, and 0.1% vitamin E. These pellets were obtained from Rat Bio® (Citra Ina Feedmill Ltd, Jakarta, Indonesia). Pellets were kept out of direct sunlight and were kept cool and dry according to the manufacturer's recommendations.

The CFED diet was prepared following earlier research [13,20]. Cholic acid (1%), cholesterol powder (2%), animal fat (20%), and maize oil (2%) were added to dry, normal pellets. After the ingredients had been homogenized, 1 L of distilled water was added to the mixer, where the pellets were subsequently shaped into smaller pieces. To reduce oxidation, the pellets were first dried under sterile conditions at ambient temperature before storage at 4 °C. Specifically, 43.6% of CFED is composed of carbohydrates, while 12.4% is protein, 4.7% is fiber, 3.2% is fat, 2% is cholesterol, 1% is cholic acid, 20% is animal fat, 4% is total ash, 2% is maize oil, and the remainder is moisture.

2.4.4. Biomedical Analysis of Collected Blood Samples

Blood was taken six weeks after the mice underwent interventional feeding. The night before blood was obtained, the animals were fasted and administered ketamine as an anesthetic. Blood was drawn from the venous sinus, and after being placed in a sterile, dry tube devoid of any anticoagulant, it was allowed to coagulate at room temperature. The serum was then obtained after 20 min of centrifugation (3000 rpm). Low-density lipoprotein (LDL), triglycerides (TG), high-density lipoprotein (HDL), total cholesterol (TC), and blood glucose (BG) biomedical analyses were carried out using the COBAS Integra® 400 Plus Analyzer (Roche Diagnostics, Basel, Switzerland). Blood was also taken from the heart tissue to evaluate other biomarkers such as superoxide dismutase (SOD) enzyme activities using the SOD Assay Kit from Sigma-Aldrich, serum lipase levels using the Mouse Pancreatic Lipase ELISA Kit (Merck KGaA, Darmstadt, Germany), and serum amylase levels using the Mouse Pancreatic Amylase ELISA Kit. Inflammatory biomarkers, namely PGC-1α (peroxisome proliferator-activated receptor-gamma coactivator-1 alpha), TNF-α (tumor necrosis factor-alpha), and IL-10 (interleukin 10), were quantified using a PGC-1α Mouse ELISA Kit (Sunlong Biotech Co., Ltd.; Zhejiang, China), a Mouse Tumor Necrosis Factor-α (TNF-α) Kit (Sunlong Biotech Co., Ltd.; Zhejiang, China), and an IL-10 ELISA Kit (Abcam), respectively. For the cardiometabolic biomarkers, both PRMT-1 (protein arginine N-methyltransferase 1) and DDAH-II (dimethylarginine dimethylaminohydrolase 2) were quantified using an LS-F65223 ELISA Kit and an LS-F14238 ELISA Kit, both from LSBio (Seattle, WA, USA). ADMA (asymmetric dimethylarginine) was evaluated directly using an ALX-850-327-KI01 ADMA Direct Mouse ELISA Kit from Enzo Life Sciences, Inc. (New York, NY, USA). Digital scales were used to determine the body weights of the mice.

2.5. Gut Microbiota Sequencing and Analysis of the 16S rRNA Gene in Mice Feces

Microbiological genomes of intestinal bacteria were extracted from excrements using OMG soil extraction kits from Shanghai Meiji Biopharmaceutical Technology Co., Ltd (Shanghai, China). Polymerase chain reaction (PCR) amplification of the V3–V4 variable region of the 16S rRNA gene was performed using primers 338F (5′-ACTCCTACGGGAGGCAGCAG-3′) and 806R (5′-GGACTACHVGGGTWTCTAAT-3′). Sequencing was carried out using the Illumina Miseq PE300 platform. The raw sequences were controlled with FAST software, cut with FLASH software, and qualified reads were clustered with UPARSE software to generate Operational Taxonomic Units (OTUs) with 97% similarity. Chimera sequences were removed using the search software. Each sequence was classified as a species using ribosomal database project (RDP) classification, and a 70% comparison threshold to the Silva 16S rRNA database (Version 138 by Max Planck Institute for Marine Microbiology and Jacobs University, Bremen, Germany) was set.

2.6. Data Analysis and Management

An unpaired *t*-test was used to statistically assess the data from in vitro experiments, including antioxidant inhibition of ABTS and DPPH and lipase, α-amylase, and α-glucosidase inhibitory activities. Experiments were performed in triplicate. Each EC_{50} data set was created using nonlinear regression formulas. In vivo lipid profile (LDL, HDL, TG, TC, and BG), inflammatory biomarkers (IL-10, TNFα, and PGC-1α), enzymatic assays (SOD cardio, serum lipase, and serum amylase), and cardiometabolic biomarkers (PRMT-1, DDAH-II, and ADMA) were analyzed using multivariate ANOVA. To identify significant variations between the starting and ending body weights (g) in each group, paired t-tests or dependent t-tests were used. In addition, one-way ANOVA was conducted to find the differences between each secondary parameter (water intake (mL), food intake (g), the food efficiency ratio (FER), and the beginning, final, and daily weight gain (g/day)) for each group. All data were provided in the form of mean ± standard error of the mean (SEM) with a 95% confidence level. On MacBook computers, GraphPad Prism version 9.4.1 software (Boston, MA, USA) was used for all in vitro and in vivo data analyses.

3. Results

3.1. In Vitro Activities of the Aqueous Extract of Caulerpa racemosa (AEC)

The in vitro activities of extracts and compounds can provide an indication of their properties in biological systems. As such, the antioxidant activities (DDPH and ABTS) and enzyme-inhibitory properties (α-glucosidase, α-amylase, and lipase) of the AEC extract were obtained prior to in vivo tests. Data reported as half-maximal effective concentration (EC_{50}) or half-maximal inhibitory concentration (IC_{50}) values are shown in Figure 1.

In the 2,2-diphenyl-1-picrylhydrazyl (DPPH) antioxidant assay, glutathione (GSH, control) had a greater inhibitory effect than AEC at a concentration of 100 μg/mL ($p < 0.05$; Figure 1A). However, at other concentrations, there were no significant differences ($p > 0.05$). DPPH overall suggests that there is no difference in the scavenging power of the AEC extract relative to GSH. Furthermore, the EC_{50} value of AEC (116.9 μg/mL) was lower than that of GSH (150.9 μg/mL), suggesting that AEC is more effective in inhibiting DPPH than GSH (Figure 1A).

Trolox (control) had greater inhibitory activity against ABTS compared to AEC at all concentrations (100–250 μg/mL). Nevertheless, scavenging activities were comparable ($p > 0.05$; Figure 1B). Similar to the DPPH inhibition results, the EC_{50} AEC values are more potent and active together with Trolox, with values of 121.7 μg/mL and 114.5 μg/mL, respectively (Figure 1B).

The abilities of the AEC extract to inhibit α-glucosidase (Figure 1C) and α-amylase (Figure 1D) were both compared to the reference inhibitor acarbose. At all concentrations (50–250 μg/mL), the inhibition of α-glucosidase by AEC was not significantly different compared to acarbose ($p > 0.05$), which indicates that AEC has an activity equivalent to that of the acarbose control (Figure 1C). Regarding α-amylase, AEC and acarbose had equivalent inhibition at 50 μg/mL, 100 μg/mL, and 250 μg/mL (Figure 1D), while acarbose was superior at the other two concentrations. For both enzymes, the EC_{50} of AEC was greater than that of the control acarbose.

The inhibition of pancreatic lipase by AEC did not differ significantly from the positive control (orlistat) at 100 μg/mL to 250 μg/mL ($p > 0.05$). Nevertheless, at the lowest concentration, the positive control had greater activity (Figure 1E). Based on the EC_{50} values, AEC is more potent at inhibiting the lipase enzyme (EC_{50} AEC < EC_{50} orlistat; Figure 1E).

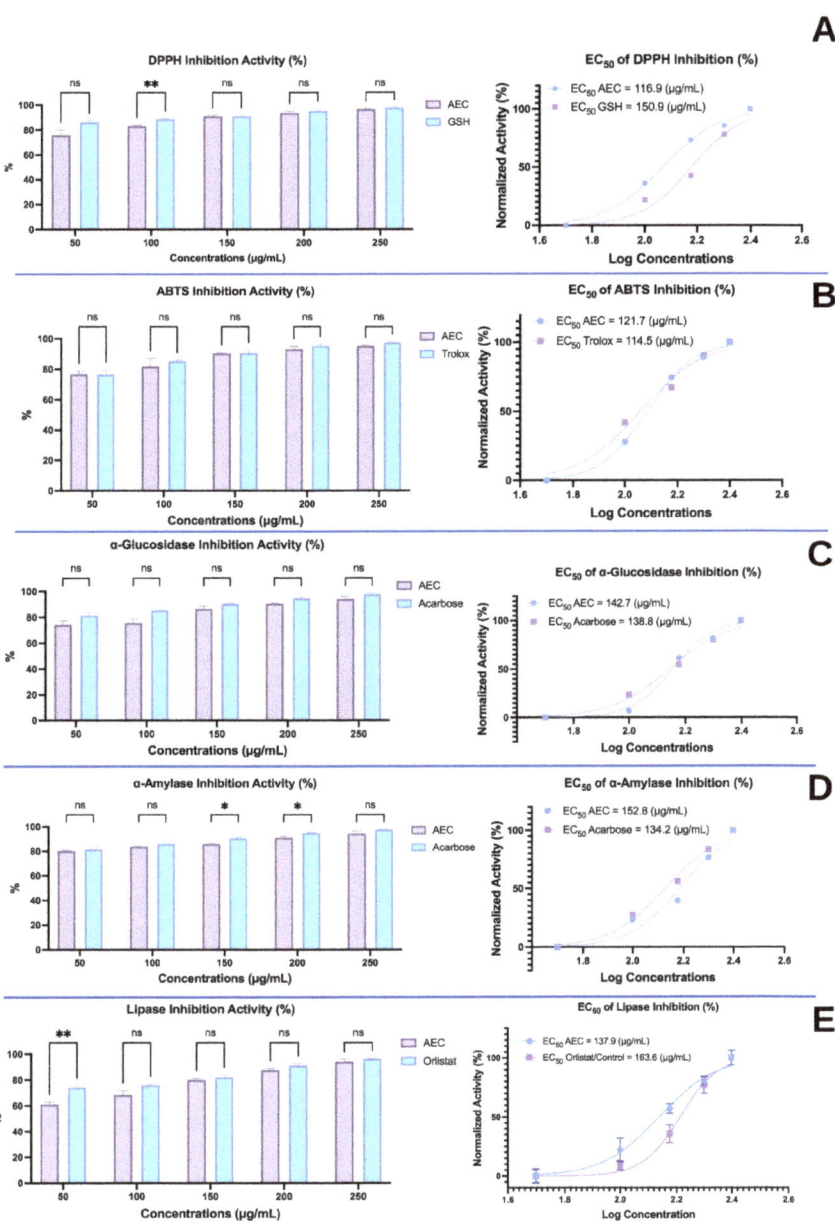

Figure 1. In vitro activities of the aqueous extract of *Caulerpa racemosa* (AEC). (**A**) DPPH radical-scavenging activity. (**B**) ABTS radical-scavenging activity. (**C**) Inhibition of the α-glucosidase enzyme. (**D**) Inhibition of the α-amylase enzyme. (**E**) Inhibition of the lipase activity; ns: $p = 0.1638$ ($p > 0.05$); *: $p = 0.0125$; **: $p = 0.0007$. Note: The EC_{50} was analyzed using the GraphPad Premium statistical analysis package "non-linear regression (log(inhibitor) vs. normalized response—variable slope". The plot bars showed that at a concentration of 50 µg/mL, all inhibition activity exceeded 50%. This may be caused by the unequal maximum and baseline effects of AEC compared to the controls. For further research, using a lower minimum dose for the controls and a higher maximum amount of AEC may result in a comparable dose response for all compounds (EC_{50}).

3.2. Effects of the Extract of Caulerpa Racemosa (AEC) on the Cardiometabolic Markers in Mice

Metabolic dysfunction was induced in mice with a cholesterol- and fat-enriched diet (CFED). The AEC extract was administered to assess its effects on various markers associated with cardiometabolic syndrome. The body weight, food intake, water intake, and FER characteristics of the mice are shown in Table 1. The effectiveness of AEC on the cardiometabolic markers is shown in Figure 2.

Table 1. Body weight, feed, water intake, and FER characteristics of experimental mice (*Mus musculus*).

Groups	Normal	CFED	C	D	p [b]
Initial body weight (g)	22.55 ± 1.717	22.05 ± 2.203	22.03 ± 1.033	22.42 ± 2.908	0.9231
Final body weight (g)	65.59 ± 3.606	82.27 ± 4.206	48.66 ± 5.509	43.18 ± 4.481	<0.0001
p [a]	*<0.0001*	*<0.0001*	*<0.0001*	*<0.0001*	
Weight gain (g/day)	0.9357 ± 0.08751	1.309 ± 0.07279	0.5789 ± 0.1116	0.4513 ± 0.1338	<0.0001
Food intake (g)	5.204 ± 0.6179	5.116 ± 0.8741	5.037 ± 1.168	5.009 ± 0.6075	0.9556
Water intake (mL)	5.758 ± 0.6237	5.752 ± 0.8913	5.349 ± 1.001	5.208 ± 0.5297	0.2954
FER (%)	18.18 ± 2.413	26.32 ± 5.064	12.00 ± 3.480	9.011 ± 2.496	<0.0001

[a] Dependent or paired *t*-test, CI 95% (0.05). [b] ANOVA CI 95% (0.05). The letter (a) behind the number in the same row indicates non-significant results. Food efficiency ratio (FER, %) = (body weight gain of experimental mice (g/day)/food intake (g/day)) × 100. CFED: cholesterol- and fat-enriched diet. C: Mice group were given a CFED diet and water ad libitum with daily supplementation of 65 of body-weight (BW) AEC. D: Mice group were given a CFED diet and water ad libitum with daily supplementation of 130 mg/kg of body-weight (BW) AEC.

Figure 2 reveals the capability of AEC in modulating cardiometabolic markers. AEC significantly ($p < 0.05$) improved the blood glucose and lipid profile of mice (for a high dose of AEC, HDL: +23.20%; LDL: −18.64%; TG: −33.00%; TC: −11.11%; BG: −7.760%; Figure 2A). AEC, particularly at a 130 mg/kg BW dose, produced greater improvements in HDL, LDL, and TG in mice that received CFED compared to Groups C and D. However, both doses of AEC had a similar effect on the TC levels. The effect of AEC on BG was similar to that of the normal diet, even though the higher dose of AEC still showed improvements in the BG levels.

The health benefits of AEC are also depicted in Figure 2B. Both AEC treatments were shown to improve cardio SOD serum levels compared to normal and CFED diets. On the other hand, 65 mg/kg BW and 130 mg/kg BW of AEC were proven to reduce amylase and lipase serum levels in mice receiving CFED, with the higher dose of AEC being similar to a normal diet. In Figure 2C, AEC treatments show improvements in the inflammatory markers PGC-1α and IL-10, which significantly increased, although the effect between both doses was similar. While both doses of AEC lowered the TNF-α levels, the higher dose of AEC showed an enhanced effect.

Figure 2D shows that AEC also exhibited positive health implications by improving the expressions of PRMT-I and DDAH-II, in particular, in mice receiving CFED supplemented with 130 mg/kg BW AEC. The higher dose of AEC also lowered ADMA concentration to a level that was similar to a normal diet.

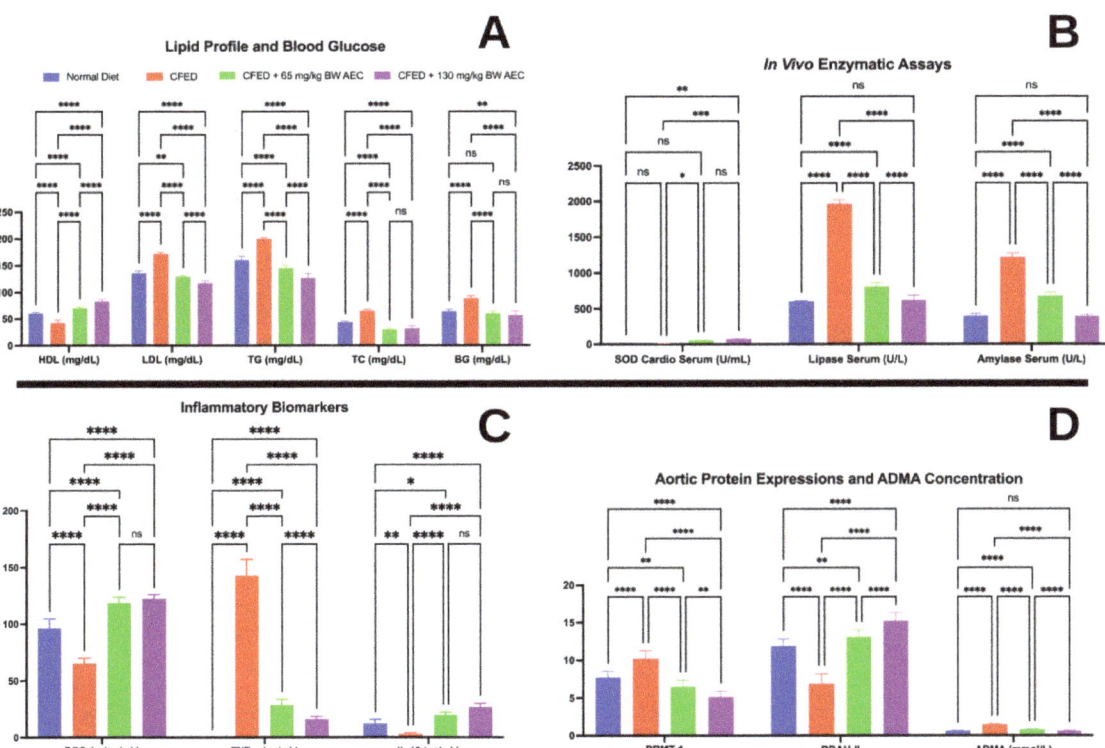

Figure 2. Effect of the aqueous extract of *Caulerpa racemosa* (AEC) on cardiometabolic markers. (**A**) Improvement of blood lipid and glucose profile of CFED mice by AEC. (**B**) Significance of improvements in SOD in cardio serum, lipase, and amylase in serum. (**C**) Improvement of inflammatory markers in CFED mice by dietary AEC. (**D**) Amelioration of cardiometabolic syndrome via regulation of PRMT-1/DDAH/ADMA pathway. ns: $p = 0.1638$ ($p > 0.05$); *: $p = 0.0125$; **: $p = 0.0067$; ***: $p = 0.0007$; ****: $p < 0.0001$. HDL = high-density lipoprotein; LDL = low-density lipoprotein; TG = triglycerides; TC = total cholesterol; BG = blood glucose; PGC-1α = peroxisome proliferator-activated receptor-gamma coactivator (PGC)-1alpha; TNF-α = tumor necrosis factor-alpha; IL-10 = interleukin 10; PRMT-1 = protein arginine N-methyltransferase 1; DDAH-II = dimethylarginine dimethylaminohydrolase 2; ADMA = plasma asymmetric dimethylarginine; CFED: cholesterol- and fat-enriched diet.

3.3. Gut Microbiome Modulation in Mice Administered a Cholesterol- and Fat-Enriched Diet Supplemented with AEC

3.3.1. Effect of AEC on Gut Microbiota Composition

After performing low-count and variance filtering, the gut microbiota of the control mice was predominantly composed of *Firmicutes* at the phylum level, which accounted for 91% of the total bacteria. CFED increased the abundance of *Bacteroidota* and *Desulfobacteria* compared to the control mice (Figure 3B). Supplementation with AEC had a different and dose-dependent effect on the gut microbiota community. A low dose of AEC increased the proportion of *Campylobacterota*, while a high dose of AEC increased the proportion of *Actinobacteria* (Figure 3). At the genus level (Figure 3A), control mice were enriched with *Dubosiella* (39%), *Lactobacillus* (20%), and *Lachnospiraceae* (11%), while *Lachnospiraceae* (23%) and *Monoglobus* (11%) were enriched in mice fed a CFED diet. Mice supplemented with low AEC had a high proportion of *Monoglobus* (17%), *Dubosiella* (11%), *Lachnospiraceae* (10%), *Lachnospiraceae* NK4A136 group (9%), and *Lactobacillus* (9%), while the high AEC group had a high proportion of *Dubosiella* (16%), *Lactobacillus* (12%), *Eubacterium fissicatena* group

(12%), *Faecalibaculum* (10%), and *Lachnospiraceae* (9%). In particular, the *Bifidobacterium* genus was proportionally higher in the high-dose AEC group compared with other groups.

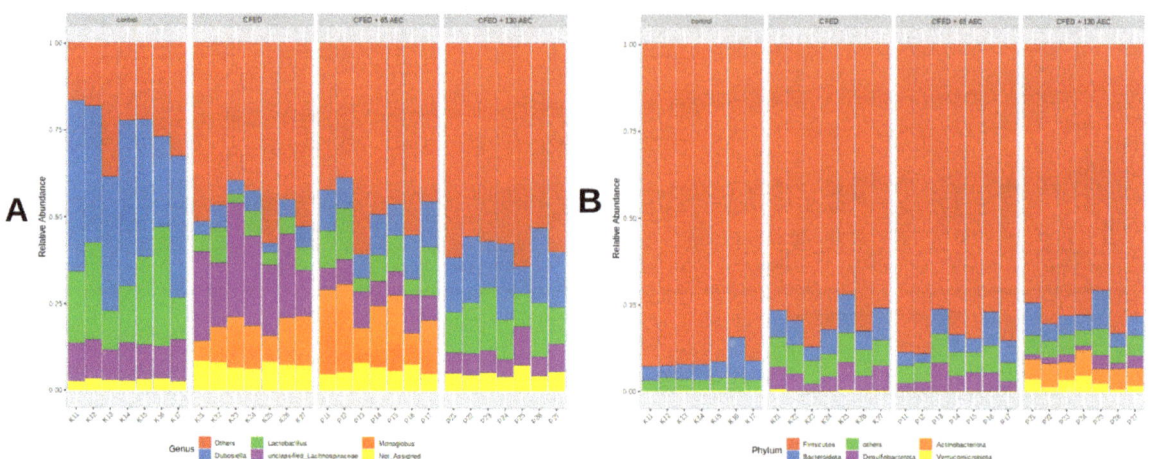

Figure 3. Taxonomic composition at the genus level (**A**) or phylum level (**B**). Each colored bar represents the percentage of each phylum or genus relative to the total microorganisms. CFED: cholesterol- and fat-enriched diet.

3.3.2. Effect of AEC on Gut Microbiota Diversity

Heatmap clustering of individual gut microbiota (bottom) according to diet groups (top) was based on Euclidean distance (Figure 4A). A significant difference ($p < 0.01$) was observed in the alpha diversity indices (Shannon, Simpson, and Chao1 indexes) according to the ANOVA test (Figure 4B). Mice fed with CFED had the highest alpha diversity index parameters compared with the other groups. A non-matrix multidimensional matrix (NMDS) using the Bray-Curtis distance was employed to compare the beta diversity among groups (Figure 4C). The results showed that gut microbiota was grouped according to the treatment groups (stress 0.05; $R^2 = 0.82$). One-way PERMANOVA analysis revealed a significant difference ($p = 0.001$), which indicated distinct gut microbiota communities among the groups.

To identify bacteria that were differentially enriched, linear discriminant analysis (LEfSe) was performed (Figure 4D). The results showed that there were 31 significant features with a log LDA score > 3 and a false discovery rate (FDR) below 0.05. *Dubosiella* and *Lactobacillus* were abundant in the control mice, whereas *Colidextribacter*, *Muribaculaceae*, *Romboutsia*, *Desulfovibrionaceae*, *Blautia*, and *Lachnospiraceae* were enriched in the CFED group. *Monoglobus*, *Lachnospiraceae* NK4A136 group, and *Oscillospiraceae* were enriched in the low-dose AEC group, while the *Eubacterium fissicatena* group, *Faecalibaculum*, and *Bifidobacterium* were enriched in the high-dose AEC group.

We performed Pearson correlation analysis to investigate the relationship between the abundances of seven significantly altered gut microbial species (FDR < 0.1) and changes in the metabolic biomarker indices in the intervention group (Figure 5). Close associations were found between glucose metabolism, lipid profile, inflammatory cytokines, and the studied microbiome species. *Dubosiella*, *Lactobacillus*, and *Eubacterium fissicatena* showed a negative association with TNF alpha, lipase, ADMA, and amylase. In particular, *Faecalibacterium* was negatively associated with TNF alpha, lipase, amylase, glucose, total cholesterol, aortic-PMRT-1, triglycerides, and LDL-cholesterol. However, *Lachnospiraceae* was positively associated with glucose, total cholesterol, aortic-PMRT-1, and LDL-cholesterol.

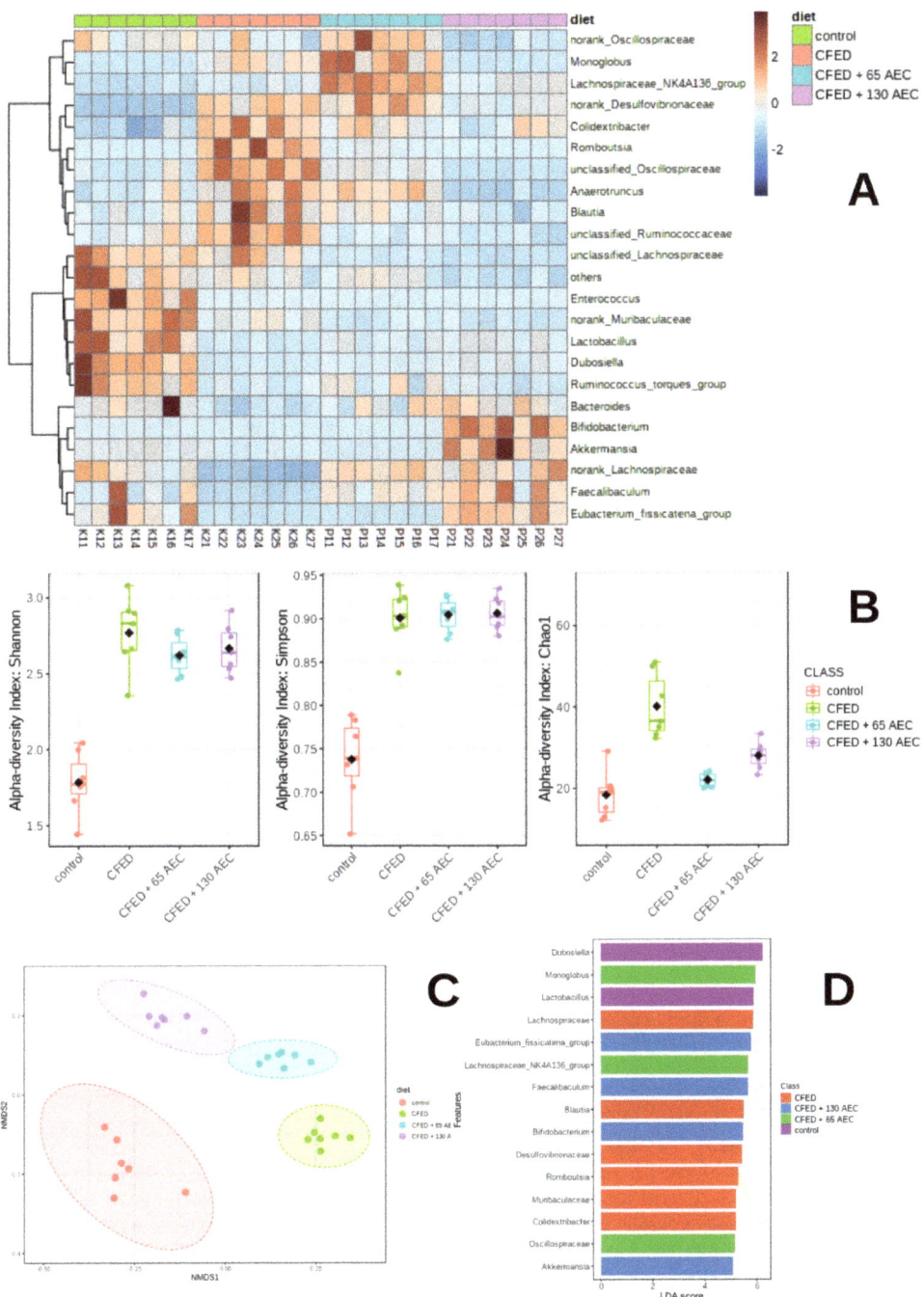

Figure 4. Clustering and community profiling of gut microbiota in mice induced with CFED. Heatmap clustering of individual gut microbiota (bottom) according to diet groups (top) based on Euclidean distance

(**A**) Boxplot of distribution of alpha diversity values (Shannon, Simpson, and Chao1) among diet groups (**B**) Non-metric multidimensional scaling (NMDS) plot of all samples using the Bray-Curtis resemblance matrix (**C**) Linear discriminant analysis (LDA) effect size (LEfSe) analyses of gut microbiota according to diet at the genus level; each colored bar indicates a genus that was significantly enriched in each consecutive group (**D**) CFED: cholesterol- and fat-enriched diet.

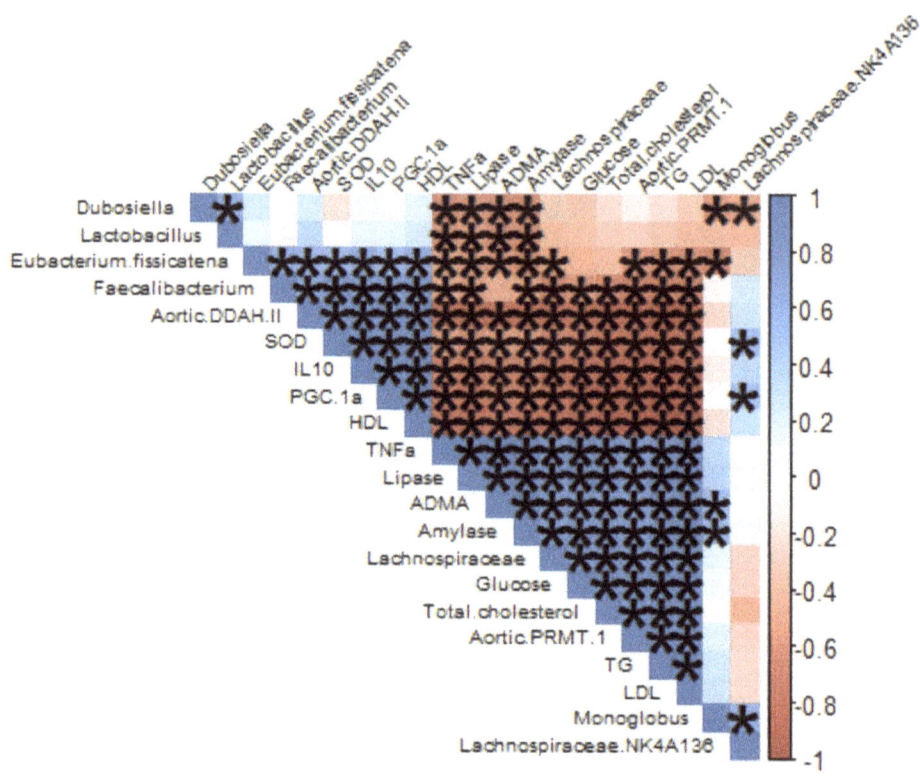

Figure 5. Heatmap of Pearson correlation between the gut microbiome and blood metabolic profiles of mice. The asterisks inside the heatmap indicate $p < 0.01$.

4. Discussion

Caulerpa racemosa is extensively used and has become one of the most popular marine fresh foods because of the various health benefits that it offers. The *Caulerpa* species are known to contain a high amount of macro- and micro-minerals, antioxidants, and secondary metabolites with attractive development or further processing prospects, supported by their distinctive taste and color [21]. Therefore, as an attempt to further advance our understanding of the potential health benefits of this marine alga, we evaluated its activity in vitro, as well as in mice models based on cardiometabolic and microbiome biomarkers. In vitro, *Caulerpa racemosa* showed potent antioxidant activity (DPPH & ABTS radical scavenging activity assays) and inhibition of α-glucosidase, α-amylase, and lipase (Figure 1). These properties are essential for mitigating and alleviating cardiometabolic syndrome. AEC showed EC_{50} values in DPPH and ABTS of 116.9 μg/mL and 121.7 μg/mL, respectively (Figure 1), which were lower than that of glutathione (often called the "master antioxidant" because of its aptitude to exploit the performance of other antioxidants) and Trolox (a water-soluble antioxidant synthesized as a vitamin E derivative with high radical scavenging potential) [22]. This study was also in line with a study by Belkacemi, where *Caulerpa racemosa* extract from Algeria exhibited an antioxidant capacity that was comparable to the controls used here [23]. The high antioxidant capacity may be due to the phytochemicals contained in *Caulerpa racemosa*, especially phenolics and flavonoids. These compounds contain hydroxyl groups, which function as hydrogen donors to stabilize free radicals [24]. Moreover, non-polar compounds such as glycolipids, phospholipids, steroids, terpenes, carotenoids, and fatty acids (especially PUFAs) are also thought to contribute to the overall radical-scavenging capacity of AEC [25]. Free radical-neutralizing capacity is essential for treating cardiometabolic syndrome because the increase in oxidative stress is deeply involved in the pathogenicity of hypertension and atherosclerosis. Pro-inflammatory adipokines caused by obesity also produce an immense amount of oxidative stress, which contributes to the progression of cardiometabolic syndrome [26]. Furthermore, this study also utilized ultrasound-assisted extraction, which is often used to increase extraction efficiency as well as natural ingredient bioactivity. Furthermore, since this technique is regarded as a "green extraction," it is environmentally friendly, requiring minimal use of solvent and time [27]. α-Amylase, α-glucosidase, and lipase are the main enzymes involved in the hydrolyzation process of carbohydrates and fat. Therefore, reacting these enzymes with AEC would cause lowered absorption of the mentioned dietary molecules, hinder carbohydrate digestion, prevent diet-induced obesity and hyperglycemia, and control diabetes, subsequently lowering the risks of micro-and macrovascular complications [28]. In addition, α-glucosidase inhibition can also aid in gastric emptying, causing satiety and weight loss, which are useful properties in obesity treatment [29]. α-Glucosidase and α-amylase inhibition by AEC was comparable to that by acarbose, an anti-diabetic drug, while lipase inhibition also showed similar results to those of orlistat, a medication used to treat obesity. This shows the potential of AEC as an alternative route of therapy.

To further advance and validate the previously mentioned results, an in vivo study using animal models was performed to assess the effect of *C. racemosa*. Data showed that the CFED diet intervention significantly increased both the final body weight and weight gain per day of mice. However, the food and water intake of the CFED mice was about the same as that of the other groups. Thus, the observed increases may be due to the significantly increased FER of the CFED-only group (Table 1). By contrast, *C. racemosa* groups experienced significantly less weight gain per day and FER compared to the other groups. This weight-loss potential is in line with other studies involving other species of *Caulerpa* (*Caulerpa sertularioides* and *Caulerpa prolifera*), which showed a significant inhibitory effect on adipogenesis of preadipocytes *in vitro*, with reductions of lipogenic transcription factors such as PPARγ, C/EBPβ, and C/EBPα mRNA [30]. Applying a similar study model, *Caulerpa lentillifera* intervention on CFED rats resulted in lower body weight post-treatment (although the results were not significant), as well as a lower FER compared to the other groups [31].

Alterations in the free fatty acid metabolism and adipose tissue dysregulation are the main suspects of hyperglycemia and dyslipidemia in cardiometabolic syndrome. The uncontrolled release of free fatty acids from adipose tissues to the bloodstream can impair the activity of insulin during muscle glucose uptake stimulation. Excess adipose tissue in obesity also causes an adipose tissue hypoxia state, which leads to insulin resistance, inflammation, and adipocyte apoptosis, as well as uncontrolled lipid secretion [32]. Furthermore, the buildup of free fatty acids in the liver (otherwise known as ectopic lipids) increases hepatic VLDL and plasma TG concentration. An increase in plasma TG leads to the transfer of TGs from VLDL to HDL, increasing HDL clearance, which in turn leads to reduced HDL and higher LDL concentrations [33]. Cardiometabolic markers were assessed in this study, and AEC intervention significantly improved the lipid profile and blood glucose in vivo. HDL increase together with LDL and TG decrease was found to be dose-dependent; however, no significant differences were found between doses in the TG and blood glucose parameters. In line with the in vitro results, lipase and amylase serum were significantly reduced in CFED mice that were given AEC, and the reduction was dose-dependent. The improvement in the lipid and blood glucose profiles can be explained by the inhibition of the digestive enzyme, as seen in vitro and in vivo. In the lipid metabolism process, inhibition of lipase by AEC prevents the conversion of ingested lipids in the form of TG into monoglycerides and fatty acids. Therefore, fewer lipid products are diffused across the intestinal cell membranes and reach the blood circulation, thus reducing excess lipid metabolism, fat deposition, and body weight and improving the lipid profile [34]. This offers the potential benefit of alleviating "the triad" of dyslipidemia, as seen in cardiometabolic syndrome, which is the increase in serum TG and LDL particles together with depressed levels of HDL. Improvement of the lipid profile can reduce the risk of atherosclerotic vascular changes, coronary artery disease, and major cardiovascular events [35]. In addition, inhibition of both α-amylase and α-glucosidase by AEC lengthens the duration of carbohydrate digestion and reduces postprandial glucose. This occurs because oligosaccharides entering the gastrointestinal tract depend on α-amylase to be broken down into smaller molecules such as maltose and maltotriose. Meanwhile, α-glucosidase carries out this process by cleaving disaccharides into digestible monosaccharides [34]. Altered glucose metabolism and CVD risk are both deeply related, as multiple studies have shown hyperglycemia to be a key risk factor for cardiovascular and all-cause mortality [36]. The control of blood glucose that is offered by AEC can be beneficial, preventing continuous hyperglycemia that leads to micro (neuropathy, nephropathy, retinopathy) and macrovascular complications (peripheral vascular disease, myocardial infarction, and stroke) [37].

The antioxidant status of mice treated with AEC, determined in vitro, was supported by in vivo findings of a significant SOD cardio serum increase in the AEC groups, although no significant difference was found between the dose groups. SODs are recognized as the "front line" of defense against reactive oxygen species (ROS)-mediated injury. These metalloenzymes catalyze the conversion of the superoxide anion (O_2^-) free radical into hydrogen peroxide (H_2O_2) and molecular oxygen [38]. In a hyperglycemic state, endothelial cells increase the production of O_2^- while immoderate amounts of O_2^- lead to the inhibition of glyceraldehyde 3-phosphate dehydrogenase (a glycolytic pathway enzyme). This causes glucose accumulation as well as increased shifts to various alternative pathways of glucose metabolism, eventually leading to the production of advanced glycation end products [39]. Moreover, ROS are also responsible for pathological processes in the vasculature, causing endothelial dysfunction through the interruption of vasoprotective pathways such as NO signaling, as well as triggering inflammasome and cytokines such as IL-1β and IL-8 via activation of caspase-1. The mechanisms above trigger atherosclerosis [40]. By increasing SOD in serum, the aforementioned consequences of cardiometabolic syndrome can potentially be prevented.

Inflammatory biomarkers were evaluated in this study. TNF-α was significantly reduced by AEC intervention. Reduction in TNF-α was dose-dependent, and a significant increase in IL-10 and PGC-1α was found. However, no significant differences in IL-10 and PGC-1α were found between the dose groups. PGC-1α is known as the master regulator of mitochondrial processes such as oxidative phosphorylation and ROS detoxification [41]. Furthermore, PGC-1α also regulates mitochondrial antioxidant gene expression, even though its dysregulation at low levels triggers an inflammatory response as well as oxidative stress and promotes the NF-κB pathway, which is responsible for inducing pro-inflammatory genes [42]. Various inflammatory markers have been determined to be deeply associated with significant risks of diabetes and cardiovascular disease. Obesity itself, as one of the main features of cardiometabolic syndrome, promotes the generation of pro-inflammatory factors, including TNF-α, in turn promoting insulin resistance [43]. Moreover, inflammatory cytokines also act on the liver and increase VLDL production, deactivating liver X receptors and causing increased cholesterol accumulation [44].

A possible mechanism implied in the development of endothelial dysfunction and oxidative stress is an increase in the levels of asymmetrical dimethylarginine (ADMA). ADMA circulation levels are increased in endothelial dysfunction-related diseases such as hypertension, hyperlipidemia, and diabetes [45]. ADMA itself is classified as a major endogenously derived methylated arginine residue that acts by inhibiting nitric oxide synthase (NOS). Nitric oxide is a well-known and potent vasodilator that is essential in cardiovascular homeostasis by exerting anti-atherogenic and anti-proliferative activities on the vasculature [46]. Furthermore, ADMA is also known to elevate ROS levels, causing oxidative stress. ADMA is synthesized in the heart, smooth muscle, and endothelial cells by PRMT-1, which is a group of enzymes that performs the methylation process [47]. Meanwhile, most (80–90%) of ADM is metabolized by DDAH, which is relevant to this study. DDAH-2 is highly expressed in vascular muscle cells and the endothelium, especially in tissues containing NOS [48]. This study also evaluated the PRMT-DDAH-ADMA metabolic axis expression in response to the CFED and AEC intervention. PRMT-1 expression and ADMA concentrations were significantly lowered in CFED mice given AEC, while DDAH-2 was significantly increased in the AEC groups, with dose-dependent effects in all parameters. Decreased DDAH activity is closely related to endothelial dysfunction and is suspected to be the mechanism responsible for ADMA-mediated NOS impairment [46]. Therefore, AEC has the potential to ameliorate the mentioned pathological metabolic axis and prevent the development and progression of cardiometabolic syndrome.

Our study also found that AEC supplementation affects gut microbiome diversity. Furthermore, at the taxa levels, the gut microbiota composition also differed significantly. *Dubosiella* and *Lactobacillus* were abundant in the control mice, whereas *Colidextribacter*, *Muribaculaceae*, *Romboutsia*, *Desulfovibrionaceae*, *Blautia*, and *Lachnospiraceae* were enriched in the CFED group. *Lachnospiraceae* comprises 58 genera [49]. All microbiota members of *Lachnospiraceae* are characterized by anaerobic, fermentative, and chemoorganotrophic features, and some display strong hydrolyzing activities (e.g., through the activity of β-xylosidase, α- and β-galactosidase, α- and β-glucosidase, or α-amylase) [50]. Several studies have demonstrated that *Lachnospiraceae* (including *Blautia*) are upregulated during diabetes-associated obesity [51] and during the development of non-alcoholic fatty liver disease (NAFLD) [52]. The increase in *Lachnospiraceae* (including *Blautia*) in these metabolic disorders may be partly explained by hyperglycemia that often occurs during obesity-related diabetes as well as NAFLD [51,53]. Likewise, our correlation analysis indicates that *Lachnospiraceae* was positively associated with fasting glucose levels.

Monoglobus, *Lachnospiraceae* NK4A136 group, and *Oscillospiraceae* were enriched in the low-dose AEC group, while the *Eubacteria* group, *Faecalibaculum*, and *Bifidobacterium* were enriched in the high-dose AEC group. These results suggest that the effect of AEC on the gut microbiome might be dose-dependent. A study suggested that *Caulerpa racemosa* exhibits antimicrobial activity that may inhibit pathogenic bacteria [54]. In this study, a high dose of AEC increased the SCFA producers such as *Faecalibacterium* and *Bifidobacterium*. In addition, these increases were negatively associated with the inflammatory marker (TNF-α), ADMA, and lipid profiles and positively associated with an increase in the antioxidant capacity (SOD levels) and PGC-1α levels in the blood. This suggests that the AEC effect on the regulation of inflammation-associated pathways as well as lipid-glucose regulation, may also be mediated by the modulation of *Faecalibacterium* and *Bifidobacterium* [55–57]. This shows that the Caulerpa genus has the potential to become a superfood, in line with a recent study showing its potential anti-non-communicable diseases properties, such as obesity-related diseases [58].

5. Conclusions

The aqueous extract of *Caulerpa racemosa* (AEC) exhibited potential antioxidant properties in vitro. Lipase inhibition, α-amylase, and α-glucosidase activities were observed. Thus, AEC is a promising functional ingredient with potential anti-cardiometabolic syndrome effects. The observed trends of the PRMT-1/DDAH/ADMA pathway and gut modulation of the microbiota demonstrated positive effects against cardiometabolic syndrome, achieved by dietary supplementation with a high dose (130 mg/kg Body Weight [BW]) of AEC. Human clinical trials are still needed and are being planned for the foreseeable future.

6. Patents

The preparation method and formulation of an aqueous extract of *Caulerpa racemosa* (AEC) resulting from the work reported in this study have been registered as a patent in Indonesia with number S00202211473 (Fahrul Nurkolis is a patent holder of the AEC Extract).

Supplementary Materials: The following supporting information can be downloaded at: https://www.mdpi.com/article/10.3390/nu15040909/s1, Table S1. High-Performance Liquid Chromatography-Mass Spectrometry (HPLC-MS) of Caulerpin in Aqueous Extract of *Caulerpa racemosa* (AEC).

Author Contributions: Conceptualization, F.N. and N.A.T.; investigation, F.N. and N.A.T.; formal analysis, F.N. and N.A.T.; methodology, F.N., H.H. and N.A.T.; data curation, F.N., R.K., D.S., W.B.G., V.M.Y. and R.J.K.; resources, F.N. and N.M.; project administration, F.N. and N.M.; writing—original draft preparation, F.N., N.A.T., R.K., D.S., W.B.G., V.M.Y. and R.J.K.; writing—review and editing, F.N., A.T., B.K., T.E.T., A.P., B.K., N.M., H.H., A.Y.S., V.M.Y., S.K., W.B.G. and N.A.T.; Software, F.N.; visualization, F.N., W.B.G., V.M.Y. and R.J.K.; supervision, N.A.T., H.H., B.K., A.Y.S., N.M., T.E.T. and A.T.; validation, N.A.T., H.H., B.K., A.Y.S., S.K., N.M., T.E.T., A.T. and A.P.; formal analysis, N.A.T., H.H., B.K., A.Y.S., S.K., N.M., T.E.T., A.T. and A.P.; writing—review and editing, F.N., N.A.T., H.H., B.K., A.Y.S., S.K., N.M., T.E.T., A.T. and A.P. All authors have read and agreed to the published version of the manuscript.

Funding: This research received no external funding. However, the APC was funded by Nurpudji Astuti Taslim (Clinical Nutrition, Faculty of Medicine, Hasanuddin University, Makassar, Indonesia).

Institutional Review Board Statement: The animal use research protocol makes mention of the Declaration of Helsinki and the Council of International Organizations of Medical Sciences (CIOMS). Additionally, all procedures involving animal research adhere to the Guidelines for Reporting In Vivo Experiments (ARRIVE) and have passed approval from the ethics board of the International Register of Preclinical Trial Animal Studies Protocols (preclinicaltrials.eu; 7 October 2022) with registration number PCTE0000329.

Informed Consent Statement: Not applicable.

Data Availability Statement: The data datasets generated and/or analyzed in this study are available on request from the corresponding author.

Acknowledgments: The authors express gratitude to all contributors, who they cannot mention one by one, for their amazing contribution to doing the research and writing the paper. We also want to express our respects to our amazing people who have given input and motivated us to keep our research passion during the pandemic, especially on the writing processes of this article: 1. Hardinsyah; 2. Nurpudji Astuti Taslim; 3. Apollinaire Tsopmo; 4. Trina E. Tallei; 5. Bonglee Kim, and Sojin Kang. Thanks also to UIN Sunan Kalijaga for granting research permission.

Conflicts of Interest: The authors declare no conflict of interest.

References

1. Kirk, E.P.; Klein, S. Pathogenesis and pathophysiology of the cardiometabolic syndrome. *J. Clin. Hypertens.* **2009**, *11*, 761–765. [CrossRef] [PubMed]
2. Magon, N.; Chauhan, M. Pregnancy and the Formative Fifteen of Diabetes. *J. Obstet. Gynecol. India* **2014**, *64*, 440–441. [CrossRef] [PubMed]
3. Kalra, S.; Chawla, R.; Madhu, S. The dirty dozen of diabetes. *Indian J. Endocrinol. Metab.* **2013**, *17*, 367. [CrossRef] [PubMed]
4. Giacco, F.; Brownlee, M. Oxidative stress and diabetic complications. *Circ. Res.* **2010**, *107*, 1058–1070. [CrossRef]
5. Association, A.D. Standards of Medical Care in Diabetes—2022 Abridged for Primary Care Providers. *Clin. Diabetes* **2022**, *40*, 10–38. [CrossRef]
6. Flood, D.; Seiglie, J.A.; Dunn, M.; Tschida, S.; Theilmann, M.; Marcus, M.E.; Brian, G.; Norov, B.; Mayige, M.T.; Gurung, M.S.; et al. The state of diabetes treatment coverage in 55 low-income and middle-income countries: A cross-sectional study of nationally representative, individual-level data in 680 102 adults. *Lancet Healthy Longev.* **2021**, *2*, e340–e351. [CrossRef]
7. Latifah, S.; Hartini, K.S.; Sadeli, A. Yuandani Identification of medicinal plants used by the community for indigenous poultry health management. *IOP Conf. Ser. Mater. Sci. Eng.* **2021**, *1122*, 012045. [CrossRef]
8. Mandlik, R.V.; Naik, S.R.; Zine, S.; Ved, H.; Doshi, G. Antidiabetic Activity of Caulerpa racemosa: Role of Proinflammatory Mediators, Oxidative Stress, and Other Biomarkers. *Planta Medica Int. Open* **2022**, *9*, e60–e71. [CrossRef]

9. Yang, P.; Liu, D.Q.; Liang, T.J.; Li, J.; Zhang, H.Y.; Liu, A.H.; Guo, Y.W.; Mao, S.C. Bioactive constituents from the green alga Caulerpa racemosa. *Bioorg. Med. Chem.* **2015**, *23*, 38–45. [CrossRef]
10. Cao, M.; Li, Y.; Famurewa, A.C.; Olatunji, O.J. Antidiabetic and nephroprotective effects of polysaccharide extract from the seaweed caulerpa racemosa in high fructose-streptozotocin induced diabetic nephropathy. *Diabetes Metab. Syndr. Obes. Targets Ther.* **2021**, *14*, 2121–2131. [CrossRef]
11. Juturu, V. Polyphenols and Cardiometabolic Syndrome. In *Polyphenols in Human Health and Disease*; Academic Press: Cambridge, MA, USA, 2013; Volume 2, pp. 1067–1076. ISBN 9780123984562.
12. Permatasari, H.K.; Nurkolis, F.; Hardinsyah, H.; Taslim, N.A.; Sabrina, N.; Ibrahim, F.M.; Visnu, J.; Kumalawati, D.A.; Febriana, S.A.; Sudargo, T.; et al. Metabolomic Assay, Computational Screening, and Pharmacological Evaluation of Caulerpa racemosa as an Anti-obesity With Anti-aging by Altering Lipid Profile and Peroxisome Proliferator-Activated Receptor-γ Coactivator 1-α Levels. *Front. Nutr.* **2022**, *9*, 1412. [CrossRef]
13. Permatasari, H.K.; Kuswari, M.; Nurkolis, F.; Mayulu, N.; Ibrahim, F.M.; Taslim, N.A.; Wewengkang, D.S.; Sabrina, N.; Arifin, G.R.; Mantik, K.E.K.; et al. Sea grapes extract improves blood glucose, total cholesterol, and PGC-1α in rats fed on cholesterol- and fat-enriched diet. *F1000Research* **2021**, *10*, 718. [CrossRef]
14. Permatasari, H.K.; Nurkolis, F.; Mayulu, N.; Vivo, C.D.; Noor, S.L.; Rahmawati, R.; Radu, S.; Hardinsyah, H.; Taslim, N.A.; Wewengkang, D.S.; et al. Sea grapes powder with the addition of tempe rich in collagen: An anti-aging functional food. *F1000Research* **2022**, *10*, 789. [CrossRef]
15. Nagahawatta, D.P.; Asanka Sanjeewa, K.K.; Jayawardena, T.U.; Kim, H.S.; Yang, H.W.; Jiang, Y.; Je, J.G.; Lee, T.K.; Jeon, Y.J. Drying seaweeds using hybrid hot water Goodle dryer (HHGD): Comparison with freeze-dryer in chemical composition and antioxidant activity. *Fish. Aquat. Sci.* **2021**, *24*, 19–31. [CrossRef]
16. Premarathna, A.D.; Ranahewa, T.H.; Wijesekera, S.K.; Harishchandra, D.L.; Karunathilake, K.J.K.; Waduge, R.N.; Wijesundara, R.R.M.K.K.; Jayasooriya, A.P.; Wijewardana, V.; Rajapakse, R.P.V.J. Preliminary screening of the aqueous extracts of twenty-three different seaweed species in Sri Lanka with in-vitro and in-vivo assays. *Heliyon* **2020**, *6*, e03918. [CrossRef]
17. Bao, X.; Bai, D.; Liu, X.; Wang, Y.; Zeng, L.; Wei, C.; Jin, W. Effects of the Cistanche tubulosa Aqueous Extract on the Gut Microbiota of Mice with Intestinal Disorders. *Evid.-Based Complement. Altern. Med.* **2021**, *2021*, 4936970. [CrossRef]
18. Sabrina, N.; Rizal, M.; Nurkolis, F.; Hardinsyah, H.; Tanner, M.J.; Gunawan, W.B.; Handoko, M.N.; Mayulu, N.; Taslim, N.A.; Puspaningtyas, D.S.; et al. Bioactive peptides identification and nutritional status ameliorating properties on malnourished rats of combined eel and soy-based tempe flour. *Front. Nutr.* **2022**, *9*, 2196. [CrossRef]
19. Permatasari, H.K.; Nurkolis, F.; Gunawan, W.B.; Yusuf, V.M.; Yusuf, M.; Kusuma, R.J.; Sabrina, N.; Muharram, F.R.; Taslim, N.A.; Mayulu, N.; et al. Modulation of gut microbiota and markers of metabolic syndrome in mice on cholesterol and fat enriched diet by butterfly pea flower kombucha. *Curr. Res. Food Sci.* **2022**, *5*, 1251–1265. [CrossRef] [PubMed]
20. Permatasari, H.K.; Firani, N.K.; Prijadi, B.; Irnandi, D.F.; Riawan, W.; Yusuf, M.; Amar, N.; Chandra, L.A.; Yusuf, V.M.; Subali, A.D.; et al. Kombucha drink enriched with sea grapes (*Caulerpa racemosa*) as potential functional beverage to contrast obesity: An in vivo and in vitro approach. *Clin. Nutr. ESPEN* **2022**, *49*, 232–240. [CrossRef]
21. Tapotubun, A.M.; Matrutty, T.E.A.A.; Riry, J.; Tapotubun, E.J.; Fransina, E.G.; Mailoa, M.N.; Riry, W.A.; Setha, B.; Rieuwpassa, F. Seaweed Caulerpa sp. position as functional food. In *Proceedings of the IOP Conference Series: Earth and Environmental Science*; IOP Publishing: Bristol, UK, 2020; Volume 517, p. 012021.
22. Forman, H.J.; Zhang, H.; Rinna, A. Glutathione: Overview of its protective roles, measurement, and biosynthesis. *Mol. Asp. Med.* **2009**, *30*, 1–12. [CrossRef] [PubMed]
23. Belkacemi, L.; Belalia, M.; Djendara, A.; Bouhadda, Y. Antioxidant and antibacterial activities and identification of bioactive compounds of various extracts of *Caulerpa racemosa* from Algerian coast. *Asian Pac. J. Trop. Biomed.* **2020**, *10*, 87–94. [CrossRef]
24. Yap, W.F.; Tay, V.; Tan, S.H.; Yow, Y.Y.; Chew, J. Decoding antioxidant and antibacterial potentials of Malaysian green seaweeds: *Caulerpa racemosa* and *Caulerpa lentillifera*. *Antibiotics* **2019**, *8*, 152. [CrossRef]
25. de Alencar, D.B.; de Carvalho, F.C.T.; Rebouças, R.H.; dos Santos, D.R.; dos Santos Pires-Cavalcante, K.M.; de Lima, R.L.; Baracho, B.M.; Bezerra, R.M.; Viana, F.A.; dos Fernandes Vieira, R.H.S.; et al. Bioactive extracts of red seaweeds *Pterocladiella capillacea* and *Osmundaria obtusiloba* (Floridophyceae: Rhodophyta) with antioxidant and bacterial agglutination potential. *Asian Pac. J. Trop. Med.* **2016**, *9*, 372–379. [CrossRef] [PubMed]
26. Chielle, E.O.; Gens, F.; Rossi, E.M. Oxidative, inflammatory and cardiometabolic biomarkers of clinical relevance in patients with metabolic syndrome. *J. Bras. Patol. Med. Lab.* **2018**, *54*, 213–219. [CrossRef]
27. Tiwari, B.K. Ultrasound: A clean, green extraction technology. *TrAC-Trends Anal. Chem.* **2015**, *71*, 100–109. [CrossRef]
28. Spínola, V.; Llorent-Martínez, E.; Lwt, P.C. Inhibition of α-amylase, α-glucosidase and pancreatic lipase by phenolic compounds of *Rumex maderensis* (Madeira sorrel). Influence of simulated gastrointestinal digestion on hyperglycaemia-related damage linked with aldose reductase activity and protein glycation. *LWT* **2020**, *118*, 108727.
29. Chen, X.; Xu, G.; Li, X.; Li, Z.; Ying, H. Purification of an α-amylase inhibitor in a polyethylene glycol/fructose-1,6-bisphosphate trisodium salt aqueous two-phase system. *Process Biochem.* **2008**, *43*, 765–768. [CrossRef]
30. Chaves Filho, G.P.; de Paula Oliveira, R.; de Medeiros, S.R.B.; Rocha, H.A.O.; Moreira, S.M.G. Sulfated polysaccharides from green seaweed *Caulerpa prolifera* suppress fat accumulation. *J. Appl. Phycol.* **2020**, *32*, 4299–4307. [CrossRef]

31. Manoppo, J.I.C.; Nurkolis, F.; Pramono, A.; Ardiaria, M.; Murbawani, E.A.; Yusuf, M.; Qhabibi, F.R.; Yusuf, V.M.; Amar, N.; Karim, M.R.A.; et al. Amelioration of obesity-related metabolic disorders via supplementation of *Caulerpa lentillifera* in rats fed with a high-fat and high-cholesterol diet. *Front. Nutr.* **2022**, *9*, 2124. [CrossRef]
32. Sakers, A.; De Siqueira, M.K.; Seale, P.; Villanueva, C.J. Adipose-tissue plasticity in health and disease. *Cell* **2022**, *185*, 419–446. [CrossRef] [PubMed]
33. Shulman, G.I. Ectopic Fat in Insulin Resistance, Dyslipidemia, and Cardiometabolic Disease. *N. Engl. J. Med.* **2014**, *371*, 1131–1141. [CrossRef] [PubMed]
34. Gong, L.; Feng, D.; Wang, T.; Ren, Y.; Liu, Y.; Wang, J. Inhibitors of α-amylase and α-glucosidase: Potential linkage for whole cereal foods on prevention of hyperglycemia. *Food Sci. Nutr.* **2020**, *8*, 6320–6337. [CrossRef]
35. Ali, K.M.; Wonnerth, A.; Huber, K.; Wojta, J. Cardiovascular disease risk reduction by raising HDL cholesterol—Current therapies and future opportunities. *Br. J. Pharmacol.* **2012**, *167*, 1177–1194. [CrossRef]
36. Pistrosch, F.; Natali, A.; Hanefeld, M. Is hyperglycemia a cardiovascular risk factor? *Diabetes Care* **2011**, *34* (Suppl. S2), S128–S131. [CrossRef]
37. Stanley Schwartz, S. Type 2 diabetes mellitus and the cardiometabolic syndrome: Impact of incretin-based therapies. *Diabetes Metab. Syndr. Obes. Targets Ther.* **2010**, *2010*, 227–242. [CrossRef] [PubMed]
38. Rosa, A.C.; Corsi, D.; Cavi, N.; Bruni, N.; Dosio, F. Superoxide dismutase administration: A review of proposed human uses. *Molecules* **2021**, *26*, 1844. [CrossRef]
39. Younus, H. Therapeutic potentials of superoxide dismutase. *Int. J. Health Sci.* **2018**, *12*, 88–93.
40. Akhigbe, R.; Ajayi, A. The impact of reactive oxygen species in the development of cardiometabolic disorders: A review. *Lipids Health Dis.* **2021**, *20*, 23. [CrossRef]
41. Chen, L.; Qin, Y.; Liu, B.; Gao, M.; Li, A.; Li, X.; Gong, G. PGC-1α-Mediated Mitochondrial Quality Control: Molecular Mechanisms and Implications for Heart Failure. *Front. Cell Dev. Biol.* **2022**, *10*, 871357. [CrossRef] [PubMed]
42. Rius-Pérez, S.; Torres-Cuevas, I.; Millán, I.; Ortega, Á.L.; Pérez, S.; Sandhu, M.A. PGC-1 α, Inflammation, and Oxidative Stress: An Integrative View in Metabolism. *Oxid. Med. Cell. Longev.* **2020**, *2020*, 1452696. [CrossRef]
43. Esser, N.; Paquot, N.; Scheen, A.J. Inflammatory markers and cardiometabolic diseases. *Acta Clin. Belgica Int. J. Clin. Lab. Med.* **2015**, *70*, 193–199. [CrossRef]
44. Brenner, D.R.; Arora, P.; Garcia-Bailo, B. The Relationship between Metabolic Syndrome and Markers of Cardiometabolic Disease among Canadian Adults. *J. Diabetes Metab.* **2011**, *S2*, 003. [CrossRef]
45. Chen, Y.; Xu, X.; Sheng, M.; Zhang, X.; Gu, Q.; Zheng, Z. PRMT-1 and DDAHs-induced ADMA upregulation is involved in ROS- and RAS-mediated diabetic retinopathy. *Exp. Eye Res.* **2009**, *89*, 1028–1034. [CrossRef]
46. Pope, A.J.; Karuppiah, K.; Cardounel, A.J. Role of the PRMT-DDAH-ADMA axis in the regulation of endothelial nitric oxide production. *Pharmacol. Res.* **2009**, *60*, 461–465. [CrossRef]
47. Fulton, M.D.; Brown, T.; George Zheng, Y. The biological axis of protein arginine methylation and asymmetric dimethylarginine. *Int. J. Mol. Sci.* **2019**, *20*, 3322. [CrossRef] [PubMed]
48. Cao, Y.; Mu, J.J.; Fang, Y.; Yuan, Z.Y.; Liu, F.Q. Impact of high salt independent of blood pressure on PRMT/ADMA/DDAH pathway in the aorta of dahl salt-sensitive rats. *Int. J. Mol. Sci.* **2013**, *14*, 8062–8072. [CrossRef]
49. Sayers, E.W.; Barrett, T.; Benson, D.A.; Bolton, E.; Bryant, S.H.; Canese, K.; Chetvernin, V.; Church, D.M.; Dicuccio, M.; Federhen, S.; et al. Database resources of the National Center for Biotechnology Information. *Nucleic Acids Res.* **2010**, *38*, D5–D16. [CrossRef]
50. Vacca, M.; Celano, G.; Calabrese, F.M.; Portincasa, P.; Gobbetti, M.; De Angelis, M. The controversial role of human gut lachnospiraceae. *Microorganisms* **2020**, *8*, 573. [CrossRef]
51. Kameyama, K.; Itoh, K. Intestinal colonization by a lachnospiraceae bacterium contributes to the development of diabetes in obese mice. *Microbes Environ.* **2014**, *29*, 427–430. [CrossRef] [PubMed]
52. Shen, F.; Zheng, R.D.; Sun, X.Q.; Ding, W.J.; Wang, X.Y.; Fan, J.G. Gut microbiota dysbiosis in patients with non-alcoholic fatty liver disease. *Hepatobiliary Pancreat. Dis. Int.* **2017**, *16*, 375–381. [CrossRef] [PubMed]
53. Zhai, B.; Zhang, C.; Sheng, Y.; Zhao, C.; He, X.; Xu, W.; Huang, K.; Luo, Y. Hypoglycemic and hypolipidemic effect of S-allyl-cysteine sulfoxide (alliin) in DIO mice. *Sci. Rep.* **2018**, *8*, 3527. [CrossRef]
54. Nagaraj, S.R.; Osborne, J.W. Bioactive compounds from Caulerpa racemosa as a potent larvicidal and antibacterial agent. *Front. Biol.* **2014**, *9*, 300–305. [CrossRef]
55. Salazar, N.; Neyrinck, A.M.; Bindels, L.B.; Druart, C.; Ruas-Madiedo, P.; Cani, P.D.; de los Reyes-Gavilán, C.G.; Delzenne, N.M. Functional effects of EPS-producing bifidobacterium administration on energy metabolic alterations of diet-induced obese mice. *Front. Microbiol.* **2019**, *10*, 1809. [CrossRef]
56. Ma, L.; Zheng, A.; Ni, L.; Wu, L.; Hu, L.; Zhao, Y.; Fu, Z.; Ni, Y. Bifidobacterium animalis subsp. lactis lkm512 Attenuates Obesity-Associated Inflammation and Insulin Resistance through the Modification of Gut Microbiota in High-Fat Diet-Induced Obese Mice. *Mol. Nutr. Food Res.* **2022**, *66*, 2100639. [CrossRef] [PubMed]

57. Maioli, T.U.; Borras-Nogues, E.; Torres, L.; Barbosa, S.C.; Martins, V.D.; Langella, P.; Azevedo, V.A.; Chatel, J.M. Possible Benefits of Faecalibacterium prausnitzii for Obesity-Associated Gut Disorders. *Front. Pharmacol.* **2021**, *12*, 740636. [CrossRef] [PubMed]
58. Nurkolis, F.; Taslim, N.A.; Qhabibi, F.R.; Kang, S.; Moon, M.; Choi, J.; Choi, M.; Park, M.N.; Mayulu, N.; Kim, B. Ulvophyte Green Algae *Caulerpa lentillifera*: Metabolites Profile and Antioxidant, Anticancer, Anti-Obesity, and In Vitro Cytotoxicity Properties. *Molecules* **2023**, *28*, 1365. [CrossRef]

Disclaimer/Publisher's Note: The statements, opinions and data contained in all publications are solely those of the individual author(s) and contributor(s) and not of MDPI and/or the editor(s). MDPI and/or the editor(s) disclaim responsibility for any injury to people or property resulting from any ideas, methods, instructions or products referred to in the content.

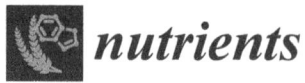

Article

SnackTrack—An App-Based Tool to Assess the Influence of Digital and Physical Environments on Snack Choice

Eva Valenčič [1,2,3,4,*], Emma Beckett [2,5], Clare E. Collins [1,2], Barbara Koroušić Seljak [3,4] and Tamara Bucher [2,5]

1. School of Health Sciences, College of Health, Medicine and Wellbeing, University of Newcastle, Callaghan, Newcastle, NSW 2308, Australia
2. Food and Nutrition Program, Hunter Medical Research Institute, New Lambton Heights, Newcastle, NSW 2305, Australia
3. Computer Systems Department, Jožef Stefan Institute, 1000 Ljubljana, Slovenia
4. Jožef Stefan International Postgraduate School, 1000 Ljubljana, Slovenia
5. School of Environmental and Life Sciences, College of Engineering, Science and Environment, University of Newcastle, Callaghan, Newcastle, NSW 2308, Australia
* Correspondence: eva.valencic@uon.edu.au

Abstract: As food choices are usually processed subconsciously, both situational and food environment cues influence choice. This study developed and tested a mobile app to investigate the association between physical and digital environments on snack choices. SnackTrack was designed and used to collect data on the snack choices of 188 users in real-life settings during an 8-week feasibility trial. The app asks users to take a photo of the food they are planning to consume and to provide additional information regarding the physical environment and context in which this food was eaten. The app also displayed various user interface designs (i.e., different background images) to investigate the potential effects of images on snack choice. Preliminary results suggest that the time of snack obtainment did not have a significant effect on the healthfulness of the snacks chosen. Conversely, it was found that unhealthy background images appeared to encourage healthier snack choices. In conclusion, despite consumers having the knowledge to make healthy choices, environmental cues can alter food choices. SnackTrack, a novel tool to investigate the influence of physical and digital environments on consumers' food choices, provides possibilities for exploring what encourages (un)healthy eating behaviours.

Keywords: digital nudging; user interface; food environment; choice behaviour; snacks; snack choice; food choice

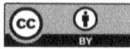

1. Introduction

Consumer behaviour, including food and nutrition choices, is influenced by factors at the individual and environmental levels. However, the DONE interactive framework [1] demonstrates that environmental factors have the greatest influence on food choices, and importantly, they can be modified. Therefore, strategies to improve dietary habits that are linked with food choices need to focus not only on individual behaviours but also on the food environment and the conditions in which people live and make food choices [2].

Some environmental factors shown to influence food choice and amounts consumed include availability, the effort required for consumption [3], the variety [4] and portion sizes [5] of food presented. Hence, strategically restructuring physical and digital food choice environments appears to be a promising avenue to improve dietary habits and promote population health [6,7]. Modifying the environment by making healthier choices easier and more accessible may have a positive influence on consumers' food choices. This approach has been described as nudging, which is defined as "any aspect of the choice architecture that alters people's behaviour in a predictable way without forbidding any options or significantly changing their economic incentives." [6].

An individual's health behaviour is determined by conscious and systematic intentions, as well as by automatic, nonintentional and subconscious processes [8]. While habits, including eating habits, can be difficult to change at the individual level, they are affected by environmental cues, such as the visibility of food, which are frequently processed unconsciously. Thus, environmental cues, which are processed outside of conscious awareness, could help in targeting automatic, effortless and spontaneous processes and therefore nudge healthier food choices [9–12]. One such potential cue is imagery, which carries messages which viewers decode and react to [13]. Food imagery, particularly, may increase food-related thoughts, cravings, hunger, guilt, appetitive appeal, and motivation to eat [11]. It has been shown that images influence consumers' trust and ease of use of websites [14]. However, to date, few studies have investigated if and how imagery influences food choices [15–19].

In recent years, the consumers' everyday food choice environments shifted, with food choices now regularly conducted in digital settings, such as online grocery stores, pre-ordering systems, food delivery services, etc. In contrast to traditional food choice environments, the perception of visual cues in a digital setting is entirely mediated through a user interface (UI). As such, UI design may play an important role in consumer perception and food selection. This raises the importance of research in digital nudging, which is defined as "the use of user-interface design elements to guide people's behaviour in digital choice environments" [20]. A recent review showed that digital nudging is a rapidly growing field, increasingly investigated in food and health contexts [21]. Therefore, the scope of a feasibility study presented in this paper pertains specifically to the imagery used in digital UI and its influence on users.

To date, little is known about how people make food choices within digital environments and which key elements of the UI influence food perception, selection and purchase [7]. Although information and communication technologies are commonly used in the healthy-eating context, research on online tools for guiding consumers' decision-making processes in the context of healthy food choices is lacking [22]. Additionally, the lack of empirical evidence limits our understanding of how imagery could be used to nudge healthy food choices and if it may even lead to unhealthy food choices.

The frequency of snacking [23] and the contribution of snacks to total energy intake has increased. Research shows that more than 30% of energy comes from snack occasions among Australian children [24] and that snacking contributes to almost one-quarter of total energy intake among Canadian adults [25]. Since the impact of snacking on the overall diet quality depends on their nutritional composition [26], in this study, we specifically focused on snack choices. Snacking is typically defined as the consumption of food or drink between main meals [27]. However, the interpretation of the terms 'snacks' and 'snacking' may vary by country [28].

In order to understand the contribution of environmental factors and determine the triggers for snack choices, we were interested in tools allowing participants to repeatedly report their experiences in real-time and real-world settings. This kind of report is called Ecological Momentary Assessment [29]. As we could not find a publicly available tool to efficiently investigate environmental and nudging impacts on food choices, the aim of this study was to develop and test a mobile app [30] to assess the contribution of physical and digital environments (i.e., digital nudging). The app allows users to track their snacks while exposing them to different UI designs (implemented as mobile app backgrounds).

2. Materials and Methods
2.1. Study Design

The feasibility study aimed to design, test and assess a mobile application, and to investigate associations between the digital and the physical environment with snack choices. A mobile app called SnackTrack was designed and developed by the University of Newcastle, Australia, in collaboration with the Computer Systems Department, Jožef Stefan Institute (JSI). SnackTrack was used to collect data on consumers' snack choices in real-life settings, and the study involved an 8-week feasibility trial to investigate which environmental factors are associated with snack choices. The app enables users to take a photo of the food they are planning to consume via the phone's camera and allows individuals to provide additional information regarding the physical environment and context in which the food was consumed by selecting pre-set options (e.g., when and how was it obtained, where was eaten, etc.). The whole process of submitting photo(s) and additional information was developed to be as intuitive as possible and not too demanding for app users. For example, participants did not have to enter text or write the answers; they only had to select the most appropriate ones.

The development of SnackTrack focussed on designing a mobile app with a variable UI (in this case, background images) to investigate whether UIs can be used to nudge consumers/app users. In the present study, the goal was to create an app which could be used to investigate whether different mobile backgrounds could nudge consumers towards selecting healthier snack options. Four different backgrounds were implemented and randomised to participants in the intervention conditions. The backgrounds were real-life photos related to either healthy (fruits, vegetables) or unhealthy (sweets, salty snacks) foods (See Figure S1 in Supplementary Materials). These photos were selected because if we wanted to ensure primes will influence consumers and encourage healthy behaviours, environmental cues need to be congruent with health-relevant concepts and products and need to complement the other components in the triggered environment [11]. As nudging should be subconscious, there was no mention of or emphasis on the presence of the backgrounds. Participants allocated to the Control condition used the app without an image background (grey plain-coloured background).

Ethical approval for this study was obtained from the University of Newcastle Human Research Ethics Committee (Approval number H-2020-0267).

2.2. Participants and Procedure

Participants were recruited in the period from February to April 2022 via social media and printed posters (displayed at JSI and on campus at the University of Newcastle). Individuals interested in participating in the study scanned a QR code on the recruitment material to download the mobile app SnackTrack from either the Apple App store or Google Play. SnackTrack was only available in the app stores in Australia (English version) and Slovenia (Slovenian version). After downloading the app, participants received a study information statement, and consent was obtained online prior to the data collection. Each participant received a unique code to protect their privacy; thus, no information on identity was recorded during the research study. Before being able to use the app, participants provided information about their sex and year of birth. Only participants aged 18 years or older were eligible to participate.

Participants were randomised into 5 conditions (4 intervention conditions; mobile background containing photos of either (i) fruits, (ii) vegetables, (iii) salty snacks or (iv) sweets, and a Control condition (v); grey-coloured background). Randomisation was performed directly in the app, using an algorithmic approach for randomisation to avoid any subjective decision. Each background was assigned once per cycle; therefore, each 5th participant downloading the app was allocated to the Control condition. Participants were asked to take photos of the snacks they consumed or were planning to consume throughout the day. Participants were instructed to capture the photo of the foods as close as possible and to make sure that the food was clearly visible. Photos could be taken of the snacking occasion (e.g., multiple food items on one photo,) or each food item could be captured separately. Photos submitted at the same time were treated as one snacking occasion. Together with photos of snacks, additional data about snacking choices, such as how and when the snack was obtained and where and in the company of how many people the snack was consumed, were collected. A screenshot of the additional data screen with the vegetable background is shown in Figure S2 in Supplementary Material. Participants were asked to upload at least 15 photos over 15 days between February and April 2022. Therefore, they were asked to use the app at least once a day for at least 15 days (no need to be consecutive). Participants who submitted at least 15 photos of actual foods were eligible to be included in a prize draw for either a $50AUD gift card (Australian participants) or a €10 gift card (Slovenian participants).

2.3. Sample Size

We aimed to recruit 500 participants (250 from each country, 50 in each condition), which is the number needed to detect medium to large effect sizes. We anticipated recruiting as many participants as possible within the eight weeks of the intervention.

2.4. Measures

After data collection was completed, we checked all the photos and removed duplicates. Duplicates could have been uploaded if the internet connection was lost while submitting the photo (this resulted in uploads of multiple of the same photos on the server). In some cases, the photos were not uploaded to the server correctly, and we could not open and see the photos. These photos were also removed from the analysis. After the removal of duplicates and 'broken' photos, we annotated and described each photo (snack). We annotated the name of the food on the photo (e.g., chocolate bar), the Nutri-Score (NS) [31] of the foods, and the food group the food corresponds to. The food groups used, together with examples based on submitted photos, are shown in Table 1.

Table 1. Food groups with examples of foods corresponding to them.

Food Group	Examples of Foods in the Food Group
Fruits	Fresh fruits, fruit-only containing smoothies, dried fruits
Vegetables	Fresh and pickled vegetables
Salty snacks	Chips, tortilla chips, popcorn, salty crackers, salty sticks/pretzels
Sweets	Chocolate bars, cookies, candy, granola/muesli/protein/nut/fruit bar, sweet pastries, cakes, waffles, etc.
Grains	Bread bun, sour pastries, rice cakes, etc.
Dairy and dairy substitutes	Yoghurt (natural or flavoured), quark, puddings, plant-based yoghurt
Meat, fish & egg	Cold cuts, jerky, salmon, eggs
Beverage	Juices, coffee/tea (with milk), carbonated drinks, energy drinks, alcoholic beverages
Nut	Nuts (plain, roasted, salted), nuts with dried fruits
Mixed dishes and other foods	Sandwich, toast with spread, soup, pizza, fries, porridge, breaded vegetables, pancakes with spreads, peanut butter, honey, etc.

The primary outcome variable was the average NS [31–33], which is a colour-coded index of overall diet quality ranging from A (healthiest) to E (least healthy) based on the British Food Standard Agency Nutrient Profiling System. For each snack (photo), we applied the standard Nutri-Score algorithm to assign a score from A to E based on nutritional quality. Later, we recorded the scores as numbers from 5 (A: the healthiest) to 1 (E: the least healthy). We calculated an average score for the snacking occasion in the following cases: when the photo contained multiple foods (e.g., mandarins and chocolate bar) as a part of one snacking occasion or if participants submitted more than 1 photo, but it was clear that the photos were part of one snacking occasion (e.g., on 1 photo a hot cross bun, and on the other a handful of nuts; both photos were submitted together).

In addition, two independent accredited dietitians (one from Slovenia and one from Australia) were asked to assess the healthiness of the photos. They assigned a score from 1 (very unhealthy) to 5 (very healthy). The dietitian's holistic assessment score (DA) was needed because NS could not be applied to all of the snacks, as some photos did not contain the information needed to assign the score. For example, foods prepared and self-packed in advance did not contain the dietary labels needed to calculate the NS (e.g., we could not distinguish the fat content of dairy products).

2.5. Data Analysis

Descriptive statistics were used to describe the properties of participants and the additional data about snacking choices (when and where the snacks were obtained, where they were eaten and with whom) using Microsoft Excel and R software [34] (v. 4.2.0, for iOS). Demographic details were summarised with frequencies, means, and standard deviations (SD) as appropriate. The time of the photo submission was considered as the time of the snack consumption. For data analysis, time was corrected to correspond to either CEST or AEST time zone (Daylight saving time change was taken into consideration), depending on the participant's location.

Data were tested for normality with the Shapiro–Wilk test, and the homogeneity of variances was tested using Levene's test, using R software; p-values <0.05 were considered statistically significant. Statistical comparison of the differences in NS and DA between conditions was performed using a Kruskal–Wallis test, followed by Dunn's posthoc test (p-value adjustment method; Benjamini and Hochberg). A chi-squared test was used to compare the proportions of food groups in the 5 conditions.

3. Results

3.1. Participants

A total of 284 adults downloaded the app; of those, 80 were from Australia and 204 from Slovenia. Of the 284, 95 people had not submitted any photo, and one person entered invalid data for their year of birth. Therefore, data from 188 people (52 from Australia and 136 from Slovenia) were included in the final analysis. Out of those, 64 people submitted 15 photos or more, and the average number of days participants were using the app was 5.02. Participants were randomised in Control (n = 36), 'Fruit' (n = 47), 'Vegetable' (n = 34), 'Salty snacks' (n = 36), and 'Sweets' condition (n = 35). Participants in the Control condition submitted 353 photos; in the 'Fruit' condition, 441 photos; in the 'Vegetable' condition, 297 photos; in the 'Salty snacks' condition, 354 photos; and in the 'Sweets' condition, they submitted 318 photos.

The mean age of the participants was 35.5 years (±12.8); of those, 72.3% identified themselves as female (n = 135), 25% as male (n = 47), 2.1% as other (n = 4), and 1.1% declined to answer (n = 2).

3.2. Feasibility Outcomes

During the intervention, participants submitted a total of 1763 (1297 from Slovenia and 466 from Australia) photos of snacks. Of those, 76.1% (n = 1343) were obtained at the moment of consumption (80.3% (n = 1042) from Slovenia and 64.6% (n = 301) from Australia) and 23.8% (n = 420) were obtained more than one-hour prior consumption (19.7% (n = 255) from Slovenia and 35.4% (n = 165) from Australia). Most snacks were purchased by the participants themselves (66.3%; n = 1169), whereas 33.7% (n = 594) of snacks were purchased by someone else, or participants got them for free. The majority of snacks were consumed when participants were by themselves (74.9%; n = 1322), followed by when they were accompanied by one additional person (14.5%; n = 257), more than two people (6.5%; n = 114), or by exactly two people (4.0%; n = 70). Overall, the most snacks were consumed at the dining table (26.6%; n = 469), followed by on the sofa (21.6%; n = 382), at the working desk (21.3%; n = 375), in the workplace (15.0%; n = 265), on the go (7.3%; n = 129), in restaurants/cafés (1.2%; n = 22), and "other" was selected for 6.9% of the snacks. The majority of snacks consumed by Australian participants were eaten at the working desk (35%; n = 163), while Slovenian participants consumed the most snacks at the dining table (31.8%; n = 412). See Figure 1 for more details.

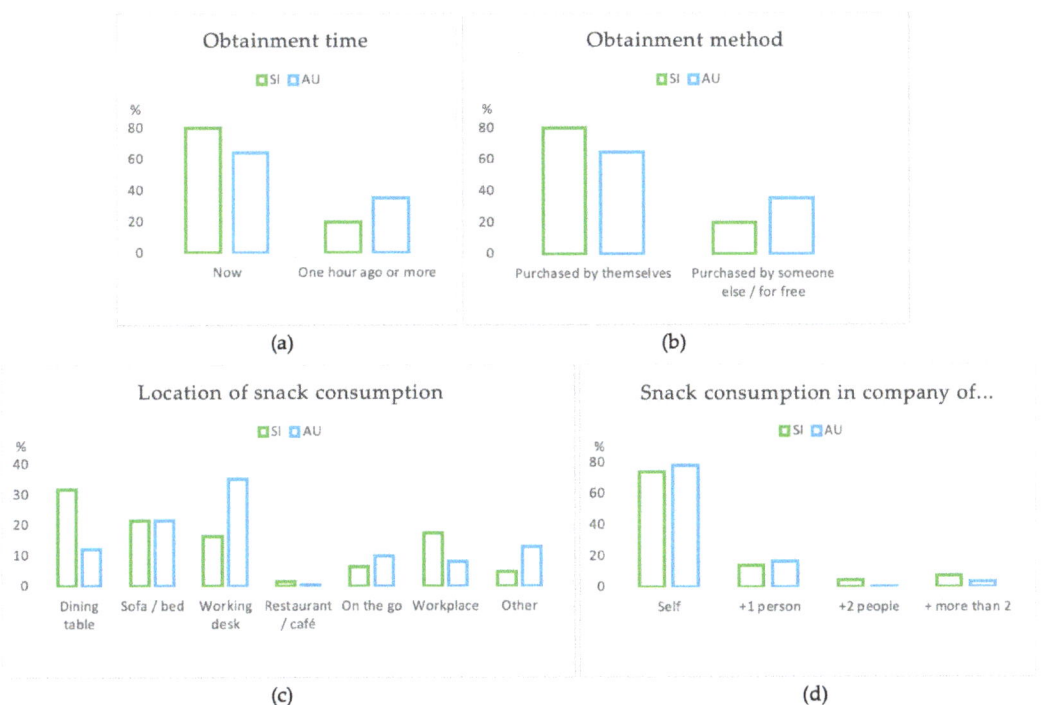

Figure 1. Results on the context of snack consumption: (**a**) Time of snack obtainment; (**b**) Method of snack obtainment; (**c**) Location of snack consumption; (**d**) How many people participants were with while eating the snacks.

When the time of the day of the snacking occasion was considered, it was found that 37.6% (n = 663) of reported snacks were consumed in the morning (from 5 a.m. to 12:59 p.m.), 36.9% (n = 652) in the afternoon (from 1 p.m. to 5:59 p.m.), and 25.4% (n = 448) in the evening/at night (from 6 p.m. to 4:59 a.m.). Slovenian participants submitted the most pictures of snacks between 5–6 p.m., while Australian participants between 4–5 p.m. We found that photos of snacks submitted by men are more likely to be consumed in the evening (24.9%) than those of women (18.1%).

The mean NS of all submitted snacks was 2.7 ± 1.6 out of five, and the mean DA was 2.5 ± 1.6 out of five. The nutritional quality of snacks among men was slightly poorer (NS: 2.5 ± 1.7 and DA: 2.4 ± 1.6) compared to women (NS: 2.7 ± 1.6 and DA: 2.5 ± 1.6) but not statistically different (NS: p = 0.66; DA: p = 0.32). Additionally, the difference in NS and DA between Australians (NS: 3.1 ± 1.6; DA: 2.6 ± 1.6) and Slovenians (NS: 2.5 ± 1.6; DA: 2.4 ± 1.5) was significant (NS: $t(763)$ = 6.0612, p < 0.001; DA: $t(785)$ = 2.6708, p = 0.008), meaning that Australians consumed healthier snacks. In addition, the results showed that the difference in NS and DA between snacks obtained at the moment of consumption (NS: 2.7 ± 1.6 and DA: 2.5 ± 1.5) and the ones obtained more than 1 hour before consumption (NS: 2.7 ± 1.7 and DA: 2.5 ± 1.6) was not significant (NS: $t(697)$ = 0.45216, p = 0.65; DA: $t(673)$ = −0.10023, p = 0.92), which means that the time of snack obtainment did not affect healthfulness of snacks. Moreover, snacks eaten when participants were alone were significantly healthier that when participants were in company with others (NS: $t(759)$ = −7.3674, p < 0.001; DA: $t(885)$ = −7.9996, p < 0.001).

Regarding the time of snacking, a Kruskal–Wallis H-test showed that there was a statistically significant difference in NS and DA between the times of day the snacks were consumed (NS: $\chi^2_{(2)}$ = 23.85, p < 0.001; DA: $\chi^2_{(2)}$ = 51.29, p < 0.001) with a mean

NS/DA score of 2.9/2.7 for morning snacks, 2.7/2.5 for afternoon snacks and 2.4/2.1 for evening snacks.

As the purpose of the app is to assess whether UI design (background) has an impact on the healthfulness of the snacks consumed, we first checked the mean NS and DA for all five backgrounds. The mean NS and DA scores were the lowest in the Control condition (NS: 2.4 ± 1.5; DA: 2.2 ± 1.5) and the highest in the 'Sweets' condition (NS: 2.9 ± 1.7; DA: 2.7 ± 1.6) as seen in Table 2. When analysing differences between the conditions (data were not normally distributed ($p < 0.001$) and did not have equal variance (NS: $p < 0.001$; DA: $p < 0.005$)) results showed that there was a statistically significant difference in NS ($\chi^2_{(4)} = 21.418$, $p = 0.0003$) and DA ($\chi^2_{(4)} = 18.392$, $p = 0.001$) as presented in Table 2. The posthoc test indicated significant differences in NS of snacks between Control and 'Fruit' ($p = 0.04$), Control and 'Salty snack' ($p = 0.004$), Control and 'Sweets' ($p = 0.0002$), and between 'Vegetable' and 'Sweets' ($p = 0.04$). See Table 2 for more details and for the condition differences between DA scores.

Table 2. Nutri-Score and Dietitian's Assessment Score per condition.

	Conditions	n	Mean (SD)	df	χ^2	p	Comparison condition	Mean (SD)	df	χ^2	p	Comparison condition
				4	21.418	<0.001			4	18.392	0.001	
Healthy conditions	Fruit	441	2.7 (1.6)			0.59	Vegetable	2.4 (1.5)			0.39	Vegetable
						0.34	Salty snacks				0.30	Salty snacks
						0.06	Sweets				0.29	Sweets
	Vegetable	297	2.6 (1.7)			0.17	Salty snacks	2.4 (1.6)			0.10	Salty snacks
						0.04 *	Sweets				0.10	Sweets
Unhealthy conditions	Salty snacks	354	2.8 (1.7)			0.30	Sweets	2.6 (1.6)			0.98	Sweets
	Sweets	318	2.9 (1.7)					2.7 (1.6)				
Control condition	Control	353	2.4 (1.5)			0.04 *	Fruit	2.2 (1.5)			0.03 *	Fruit
						0.16	Vegetable				0.25	Vegetable
						0.004 **	Salty snacks				0.003 **	Salty snacks
						<0.001 ***	Sweets				0.002 **	Sweets
	Total	1763	2.7 (1.6)					2.5 (1.6)				

SD, standard deviation; χ^2, results from Kruskal-Wallis test; df, degree of freedom; * $p < 0.05$; ** $p < 0.01$; *** $p < 0.001$.

In addition, which food groups were most represented among the conditions was evaluated. Interestingly, among all five conditions, the majority of photos of snacks corresponded to the sweets food group, followed by fruits. See Table 3 for more details. This indicated that the majority of snacks consumed were chocolate, cookies, candy, fruit/nut/granola/protein bars or similar, followed by different types of fresh fruits, fruit-only smoothies or dried fruits. When comparing between countries, the Slovenian participants submitted more sweet snacks (46.7%) than Australian participants (35%). In addition, one-quarter of Slovenians and over 22% of Australians had fruits as a part of their snacking occasions, and less than 3% of Australians and less than 2% of Slovenians consumed vegetables as snacks. Moreover, background images had a significant effect on snack choices ($\chi^2_{(45)} = 100.95$, $p < 0.001$), and from the visual presentation in Figure S3 in Supplementary Materials, it can be seen that in the 'Fruit' condition, more photos of 'Mixed meals and other' were submitted, and in 'Sweets' condition more photos of 'Beverages' were submitted. Post-hoc analysis indicated that only the proportion of snacks within the 'Mixed meals and other' condition (Table 1 for more details) food group is significant ($p = 0.02$). There was no significant difference between other intervention groups.

Table 3. Food groups of snacks per condition.

	All photos n (%)	Healthy Conditions		Unhealthy Conditions		Control Condition
		Fruit n (%) $n^p = 47$ (AU = 13; SI = 34)	Vegetable n (%) $n^p = 34$ (AU = 11; SI = 23)	Salty snacks n (%) $n^p = 36$ (AU = 9; SI = 27)	Sweets n (%) $n^p = 35$ (AU = 9; SI = 26)	Control n (%) $n^p = 36$ (AU = 10; SI = 26)
Fruits	412	103 (25)	67 (16.3)	92 (22.3)	82 (19.9)	68 (16.5)
Vegetables	35	5 (14.3)	8 (22.9)	5 (14.3)	13 (37.1)	4 (11.4)
Dairy	169	50 (29.6)	25 (14.8)	44 (26.0)	35 (20.7)	15 (8.9)
Grains	41	11 (26.8)	6 (14.6)	13 (31.7)	4 (9.8)	7 (17.1)
Meat, fish and eggs	18	4 (22.2)	1 (5.6)	7 (38.9)	0 (0.0)	6 (33.3)
Nut	130	26 (20.0)	16 (12.3)	27 (20.8)	38 (29.2)	23 (17.7)
Salty snacks	158	33 (20.9)	40 (25.3)	31 (19.6)	15 (9.5)	39 (24.7)
Sweets	770	190 (24.7)	129 (16.8)	136 (17.7)	141 (18.3)	174 (22.6)
Beverages	94	23 (24.5)	7 (7.4)	15 (16.0)	31 (33.0)	18 (19.1)
Mixed meals and other	166	64 (38.6)	21 (12.7)	28 (16.9)	20 (12.0)	33 (19.9)

n = number of submitted photos; n^p = number of participants from Australia or Slovenia.

We also investigated whether background images were associated with the selection of foods present in this image. For example, whether fruity background images stimulate fruit consumption. We found only in the 'Sweets' condition that the percentage of sweets containing photos was the highest (41.2%) compared to other conditions. For this purpose, all photos containing food(s) corresponding to the background foods were considered. This means that if fruit and cookies were consumed as a part of one snacking occasion, the cookies were considered in the 'Sweets' condition, even if not solely cookies were in the photo.

4. Discussion

Innovative interventions are needed to understand how people make food choices within digital environments and which (if any) UI features influence the selection the most. This study explored the feasibility of an app-based tool to investigate (physical and digital) environmental influences on snack choice.

In the existing literature [35], it is seen that monitoring dietary intake can be very demanding for people; thus, we wanted to develop an easy-to-use and intuitive app. Hence, we intentionally removed the burden of taking pictures of separated foods or ingredients when consuming a composite dish (e.g., all the ingredients used to prepare the sandwich) and providing additional information by typing. Instead, the app allows selecting pre-set options.

Contrary to the studies suggesting that meal planning and food prepared at home is healthier (e.g., [36–38]), in our study, we found that the average NS or DA did not significantly change between snacks obtained immediately prior to consumption and the ones obtained more than one hour before consumption. This may be due to the fact that the intervention was performed during the COVID-19 pandemic when people worked remotely or mainly from home. This would also justify that more than 75% of snacks were obtained at the moment of consumption, as participants did not need to prepare the foods in advance. Similarly, it would explain the fact that the majority of snacks were eaten at the dining table (Slovenians) or at the working desk (Australian). In addition, 75% of snacks were consumed when participants were by themselves, which can again be a consequence of the working-from-home requirement. However, in contrast to a study by Chae et al. [39], we found that the food quality of these snacks was higher compared to snacks eaten in the company of others (either one, two, or more people).

We found that among participants from both countries, the majority of snack photos contained some sort of sweets, but photos submitted by Slovenians contained more of these compared to photos from Australians. This might be due to the holiday season in Slovenia, which took place during the data collection when fried sweet pastries are traditionally consumed. In addition, surprisingly, one-quarter of Slovenians and a bit more than 22% of Australians had fruits as a part of their snacking occasions. In contrast, only less than 3% of Australians and less than 2% of Slovenians consumed vegetables as a part of the snacking occasions. A very recent study showed that the majority of Polish adults are aware of the importance of vegetable and fruit intake, the negative effects of the consumption of sugar and salt, and the related dietary risk factors [40]. Nevertheless, many people still do not meet the recommended fruit and vegetable intakes (e.g., [41–43]), even though research is consistent that fruits and vegetables have beneficial effects on our overall physical and mental health [44–46]. This calls for innovative strategies to promote nutritious snacks and overall food consumption, which can be challenging as people have difficulties assessing snacks' nutritiousness when snacks contain healthy and less healthy components (e.g., fruit yoghurt containing large amounts of sugar or nuts with high energy and/or salt content) [47]. Despite the widespread knowledge about the impact of diet on health, people still have difficulties consuming and selecting nutritious foods. Hence, promoting nutritious snack consumption of, for example, snack-sized vegetables (such as mini carrots, which can be found in any well-stocked Australian store) and making them more accessible could increase vegetable intake and reduce health-related risks.

In addition, findings here are consistent with results from other studies suggesting that women make healthier food choices than men (e.g., [48]). Moreover, in agreement with previous studies on adults in France and Australia, our findings suggest that snacks consumed in the morning are healthier than the ones consumed later in the day [49,50]. Further research needs to investigate what drives these behaviours to promote healthier snacking behaviours and choices.

The nudging theory suggests that manipulating the consumer's environment can change behaviour in a predictable way. Hence, it could be expected that people who are exposed to healthy images would be nudged to choose healthier food [51]. However, our results showed that NS and DA were the highest (i.e., more healthful) in the 'Sweets' condition. Moreover, the DA score was the lowest in the 'Fruit' and 'Vegetable' conditions. This suggests that presenting images containing healthy foods can encourage unhealthy food choices and vice versa; images of unhealthy foods (sweets) may nudge consumers towards healthier food choices. While this is inconsistent with the previous results of other studies conducted in real-life settings (not online) (e.g., [15]), there is literature supporting our findings that healthy cues can lead to unhealthy choices (e.g., [52,53]). In the study by Wilcox et al. [52], consumers that saw a healthy food option on a menu were more likely to choose the least healthy option compared to when a healthy option was not included. This effect is called vicarious goal fulfilment, where the mere presence of healthy options fulfils the need to make healthy food choices and provides the individual with a rationale for unhealthy choices. Therefore, it may be possible that seeing unhealthy foods fulfilled participants' desire to indulge and select unhealthy snack and thus they felt satisfied enough to make a healthy choice. However, the small sample size within each condition may have influenced these results, which should be interpreted with caution. Additional studies are warranted to determine whether these findings can be repeated in a larger sample size, and our findings provide a rationale for investigating this.

Moreover, results here showed that participants in the 'Sweets' condition submitted more than 40% of snacks that corresponded to the sweet confectionary food group. These conflicting results need further investigation, and future research should examine whether the positive benefits of nudging strategies used in real-life settings have the same effect in online settings. For example, can repositioning foods in online settings influence food choices the same as it does in field studies [3]? In addition, as UIs can easily be modified in an online environment, it may be beneficial for our understanding of UI impact on consumers to test different types of imagery. In our study, we used food imagery; however, the potential impact of using nature imagery or warning graphic images (as seen on cigarette packages) in an online setting still needs to be addressed. Hence, SnackTrack is an open-source mobile app, and its source code is freely available (See Computer Codes S1–S3 in Supplementary Materials) for use and modification required for any research purposes (CC-BY-NC, i.e., the Creative Commons Attribution-NonCommercial).

Limitations

The current study has some limitations that need to be acknowledged. Firstly, the small sample size prevented us from detecting small effects. Participants overall submitted fewer photos per person than anticipated, impacting the ability to assess the overall impacts of the image-based nudging. This feasibility study confirmed that food intake monitoring could be a burden to consumers, as participants were struggling with tracking their snack intakes for 15 days. This might also be due to the fact that 25% of apps are used only once after being downloaded [54]. Furthermore, sending reminders to participants to encourage them to track food intake would be advisable, although this cannot guarantee photo acquisition, as reminders are sent automatically and not necessarily immediately before snacking occasion. In addition, the NS nutrient profiling system, as well as the developed app, did not consider the portion size of foods. Since SnackTrack is not a dietary assessment application, portion size estimation was beyond the scope of the study, which was to assess the impact of the UI on food choices. Future research should incorporate portion size into a nutrient profiling system and/or the app and compare nutrient profile scores relative to nudging strategies.

Another limitation may be the understanding of the definition of snacking and the perception of what is considered a snack. For example, in Slovenia, a lot of companies offer warm meals for employees during working hours. Therefore, people frequently eat a multi-course meal (e.g., soup, potatoes with meat and salad) between breakfast and lunchtime. Even though we did not receive many photos of meals like this, we do have to emphasise that 'a meal between main meals' might mean different things for different people, cultures, etc.

Lastly, investigating the ability of imagery to nudge consumers over time is warranted. As environmental cues affect eating habits and are processed subconsciously, consumers might have been nudged the first time using the app. Currently, there is no strong evidence of how much time it takes to influence consumers to change their dietary behaviours; therefore, future research should seek to address this. For example, investigating how long the exposure should be for (food) imagery to target and increase cravings and motivation to eat certain foods (e.g., healthy foods) and if the exposure time is different for different types of foods (e.g., healthy vs unhealthy) or during the day. In addition, how the healthfulness of foods or diet quality changes over time while exposed to nudges (e.g., if more and more unhealthy choices were made in the unhealthy condition) needs further investigation. In order to investigate this, monitoring dietary intake and tracking behavioural changes or nutritional quality of the snacks over a period of time is needed. Hence, finding a solution to motivate participants to track their food intake is warranted. A potential solution could be automatic food image recognition [55,56], which can further contribute to the development of automated dietary assessment. Future research should seek to address this. Lastly, we would like to emphasise that during the recruitment period, COVID-19 lockdown restrictions were in place in both countries.

5. Conclusions

This pilot study demonstrates that food (online) environments play an important role, and innovative strategies are needed for behavioural changes. Since promoting healthy foods can impact consumer choices and have the opposite effect than intended, our findings suggest that future research needs to address this, especially in an online context. Further, a clear description of implemented UI elements to investigate and quantify the effect on consumers' food choices is needed. In addition, while consumers have the knowledge to make a healthy choice, the plethora of environmental stimuli influencing them is evidently altering food choices. Although the current study has a relatively small sample size, it still provides some interesting findings, such as insights into the healthy cues leading to unhealthy choices and the time of food obtainment not having an effect on the healthfulness of selected foods.

Supplementary Materials: The following supporting information can be downloaded at: https://www.mdpi.com/article/10.3390/nu15020349/s1. Figure S1: Background images used in four conditions; Figure S2: A screenshot of Take a photo screen and the additional info screen with the vegetable background; Figure S3: Visual presentation of standard residuals; Source code S1: SnackTrack–iOS version; Source code S2: SnackTrack–Android version and Source code S3: SnackTrack–Server.

Author Contributions: Conceptualisation, E.V., E.B., C.E.C., B.K.S. and T.B.; methodology, E.V., E.B., C.E.C., B.K.S. and T.B.; formal analysis, E.V., E.B. and T.B.; writing—original draft preparation, E.V.; writing—review and editing, E.V., E.B., C.E.C., B.K.S. and T.B.; supervision, E.B., C.E.C., B.K.S. and T.B.; funding acquisition, B.K.S. and T.B. All authors have read and agreed to the published version of the manuscript.

Funding: This research was supported by the Australian Research Council (ARC DP210100285) and the Hunter Medical Research Institute. Additionally, this work was undertaken within the OPKP ('Upgrade of the Open platform for clinical nutrition with a mobile app') project, which has received funding from the Ministry of Health of Slovenia under Grant Agreement No. C2711-19-185021, from the COMFOCUS project, which has received funding from the European Union's Horizon 2020 research and innovation program under Grant Agreement No. 101005259, and from the Slovenian Research Agency [P2-0098: Computer Structures and Systems]. Lastly, C.E.C. is supported by an NHMRC Leadership Research Fellowship (L3, APP2009340).

Institutional Review Board Statement: The study was conducted in accordance with the Declaration of Helsinki and approved by The University of Newcastle Human Research Ethics Committee (H-2020-0267).

Informed Consent Statement: Informed consent was obtained from all subjects involved in the study.

Data Availability Statement: The data presented in this study are available on request. The data are not publicly available due to privacy and ethical restrictions.

Acknowledgments: The authors wish to thank Matevž Ogrinc, Andraž Simčič, Robert Modic, Gordana Ispirova, Simon Mezgec and Peter Novak for their contribution to the design and development of SnackTrack. In addition, we would like to thank Tammie Jakstas and Julija Repolusk for their contribution to the study.

Conflicts of Interest: The authors declare no conflict of interest. The funders had no role in the design of the study; in the collection, analyses, or interpretation of data; in the writing of the manuscript, or in the decision to publish the results.

References

1. Stok, F. Marijn; Renner Britta; Hoffmann Stefan; Volkert Dorothee DONE (Determinants of Nutrition and Eating) Framework. Available online: https://www.uni-konstanz.de/DONE/ (accessed on 3 January 2020).
2. Story, M.; Kaphingst, K.M.; Robinson-O'Brien, R.; Glanz, K. Creating Healthy Food and Eating Environments: Policy and Environmental Approaches. *Annu. Rev. Public Health* **2008**, *29*, 253–272. [CrossRef] [PubMed]
3. Bucher, T.; Collins, C.; Rollo, M.E.; McCaffrey, T.A.; De Vlieger, N.; Van der Bend, D.; Truby, H.; Perez-Cueto, F.J. Nudging Consumers towards Healthier Choices: A Systematic Review of Positional Influences on Food Choice. *Br. J. Nutr.* **2016**, *115*, 2252–2263. [CrossRef] [PubMed]
4. Bucher, T.; van der Horst, K.; Siegrist, M. Improvement of Meal Composition by Vegetable Variety. *Public Health Nutr.* **2011**, *14*, 1357–1363. [CrossRef] [PubMed]
5. Steenhuis, I.H.; Vermeer, W.M. Portion Size: Review and Framework for Interventions. *Int. J. Behav. Nutr. Phys. Act.* **2009**, *6*, 58. [CrossRef] [PubMed]

6. Thaler, R.H.; Sunstein, C.R. *NUDGE: Improving Decisions about Health, Wealth, and Happiness*; Yale University Press: New Haven, CT, USA; London, UK, 2008; ISBN 9780300122237.
7. Valenčič, E.; Beckett, E.; Collins, C.E.; Seljak, B.K.; Bucher, T. Digital Nudging in Online Grocery Stores: A Scoping Review on Current Practices and Gaps. *Trends Food Sci. Technol.* **2022**, *131*, 151–163. [CrossRef]
8. Papies, E.K. Health Goal Priming as a Situated Intervention Tool: How to Benefit from Nonconscious Motivational Routes to Health Behaviour. *Health Psychol. Rev.* **2016**, *10*, 408–424. [CrossRef] [PubMed]
9. Evans, J.S.B. Dual-Processing Accounts of Reasoning, Judgment, and Social Cognition. *Annu. Rev. Psychol.* **2008**, *59*, 255–278. [CrossRef]
10. Cohen, D.A.; Babey, S.H. Contextual Influences on Eating Behaviours: Heuristic Processing and Dietary Choices. *Obes. Rev.* **2012**, *13*, 766–779. [CrossRef]
11. Phillips, M. Store Atmospherics as a Prime to Nudge Shoppers toward Healthier Food Choices. Ph.D. Thesis, Auckland University of Technology, Auckland, New Zealand, 2017.
12. Vermeir, I.; Roose, G. Visual Design Cues Impacting Food Choice: A Review and Future Research Agenda. *Foods* **2020**, *9*, 1495. [CrossRef]
13. Geise, S.; Baden, C. Putting the Image Back Into the Frame: Modeling the Linkage Between Visual Communication and Frame-Processing Theory. *Commun. Theory* **2015**, *25*, 46–69. [CrossRef]
14. Rendell, A.; Adam, M.; Eidels, A. Towards Understanding the Influence of Nature Imagery in User Interface Design: A Review of the Literature. In Proceedings of the 52nd Hawaii International Conference on System Sciences, Maui, HI, USA, 8–11 January 2019.
15. Stöckli, S.; Stämpfli, A.E.; Messner, C.; Brunner, T.A. An (Un) Healthy Poster: When Environmental Cues Affect Consumers' Food Choices at Vending Machines. *Appetite* **2016**, *96*, 368–374. [CrossRef] [PubMed]
16. Lee, D.; Moon, J.; Rhee, C.; Cho, D.; Cho, J. The Effect of Visual and Auditory Elements on Patrons' Liquor-Ordering Behavior: An Empirical Study. *Int. J. Hosp. Manag.* **2016**, *55*, 11–15. [CrossRef]
17. Papies, E.K.; Hamstra, P. Goal Priming and Eating Behavior: Enhancing Self-Regulation by Environmental Cues. *Health Psychol.* **2010**, *29*, 384. [CrossRef] [PubMed]
18. Bell, R.; Meiselman, H.L.; Pierson, B.J.; Reeve, W.G. Effects of Adding an Italian Theme to a Restaurant on the Perceived Ethnicity, Acceptability, and Selection of Foods. *Appetite* **1994**, *22*, 11–24. [CrossRef] [PubMed]
19. Adams, J.M.; Hart, W.; Gilmer, D.O.; Lloyd-Richardson, E.E.; Burton, K.A. Concrete Images of the Sugar Content in Sugar-Sweetened Beverages Reduces Attraction to and Selection of These Beverages. *Appetite* **2014**, *83*, 10–18. [CrossRef]
20. Weinmann, M.; Schneider, C.; Brocke, J. vom Digital Nudging. *Bus. Inf. Syst. Eng.* **2016**, *58*, 433–436. [CrossRef]
21. Piper, J.; Adam Marc, T.P.; De Vlieger, N.; Collins, C.E.; Bucher, T. A Bibliometric Review of Digital Nudging within Digital Food Choice Environments. In Proceedings of the 32nd Australasian Conference on Information Systems, Sydney, Australia, 6–10 December 2021; Volume 63, pp. 1–12.
22. Bucher, T.; Keller, C. The Web-Buffet–Development and Validation of an Online Tool to Measure Food Choice. *Public Health Nutr.* **2015**, *18*, 1950–1959. [CrossRef]
23. Hunter, S.R.; Mattes, R.D. The Role of Eating Frequency and Snacking on Energy Intake and BMI. In *Handbook of Eating and Drinking*; Springer: Cham, Switzerland, 2020; pp. 659–678.
24. Wang, D.; Van der Horst, K.; Jacquier, E.F.; Afeiche, M.C.; Eldridge, A.L. Snacking Patterns in Children: A Comparison between Australia, China, Mexico, and the US. *Nutrients* **2018**, *10*, 198. [CrossRef]
25. Vatanparast, H.; Islam, N.; Patil, R.P.; Shafiee, M.; Smith, J.; Whiting, S. Snack Consumption Patterns among Canadians. *Nutrients* **2019**, *11*, 1152. [CrossRef]
26. Myhre, J.B.; Løken, E.B.; Wandel, M.; Andersen, L.F. The Contribution of Snacks to Dietary Intake and Their Association with Eating Location among Norwegian Adults—Results from a Cross-Sectional Dietary Survey. *BMC Public Health* **2015**, *15*, 369. [CrossRef]
27. Chaplin, K.; Smith, A.P. Definitions and Perceptions of Snacking. *Curr. Top. Nutraceuticals Res. Coppell* **2011**, *9*, 53–59. [CrossRef]
28. Potter, M.; Vlassopoulos, A.; Lehmann, U. Snacking Recommendations Worldwide: A Scoping Review. *Adv. Nutr.* **2018**, *9*, 86–98. [CrossRef] [PubMed]
29. Shiffman, S.; Stone, A.A.; Hufford, M.R. Ecological Momentary Assessment. *Annu. Rev. Clin. Psychol.* **2008**, *4*, 1–32. [CrossRef] [PubMed]
30. Valenčič, E.; Novak, P.; Ogrinc, M.; Simčič, A.; Modic, R.; Ispirova, G.; Mezgec, S.; Koroušić-Seljak, B. *Design, Implementation and Validation of the SnackTrac Mobile Application*; JSI Technical Report: Boston, Mam USA, 2022.
31. Nutri-Score. Available online: https://www.santepubliquefrance.fr/en/nutri-score (accessed on 30 May 2022).
32. Chantal, J.; Hercberg, S.; World Health Organization. Development of a New Front-of-Pack Nutrition Label in France: The Five-Colour Nutri-Score. *Public Health Panor.* **2017**, *3*, 712–725.
33. Julia, C.; Etilé, F.; Hercberg, S. Front-of-Pack Nutri-Score Labelling in France: An Evidence-Based Policy. *Lancet Public Health* **2018**, *3*, e164. [CrossRef]
34. Field, A.; Miles, J.; Field, Z. *Discovering Statistics Using R*; Sage publications: London, UK; Thousand Oaks, CA, USA; New Delhi, India; Singapore, 2012; ISBN 1-4462-0046-9.
35. Burke, L.E.; Wang, J.; Sevick, M.A. Self-Monitoring in Weight Loss: A Systematic Review of the Literature. *J. Am. Diet. Assoc.* **2011**, *111*, 92–102. [CrossRef]

36. Ducrot, P.; Méjean, C.; Aroumougame, V.; Ibanez, G.; Allès, B.; Kesse-Guyot, E.; Hercberg, S.; Péneau, S. Meal Planning Is Associated with Food Variety, Diet Quality and Body Weight Status in a Large Sample of French Adults. *Int. J. Behav. Nutr. Phys. Act.* **2017**, *14*, 12. [CrossRef]
37. Hanson, A.J.; Kattelmann, K.K.; McCormack, L.A.; Zhou, W.; Brown, O.N.; Horacek, T.M.; Shelnutt, K.P.; Kidd, T.; Opoku-Acheampong, A.; Franzen-Castle, L.D.; et al. Cooking and Meal Planning as Predictors of Fruit and Vegetable Intake and BMI in First-Year College Students. *Int. J. Environ. Res. Public Health* **2019**, *16*, 2462. [CrossRef]
38. Laska, M.N.; Hearst, M.O.; Lust, K.; Lytle, L.A.; Story, M. How We Eat What We Eat: Identifying Meal Routines and Practices Most Strongly Associated with Healthy and Unhealthy Dietary Factors among Young Adults. *Public Health Nutr.* **2015**, *18*, 2135–2145. [CrossRef]
39. Chae, W.; Ju, Y.J.; Shin, J.; Jang, S.-I.; Park, E.-C. Association between Eating Behaviour and Diet Quality: Eating Alone vs. Eating with Others. *Nutr. J.* **2018**, *17*, 117. [CrossRef]
40. Żarnowski, A.; Jankowski, M.; Gujski, M. Public Awareness of Diet-Related Diseases and Dietary Risk Factors: A 2022 Nationwide Cross-Sectional Survey among Adults in Poland. *Nutrients* **2022**, *14*, 3285. [CrossRef]
41. Charlton, K.; Kowal, P.; Soriano, M.M.; Williams, S.; Banks, E.; Vo, K.; Byles, J. Fruit and Vegetable Intake and Body Mass Index in a Large Sample of Middle-Aged Australian Men and Women. *Nutrients* **2014**, *6*, 2305–2319. [CrossRef]
42. Vandevijvere, S.; De Ridder, K.; Fiolet, T.; Bel, S.; Tafforeau, J. Consumption of Ultra-Processed Food Products and Diet Quality among Children, Adolescents and Adults in Belgium. *Eur. J. Nutr.* **2019**, *58*, 3267–3278. [CrossRef] [PubMed]
43. Dietary Guidelines Advisory Committee. *Scientific Report of the 2015 Dietary Guidelines Advisory Committee: Advisory Report to the Secretary of Health and Human Services and the Secretary of Agriculture*; U.S. Department of Agriculture, Agricultural Research Service: Washington, DC, USA, 2015; p. 421.
44. World Health Organization. *Healthy Diet*; No. WHO-EM/NUT/282/E; World Health Organization: Nasr City, Egypt, 2019.
45. Głąbska, D.; Guzek, D.; Groele, B.; Gutkowska, K. Fruit and Vegetable Intake and Mental Health in Adults: A Systematic Review. *Nutrients* **2020**, *12*, 115. [CrossRef] [PubMed]
46. World Health Organization. *Diet, Nutrition, and the Prevention of Chronic Diseases: Report of a Joint WHO/FAO Expert Consultation*; World Health Organization: Geneva, Switzerland, 2003; Volume 916, ISBN 92-4-120916-X.
47. De Vlieger, N.M.; Collins, C.; Bucher, T. What Is a Nutritious Snack? Level of Processing and Macronutrient Content Influences Young Adults' Perceptions. *Appetite* **2017**, *114*, 55–63. [CrossRef] [PubMed]
48. Hartmann, C.; Siegrist, M.; Horst, K. van der Snack Frequency: Associations with Healthy and Unhealthy Food Choices. *Public Health Nutr.* **2013**, *16*, 1487–1496. [CrossRef]
49. Si Hassen, W.; Castetbon, K.; Tichit, C.; Péneau, S.; Nechba, A.; Ducrot, P.; Lampuré, A.; Bellisle, F.; Hercberg, S.; Méjean, C. Energy, Nutrient and Food Content of Snacks in French Adults. *Nutr. J.* **2018**, *17*, 33. [CrossRef]
50. McNaughton, S.A.; Leech, R.; Worsley, A. Does the Nutrient Profile of Snacks Vary According to the Time of Day of Consumption? *FASEB J.* **2016**, *30*, 677.20. [CrossRef]
51. Sunstein, C.R.; Thaler, R. Libertarian Paternalism. *Am. Econ. Rev.* **2003**, *93*, 175–179. [CrossRef]
52. Wilcox, K.; Vallen, B.; Block, L.; Fitzsimons, G.J. Vicarious Goal Fulfillment: When the Mere Presence of a Healthy Option Leads to an Ironically Indulgent Decision. *J. Consum. Res.* **2009**, *36*, 380–393. [CrossRef]
53. Chiou, W.-B.; Yang, C.-C.; Wan, C.-S. Ironic Effects of Dietary Supplementation: Illusory Invulnerability Created by Taking Dietary Supplements Licenses Health-Risk Behaviors. *Psychol. Sci.* **2011**, *22*, 1081–1086. [CrossRef] [PubMed]
54. BuildFire Mobile App Download Statistics & Usage Statistics (2022). Available online: https://buildfire.com/app-statistics/ (accessed on 30 November 2022).
55. Mezgec, S.; Koroušić Seljak, B. NutriNet: A Deep Learning Food and Drink Image Recognition System for Dietary Assessment. *Nutrients* **2017**, *9*, 657. [CrossRef] [PubMed]
56. Mezgec, S.; Eftimov, T.; Bucher, T.; Koroušić Seljak, B. Mixed Deep Learning and Natural Language Processing Method for Fake-Food Image Recognition and Standardization to Help Automated Dietary Assessment. *Public Health Nutr.* **2019**, *22*, 1193–1202. [CrossRef] [PubMed]

Disclaimer/Publisher's Note: The statements, opinions and data contained in all publications are solely those of the individual author(s) and contributor(s) and not of MDPI and/or the editor(s). MDPI and/or the editor(s) disclaim responsibility for any injury to people or property resulting from any ideas, methods, instructions or products referred to in the content.

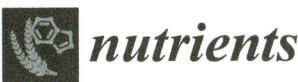

Review

Dietary Epigenetic Modulators: Unravelling the Still-Controversial Benefits of miRNAs in Nutrition and Disease

Elisa Martino [1], Nunzia D'Onofrio [1,*], Anna Balestrieri [2], Antonino Colloca [1], Camilla Anastasio [1], Celestino Sardu [3], Raffaele Marfella [3], Giuseppe Campanile [4,†] and Maria Luisa Balestrieri [1,†]

1. Department of Precision Medicine, University of Campania Luigi Vanvitelli, 80138 Naples, Italy; elisa.martino@unicampania.it (E.M.); antonino.colloca@studenti.unicampania.it (A.C.); camilla.anastasio@unicampania.it (C.A.); marialuisa.balestrieri@unicampania.it (M.L.B.)
2. Food Safety Department, Istituto Zooprofilattico Sperimentale del Mezzogiorno, 80055 Portici, Italy; anna.balestrieri@izsmportici.it
3. Department of Advanced Clinical and Surgical Sciences, University of Campania Luigi Vanvitelli, 80138 Naples, Italy; celestino.sardu@unicampania.it (C.S.); raffaele.marfella@unicampania.it (R.M.)
4. Department of Veterinary Medicine and Animal Production, University of Naples Federico II, 80137 Naples, Italy; giuseppe.campanile@unina.it
* Correspondence: nunzia.donofrio@unicampania.it
† These authors contributed equally to this work.

Abstract: In the context of nutrient-driven epigenetic alterations, food-derived miRNAs can be absorbed into the circulatory system and organs of recipients, especially humans, and potentially contribute to modulating health and diseases. Evidence suggests that food uptake, by carrying exogenous miRNAs (xenomiRNAs), regulates the individual miRNA profile, modifying the redox homeostasis and inflammatory conditions underlying pathological processes, such as type 2 diabetes mellitus, insulin resistance, metabolic syndrome, and cancer. The capacity of diet to control miRNA levels and the comprehension of the unique characteristics of dietary miRNAs in terms of gene expression regulation show important perspectives as a strategy to control disease susceptibility via epigenetic modifications and refine the clinical outcomes. However, the absorption, stability, availability, and epigenetic roles of dietary miRNAs are intriguing and currently the subject of intense debate; additionally, there is restricted knowledge of their physiological and potential side effects. Within this framework, we provided up-to-date and comprehensive knowledge on dietary miRNAs' potential, discussing the latest advances and controversial issues related to the role of miRNAs in human health and disease as modulators of chronic syndromes.

Keywords: cancer; chronic diseases; epigenetics; microRNA; nutrients

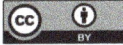

1. Introduction

Among lifestyle factors, diet displays a strong impact on human health. Over decades, unhealthy dietary habits have been responsible for the spread of many severe chronic degenerative diseases such as obesity, type 2 diabetes mellitus (T2DM), cardiovascular diseases, and cancer [1]. Food intake may modify gene expression as well as disease susceptibility through the regulation of several epigenetic modulators [1]. MicroRNAs (miRNAs) play critical roles in gene regulation and biological processes [2,3]. They are transcribed by RNA polymerase II, leading to the generation of a hairpin structure called primary microRNA or pri-miRNA, which is further processed by the RNA endonucleases located in the nucleus (Drosha) and in the cytoplasm (Dicer) to generate a duplex of 22–25 nucleotides [2]. This latter is then divided into two mature sequences associated with the Argonaute protein (AGO), resulting in the formation of the RNA-induced silencing complex (RISC), which can ultimately act as a translation repressor on target genes [3]. Gene expression regulation at intracellular and extracellular levels is improved by mature transcript encapsulation into extracellular vesicles, such as exosomes, secreted by multiple cell types as mediators of cell-to-cell communication [4]. Because of their biocompatibility and biostability, extracellular vesicles are considered regulatory cargos in a wide range of intercellular communication and crosstalk systems [5,6]. MiRNAs have been described in body fluids as blood, serum, plasma, urine, saliva, and breast milk, and changes in their circulating levels are related to a plethora of different chronic syndromes, including obesity, cardiovascular and neurodegenerative diseases, T2DM, and cancer [7,8]. Preserving the human miRNA profile could contribute to the prevention of diseases and the maintenance of good health. MiRNAs have been widely reported in plants, animals, and humans [9]. Plant-derived miRNAs bind to recipient target transcripts with quite perfect complementarity, acting as small interfering RNAs (siRNAs), while animal miRNAs interact with the host mRNA targets with imperfect complementarity, thus inducing their translational repression [10,11]. Given this imperfect complementarity, a single exogenous miRNA (xenomiRNA) is able to recognize multiple target sites and modulate different target genes in the host [10,11]. After ingestion, xenomiRNAs could modulate the gene expression by a cross-kingdom pattern or horizontal transfer of genetic information to the host [10,11]. Bioactive dietary compounds, by affecting directly and indirectly gene activity, have been related to epigenetic changes, such as DNA methylation, histone acetylation, and the modulation of miRNA expression in both physiological and pathological conditions [12,13]. However, the clinical relevance of food-derived xenomiRNAs in human diseases is still undefined. Several studies have demonstrated that the intricate interplay between miRNAs and nutrients could regulate health and chronic diseases, hence pointing to food modification as a pivotal tool in different diseases [14,15]. However, further studies to reveal the precise mode of action of dietary active compounds and how nutrients and bioactive molecules affect miRNA expression are still required. This review aims to provide an update on the role of dietary miRNAs in health and diseases by underlining the benefits, obstacles, and controversies of the relationship between food-derived miRNAs and the pathogenesis of chronic diseases.

2. Dietary XenomiRNAs in Health and Disease

XenomiRNAs represent a family of exogenous miRNAs characterized by several dietary sources, animals and vegetables, and are able to integrate into the total miRNA profile of a recipient [16]. Once in the host, these small molecules can be absorbed by the gastrointestinal tract, packaged into vesicles, released into the bloodstream, and delivered to multiple cells and tissues, thus promoting healthy state or affecting the development of chronic diseases, including cancer [17–19]. In the following sections, the role of xenomiRNAs from both animals and vegetables as regulators of several chronic conditions will be extensively discussed (Figure 1).

2.1. XenomiRNAs from Animal Sources

The following subsection is dedicated to the most studied and characterized xenomiRNAs derived from animal sources and their involvement in chronic syndromes and cancer.

2.1.1. Eggs

Analysis of RNA sequencing revealed the content of several miRNAs, such as gga-mir-2188, gga-mir-30c-5p and gga-mir-92-3p, in the edible parts of chicken eggs, suggesting these noncoding RNAs as interesting tools to take into account for the improvement of egg nutritional value [20]. More recently, Fratantonio et al. described the availability of miRNA-related exosomal vesicles from chicken eggs in mice and humans [21]. Accumulated in the brain, intestine, and lung, miRNA-exosomes regulated spatial learning and memory function in C57BL/6J mice, while egg-derived miRNA levels increased in human peripheral blood following exosomal oral administration (Figure 1) [21].

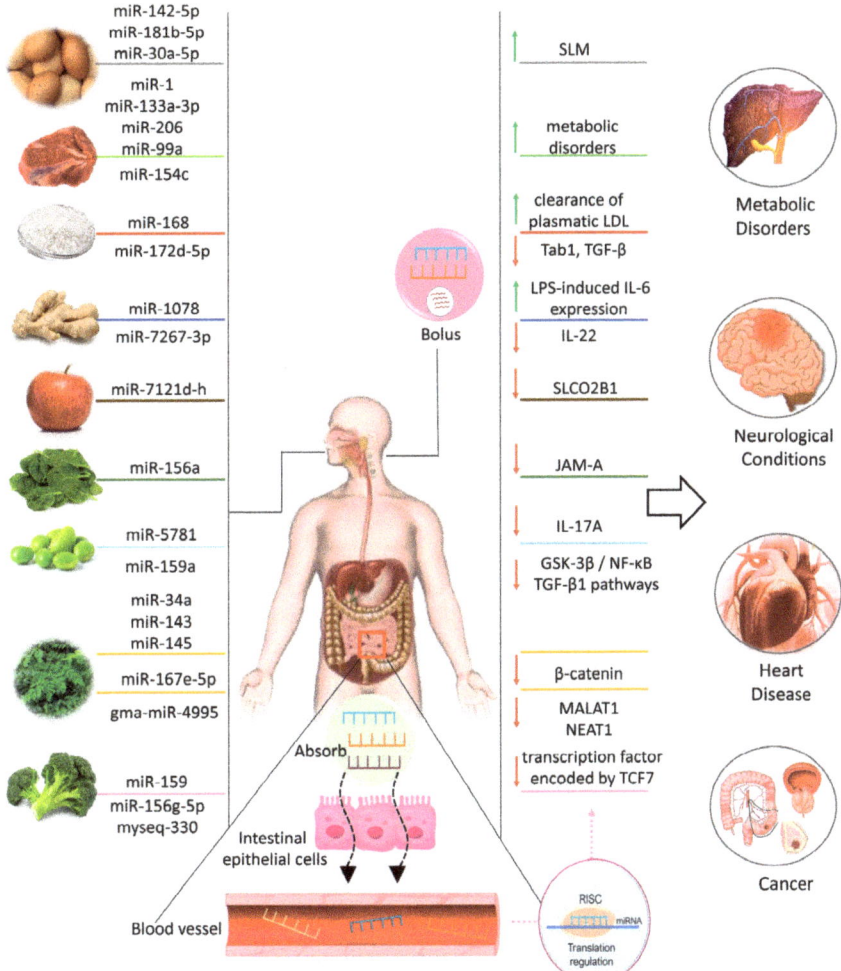

Figure 1. XenomiRNAs from animal and vegetable sources. Exogenous miRNAs from animal and vegetable sources are absorbed by the gastrointestinal tract, packaged into vesicles, and delivered via blood stream to cells and tissues. Here, exogenous miRNAs are able to regulate the development of chronic diseases, such as inflammation, fibrosis, metabolic disorders, neurological conditions, cardiovascular diseases, and cancer, by modulating different cellular pathways. The up arrows stand for upregulation, while the down ones indicate downregulation. GSK-3β, glycogen synthase kinase-3β; IL, interleukin; JAM-A, junctional adhesion molecule A; LDL, low-density lipoprotein; LPS, lipopolysaccharide; MALAT1, metastasis-associated lung adenocarcinoma transcript 1; miR/miRNA, microRNA; NEAT1, nuclear paraspeckle assembly transcript 1; NF-κB, nuclear factor kappaB; RISC, RNA-induced silencing complex; SLCO2B1, Solute Carrier Organic Anion Transporter Family Member 2B1; SLM, spatial learning and memory; Tab1, TGF-β activated kinase 1 (MAP3K7) binding protein 1; TCF7, transcription factor 7; TGF-β1, transforming growth factor-β1.

2.1.2. Meat

The effects of the chronic administration of cooked pork-derived exosomal vesicles were evaluated in mouse model [22]. The upregulated miR-1, miR-133a-3p, miR-206 and miR-99a plasma levels resulted in glucose and insulin metabolism impairment, as well as in lipid droplet accrual in mice liver, supporting the role of pork-derived miRNAs in the development of metabolic disorders (Figure 1) [22]. The bta-miR-154c has been recently characterized by comestible parts of beef. This xenomiRNA is able to contrast the human digestion processes being absorbed from Caco-2, SW480, and SW620 colorectal cancer cells [23]. However, the comprehension of the specific role of miR-154c in colorectal carcinoma requires further investigation [23].

2.1.3. Milk

The classification of milk as an "epi-nutrient", rich in bioactive compounds and functional molecules, as well as its involvement in counteracting chronic syndromes and cancer, have been recently investigated [24–28]. A total of 678 miRNAs were identified in bovine milk-derived exosomal vesicles [29,30]. These miRNAs are involved in a wide range of cell metabolic pathways, such as miR-181 and miR-155, related to the normal function and differentiation of T and B cells, miR-let-7c, miR-17, miR-92, miR-223 implied in the regulation of immunity and inflammatory cells, and miR-30a, a regulator of autophagy in post-acute myocardial infarction (Figure 2) [31–33].

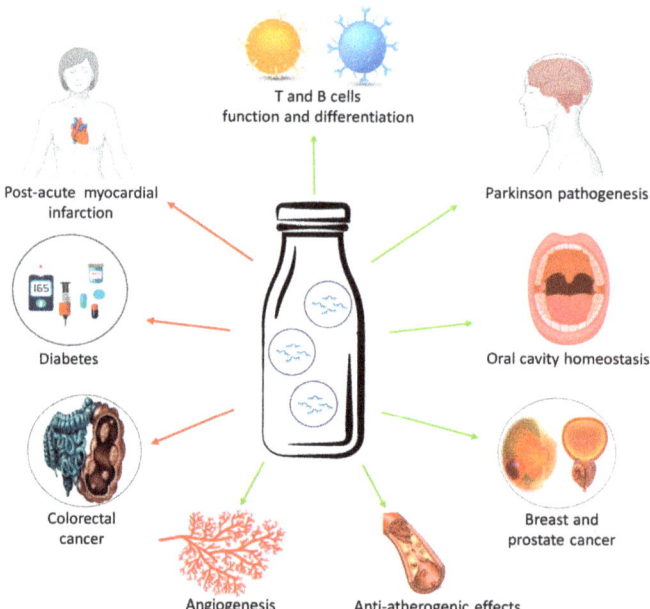

Figure 2. Milk-derived miRNAs and human health. Identified in exosomal vesicles, miRNAs contained in milk are involved in a wide range of metabolic pathways, as the normal function and differentiation of T and B cells, homeostasis of oral cavity, pathogenesis of Parkinson disease, anti-atherogenic action, promotion of angiogenesis, and breast and prostate cancer. MiRNAs contained in milk are also able to counteract diabetes and colorectal cancer development, as well as regulate autophagy in post-acute myocardial infarction. The green arrows stand for promoting activity, while the red ones indicate an opposing role.

The most abundant miRNA in milk exosomes is miR-148a, able to modulate oral cavity homeostasis as well as to inhibit 5′ AMP-activated protein kinase (AMPK) and phosphatase and tensin homolog (PTEN), both suppressors of mammalian target of rapamycin complex 1 (mTORC1), a pivotal regulator of multiple cell metabolic pathways [31–33]. Moreover, milk-derived miR-148a impairs insulin secretion with diabetogenic action through its ability to promote pancreatic β-cell de-differentiation via mTORC1-high/AMPK-low phenotype [33]. It has been reported that miR-148a and miR-21 alter the α-synuclein homeostasis, causing its overexpression and aggregation, with toxic effects on dopaminergic neurons and pancreatic β-cells, thus exerting a possible role in the pathogenesis of Parkinson disease and T2DM [34]. MiRNAs belonging to the miR-148 family affect the immune response, suppressing calcium/calmodulin-dependent protein kinase IIα (CaMKIIα) and the subsequent toll-like receptor (TLR)-mediated expression of major histocompatibility complex II (MHC II) in dendritic cells [31]. Among miRNAs derived from milk exosomes, miR-125a is involved in the modulation of immune response to bacterial and viral aggressions, while the human homolog miR-718, still involved in immune response regulating p53, also regulates vascular endothelial growth factor (VEGF) and insulin growth factor (IGF) pathways [35], and miR-146 exerts a regulatory function in TLR signaling and in the resolution of bacterial infections [36]. As bovine milk, human breast milk-derived miRNAs play a crucial role in modulating development and differentiation of immune system cells and counteracting the onset of metabolic disorders [37,38]. In the first six months of lactation, miR-181a and b, miR-155, miR-125b, and the cluster miR-17-92 actively regulate the T- and B-cell maturation and the tumor necrosis factor α (TNF-α) activation, modulating the immune response of the baby [38], while miR-22-3p counteracts the development of insulin resistance and the onset of T2DM, attenuating the Wnt pathway [37]. Milk-derived miRNAs are also involved in different pivotal metabolic pathways. The presence in milk exosomes of miR-181a-5p has been related to anti-atherogenic effects and reduced vascular inflammation, due to its ability to downregulate nuclear factor kappaB (NF-κB) levels [39]. Another miRNA characterized from milk exosomal vesicles is miR-29, capable of targeting IL-23, a cytokine involved in intestinal damage. To this aim, treatment with milk vesicles containing miR-29 stimulated intestinal stem cell proliferation and gut recovery under several pathological conditions [40], while incubation with miR-31-5p from milk-derived exosomes improved in vitro endothelial function and promoted angiogenesis and diabetic wound healing in vivo [41]. Recent studies reported that oral administration of exosomal vesicles prevented colon shortening, intestinal epithelium disruption, infiltration of inflammatory cells, and tissue fibrosis in a mouse ulcerative colitis model via inhibition of the TLR4-NF-κB signaling pathway and nucleotide-binding oligomerization domain, the NLR family pyrin domain containing 3 (NLRP3) inflammasome activation [30]. Transfection with the milk-derived miR-22 promoted cell proliferation by inhibition of CCAAT/enhancer-binding protein δ (C/EBPδ) expression and promotion of intestinal development in human intestinal epithelial cells [42]. On the other hand, the milk-exosomal miR-148a and miR-30b have been correlated to adipogenic effects, supporting a correlation between milk consumption and obesity incidence [43]. In vitro and in vivo studies reported that milk exosome-derived miRNAs also exert oncogenic or oncosuppressor properties (Figure 2). An association has been reported between cow milk consumption and large B-cell lymphoma development, sustained by miR-148a-3p and miR-155-5p/miR-29b-5p increase via let-7-5p/miR-125b-5p [44]. As oncomir, miR-21 promotes cell growth and anabolism, encouraging cell proliferation and cancer development by activating mTORC1 [45]. MiR-21 and miR-155 have been related to the most advanced stages of breast cancer progression, being involved in the development of tamoxifen resistance, metastasis formation, and worst prognosis [46]. Commercial milk consumption has been correlated to an increased risk of estrogen receptor-positive breast cancer development, due to the content of multiple oncogenic factors, as miR-148a-3p and miR-21-5p [47]. Milk-derived miRNAs have been associated with prostate cancer tumorigenesis promotion. In vitro studies have shown that milk-derived miR-148 increased prostate cancer proliferation by inhibiting cyclin-dependent kinase inhibitor 1B (CDKN1B) and promoted DNA methyltransferase 1 (DNMT1)-dependent epithelial-mesenchymal transition (EMT) [45]. Another significant milk-derived miRNA, miR-125b, increases the development of prostate xenograft cancer targeting proapoptotic genes, as p53, p53-upregulated modulator of apoptosis (PUMA), and BCL2 Antagonist/Killer 1 (BAK1) [48], and regulates several tumorigenic pathways, including NF-κB, p53, phosphatidyl inositol 3-kinase (PI3K)/protein kinase B (AKT)/mTORC1, erb-b2 receptor tyrosine kinase 2 (ERBB2), and Wnt [45]. Epidemiological studies highlighted the association between milk consumption and reduced risk of colorectal cancer [49]. The expression of miR-148a is downregulated in colorectal cancer (CRC), where it exerts a tumor-suppressor activity interfering in NF-κB and signal transducer and activator of transcription 3 (STAT3) pathways and modulating cancer related immune response via inhibition of the programmed death ligand-1 (PD-L1) levels [45]. The in vitro antineoplastic effect of miR-148a-3p overexpression also occurs through mitochondrial impairment, lipid peroxidation, and ferroptosis sustained by the Acyl CoA synthetase long-chain family member 4 (ACSL4)/transferrin receptor (TFRC)/Ferritin axis and direct solute carrier family seven-member 11 (SLC7A11) downregulation in the CRC model [50]. Another buffalo milk-derived miRNA, miR-27b, exerted antineoplastic effects on HCT116 and HT-29 CRC cells by inducing mitochondrial oxidative stress, lysosome accumulation, and apoptotic cell death mediated by endoplasmic reticulum (ER) stress [51].

2.2. XenomiRNAs from Vegetable Sources

Several miRNAs characterized from different vegetables and involved in chronic diseases, including cancer, have been evaluated (Figure 1). It has been described the ability of miR-156a, contained in different vegetables, such as cabbage, spinach, and lettuce, to target junctional adhesion molecule A (JAM-A), thus suppressing the development of atherosclerosis in human aortic endothelial cells through the inhibition of monocyte adhesion, occurring under inflammatory stress [52]. Similarly, the miR-167e-5p, characterized by *Moringa oleifera*, exerted a time- and dose-dependent anticancer action in Caco-2 cells acting on the β-catenin pathway [53]. The miR-159, particularly abundant in broccoli, is able to suppress breast tumor development, both in vitro and in vivo models [54,55]. In silico prediction identified two miRNA sequences, bra-miR156g-5p and Myseq-330, in broccoletti *Brassica rapa sylvestris*, as targeting apoptosis-related human genes, although further in vitro studies on pancreatic cancer cells did not support a miR-based modulating role in cancer growth [56].

2.2.1. Rice

An extensive study on miRNAs derived from *Oryza sativa* rice revealed their binding affinity for multiple human genes involved in cardiovascular and neurological diseases and cancer [57]. The *Oryza sativa*-derived osa-miR-172d-5p exerted in vitro beneficial effects in human lung fibroblasts, suppressing transforming growth factor (TGF)-β activated kinase 1 (MAP3K7) binding protein 1 (Tab1) and TGF-β-induced fibrotic gene expression in a bleomycin-induced lung fibrosis model [58]. Analyses on mice and human serum after rice consumption revealed miR-168 circulating levels associated with reduced clearance of plasmatic low-density lipoprotein (LDL) [59,60], while the rice aleurone-derived hvu-miR-168-3p increased the glucose transporter 1 (GLUT1) expression and reduced blood glucose levels by specifically inhibiting the electron transport chain complex I in both in vitro and in vivo models [61].

2.2.2. Ginger

The action of different xenomiRNAs from vegetable sources in the modulation of oncological pathways has been reported. A report on stomach tissues of patients with different gastric conditions, such as gastritis, metaplasia, and cancer, unveiled higher plant-derived miR-168 levels in tissues of patients affected by intestinal metaplasia [62]. In particular, the ginger-derived miR-1078, by regulating leptin, is related to lipopolysaccharide (LPS)-induced interleukin (IL)-6 expression, whereas miR-167a acts as a gut microbiota modulator targeting *Lactobacillus rhamnosus* GG SpaC pilus adhesin [63,64]. Among the different miRNAs contained in the ginger-derived exosomes-like nanoparticles (GELNs), mdo-miR-7267-3p increased the production of IL-22, thus inducing mice colitis [65], while the plant-derived miR-34a, miR-143, and miR-145 act as tumor suppressors in the mouse CRC model [66].

2.2.3. Soybean

In vitro studies showed that the soybean-derived miR-159a exerted an antitumor activity, suppressing Caco-2 proliferation and triggering apoptotic cell death [67], while gma-miR-4995 targets the transcripts of two long noncoding RNAs, metastasis-associated lung adenocarcinoma transcript 1 (MALAT1) and nuclear paraspeckle assembly transcript 1 (NEAT1), strongly expressed during the metastasis formation of several cancer types. The inhibitory action of gma-miR-4995 on MALAT1 and NEAT1 results in the attenuation of cell proliferation and apoptosis induction in CRC cell lines [68]. The soybean exosome-like nanoparticles (ELNs)-derived miR-5781 is able to modulate the inflammatory response by targeting IL-17A [62], while miR-159a might prevent hepatic fibrosis suppressing glycogen synthase kinase-3β (GSK-3β)-mediated NF-κB and TGF-β1 pathways, thus impairing TGF-β1- and platelet-derived growth factor (PDGF)-related hepatic stellate cell activation [69].

2.2.4. Fruits

The ELNs from 11 different edible fruits (blueberry, coconut, grapefruit, Hami melon, kiwifruit, orange, pea, pear, and tomato) contain several miRNAs capable of specifically targeting genes encoding inflammatory mediators [63]. The apple-derived mdm-miR-7121d-h can downregulate the intestinal solute carrier organic anion transporter family member 2B1 (SLCO2B1), thus influencing enteric macromolecules absorption in the human intestine [70].

3. Food-Derived Nutrients as miRNA Regulators in Chronic Diseases

Nutrients affect the miRNA profile through the direct or indirect modulation of gene expression. Multiple macro- and micronutrients, such as fatty acids, carbohydrates, vitamins and phytochemicals, are able to regulate miRNA levels [31], thus rendering food epigenetics more intriguing since several pathological patterns and their related pathways are still unravelled. Herein, we report the capability of many phytochemicals, belonging to the macrocategory of polyphenols (resveratrol, curcumin, quercetin, genistein, epigallocatechin gallate), and nonpolyphenols (fatty acids and vitamins), to affect miRNA expression and the involvement of these noncoding RNAs in chronic diseases and cancer (Figure 3).

3.1. Inflammatory and Degenerative Diseases

Several bioactive compounds, such as resveratrol, curcumin, polyunsatured fatty acids (PUFA), and quercetin act as antioxidants by modulating the expression of miRNA involved in crucial inflammatory pathways (Figure 3). Resveratrol displayed anti-inflammatory actions by inducing miR-663 and miR Let7A upregulation and a decrease of miR-155 in human monocytes stressed with LPS [71–73]. This polyphenolic molecule ameliorated liver fibrosis and reduced hepatocyte apoptosis by inhibiting miR-190a-5p expression, upregulated by profibrogenetic factors such as TGF-β1 and CCl_4 [74]. The reduction of miR-155 levels to counteract the LPS-induced inflammation has also been reported in macrophages treated with curcumin [75] as well as in mouse macrophages and human microvascular endothelial cells. The treatment with PUFA induced the negative regulation of inflammatory-related miRNAs levels, such as miR-146a, miR-146b, miR-21, miR-125a, and miR-155 [76]. In vitro treatment with apple-derived exosomes displayed anti-inflammatory activity via the promotion of miR-146 expression in human macrophages [77]. Recently, the potential therapeutic role of quercetin, resveratrol, curcumin, and vitamin D against the psoriasis-related inflammatory and proliferative pathogenetic pathways via miR-155, miR-146, and miR-125b regulation has been described [78]. The protective action of quercetin in endometriosis has been reported both in vitro and in vivo. Treatment with quercetin led to miR-145 upregulation, thus negatively regulating the TGF-β1/small mother against the decapentaplegic (SMAD)2/SMAD3 pathway and modulating the pathological process of endometrial fibrosis [79]. Additionally, quercetin downregulated cyclin D1 levels, opposing cell proliferation and inducing apoptosis, by enhancing miR-503-5p, miR-1283, miR-3714, and miR-6867-5p levels [80]. In Alzheimer disease, quercetin exhibited a neuroprotective role in maintaining miRNA homeostasis in neuronal cells by preventing miR-125b, miR-26a, and miR-2218 altered expression [81]. Treatment with resveratrol and selenium nanoparticles reduced metabolic dysfunction and neuroinflammation via increased amyloid-β clearance, sirtuin (SIRT)1 upregulation, and STAT3, IL-1β, and miR-143 downregulation in a rat model of Alzheimer disease [82].

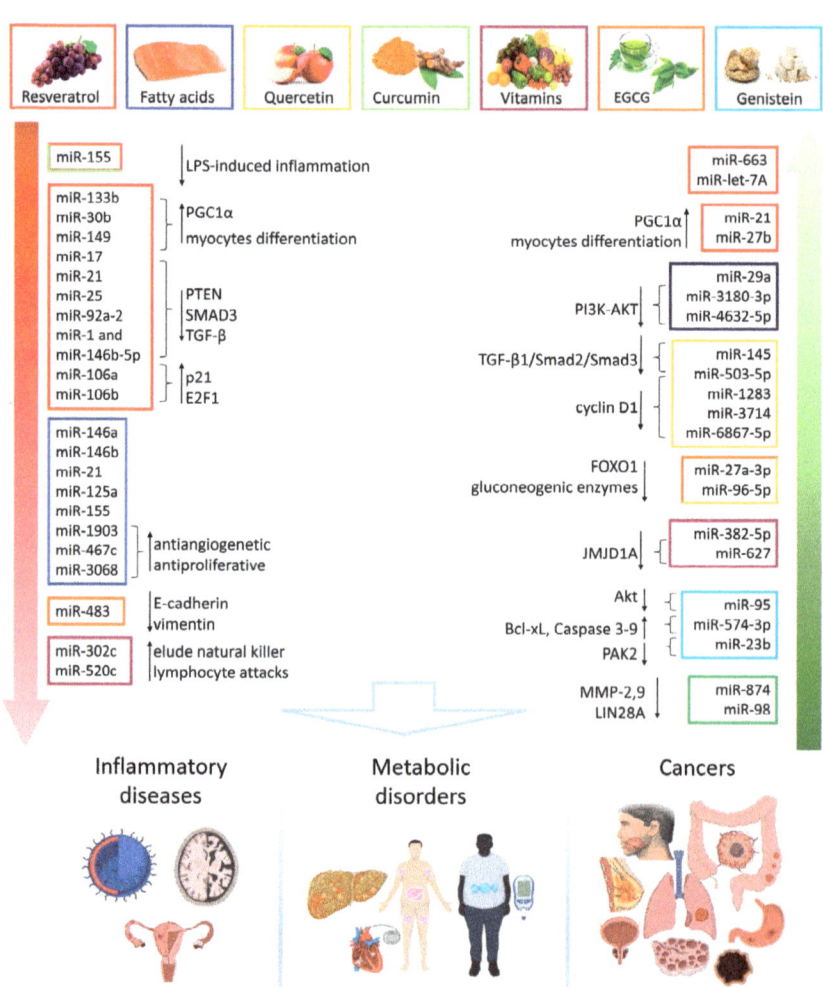

Figure 3. Diet-derived nutrients and miRNA expression. Bioactive compounds, such as curcumin, quercetin, vitamins, fatty acids, EGCG, resveratrol, and genistein, affect human miRNA expression and regulate several pathways, thus modulating the development of pathological chronic states, including inflammatory diseases, metabolic disorders, and cancer. The up arrows stand for upregulation, while the down ones indicate downregulation. AKT, protein kinase B; EGCG, epigallocatechin gallate; FOXO1, Forkhead Box O1; JMJD1A, Jumonji domain-containing 1A; LIN28A, Lin-28 Homolog A; LPS, lipopolysaccharide; miR, microRNA; PAK2, p21 activated kinase 2; MMP, matrix metalloproteinase; PGC1α, peroxisome proliferator-activated receptor gamma coactivator 1α; PI3K, phosphatidyl inositol 3-kinase; PTEN, phosphatase and tensin homolog; SMAD, small mother against decapentaplegic; TGF, transforming growth factor.

3.2. Metabolic Diseases

Many phytochemicals are able to counteract the pathogenesis of metabolic conditions by acting as miRNA regulators (Figure 3). Resveratrol exerted beneficial action on age-related alterations, as senile sarcopenia, by promoting peroxisome proliferator-activated receptor-gamma coactivator 1α (PGC1α) expression and myocyte differentiation by miR-21 and miR-27b upregulation and a decrease of miR-133b, miR-30b, and miR-149 levels [83]. In addition, the resveratrol-induced miR-21 upregulation alleviated cognitive impairment due to insulin resistance and diabetes in mice [84]. The link between saturated fatty acids (SFA) and poor health outcomes and metabolic disorders [85] is already well established; additionally, it is reported that SFA effects on human health could also depend on their influence on miRNAs [86]. Rat myoblast cells treated with palmitic acid (PA) developed insulin resistance and T2DM triggered by miR-29a increase [86]. In addition, PA decreased insulin-induced activation of the PI3K-AKT pathway, enhancing the expression of miR-3180-3p and miR-4632-5p, thus favoring insulin resistance development in HepG2 cells [87]. Stimulation with PA treatment induced mouse cardiomyocyte injuries derived from atrial arrhythmia by targeting miR-27b [88]. High fat and hypercaloric diets can modulate the levels of miRNAs involved in lipid metabolism, cell homeostasis, and fibrogenesis. Evidence demonstrates that fat-rich dietary regimens are associated with downregulation of miR-122 and upregulation of miR-200a, miR-200b, and miR-429 in liver, determining the onset of nonalcoholic fatty liver disease (NAFLD) [89,90]. Similarly, treatment with *Moringa oleifera* prevented liver damage and nonalcoholic steatohepatitis (NASH) progression via SIRT1 upregulation and miR-21a-5p, miR-103-3p, miR-122-5p, and miR-34a-5p downregulation [91]. The role of vitamins in many metabolic processes, as well as in modulating the immune system and disease prevention, has been extensively reported [92]. To this aim, recent reports revealed that treatment with the carotenoid astaxanthin has been able to promote miR-382-5p expression in hepatic stellate cells, thus opposing liver dysfunctional fibrosis [93]. The potential of vitamin D3 and all trans retinoic acid formulations in the prevention of diabetic cardiovascular complications via miR-126 upregulation has been revealed in diabetic mice [94]. Evidence described the ability of quercetin to ameliorate diabetic nephropathy damage by miR-485-5p upregulation and yes-associated protein 1 (YAP1) suppression in human mesangial cells [95] and to attenuate testosterone secretion dysfunction in diabetic rats by reducing ER stress through miR-1306-5p/hydroxysteroid 17-β dehydrogenase 7 (HSD17B7) axis modulation [96]. The combined treatment of catechin epigallocatechin gallate (EGCG) and quercetin prevented insulin resistance by increasing the expression of miR-27a-3p and miR-96-5p, which directly target Forkhead Box O1 (FOXO1), reducing the production of glucose and the transcription of gluconeogenic enzymes [97]. In addition, ECGC showed therapeutic potential in obesity inhibiting white and beige 3T3-L1 and D12 preadipocyte growth by upregulated miR-let-7a and subsequent high-mobility group AT-hook 2 (HMGA2) suppression [98] and inhibiting the MAPK7 pathway by increased miR-143 levels [99]. Clinical data from a cohort of women affected by overweight and insulin resistance revealed that blood orange juice consumption (500 mL per day) for four weeks resulted in upregulated miR-144-3p, miR-424-5p, miR-144-3p, and miR-130b-3p and decreased let-7f-5p and miR-126-3p levels in peripheral blood mononuclear cells, leading to attenuated IL-6 and NF-κB mRNA expression [100].

3.3. Cancer

Given the beneficial effects mediated by nutrients on miRNA profile, several studies dissected their use as an oncological approach in different neoplastic contexts (Figure 3).

3.3.1. Digestive System Cancers

Resveratrol exerted anti-inflammatory effects and attenuated colitis-induced tumorigenesis by increasing miR-101b and miR-455 levels [101]. In colorectal cancer, resveratrol decreased the expression levels of characterized oncomiRs, as miR-17, miR-21, miR-25, and miR-92a-2 [102], and exerted a pivotal regulation on many tumor suppressors, such as

PTEN and SMAD3, as well as on the oncogenic TGF-β pathway related to progression and metastasis of colorectal cancer by targeting the expression levels of miR-1 and miR-146b-5p [103]. The resveratrol-related modulation of the tumor promoter TGF-β1 was further associated with upregulated miR-663 levels as reported in the SW480 cell line [104]. Genistein exhibited in vitro and in vivo anticancer effect inhibiting miR-95 and its targets AKT and serum and glucocorticoid-regulated kinase 1 (SGK1) on HCT116 cells [105,106] and enhanced miR-1275 levels thus suppressing Eukaryotic Translation Initiation Factor 5A2 (EIF5A2)/PI3K/AKT pathway in hepatocellular carcinoma [107]. In mice colorectal cancer tissues, the walnut-based diet PUFAs have been associated with reduced levels of miR-1903, miR-467c, and miR-3068, along with augmented miR-297a expression levels, resulting in anti-inflammatory, antiangiogenetic, antiproliferative and pro-apoptotic effects [108,109]. In vivo studies showed that vitamin D suppressed colorectal cancer cell proliferation, downregulating histone demethylase 1A (JMJD1A) by increasing miR-627 levels [110,111]. The EGCG treatment was able to suppress miR-483 levels via hypermethylation of its promoter region, modulating the expression of metastatic markers as E-cadherin and vimentin in a mouse model of hepatocellular carcinoma [112], while resveratrol opposed the tumor progression via downregulation of miR-155-5p in gastric cancer cells [113].

3.3.2. Hormone-Dependent Cancers

Resveratrol opposed the overexpressed levels of miR-17, miR-18b, miR-20a, miR-20b, miR-92b, miR-106a, and miR-106b in prostate cancer [114,115], whilst genistein was able to restore in vivo and in vitro miR-574-3p expression levels, generally downregulated in prostate cancer cells [116,117]. Treatment with vitamin D positively regulated the levels of miR-100 and miR-125b in primary prostate cancer tissues, opposing tumor progression [118,119], while in breast cancer T47D and SK-BR-3, cell line treatment with retinoic acid strongly increased miR-10a expression and retinoic acid receptor β (RARβ), whose loss is associated with breast carcinogenesis [120]. Vitamin D was also shown to decrease breast cancer cell capacity to elude natural killer lymphocyte attacks through the reduction of miR-302c and miR-520c expression [121,122]. The effect of curcumin treatment on miR-21 was effective in inhibiting the growth of MCF-7 breast cancer cells [123]. Curcumin treatment also positively regulated miR-181b, miR-34a, miR-16, miR-15a, and miR-146b-5p and down-regulated miR-19a, and miR-19b expression in estrogen receptor-positive primary cells and several breast cancer cell lines with effects on inflammatory cascade, cell cycle progression, survival, and invasiveness [124,125]. The curcumin-dependent miR-146b-5p upregulation suppressed the transactivation of the breast stromal fibroblasts, responsible for the epithelial-to-mesenchymal transition in breast cancer stromal fibroblasts [126]. In vitro studies proved that EGCG counteracted breast cancer progression, attenuating the expression of miR-25 [127], while genistein reduced the expression levels of onco-miR-155, the regulator of several tumor suppressors as PTEN and p27, and impaired cell mobility via p21 activated kinase 2 (PAK2) and miR-23b upregulation in breast cancer cells [128,129]. Resveratrol modulated the oncosuppressor ARH-I expression and limited the "awakening" of ovarian cancer cells, reducing the oncomiR-1305 [130].

3.3.3. Respiratory Tract Cancers

In lung cancer cells, curcumin treatment was able to inhibit cell invasion via upregulation of miR-874, which directly targets matrix metalloproteinase-2 (MMP-2), and miR-98, which suppresses MMP-2 and MMP-9 pathways by targeting LIN28A [131]. In human non-small cell lung carcinoma (NSCLC) A549 cell line, curcumin-induced apoptosis and reduced migration and invasion through miR-206 upregulation and suppression of the PI3K/AKT/mTOR signaling pathway [132]. In addition, treatment with curcumin suppressed tumor progression by increasing miR-192-5p expression and c-Myc reduction in NSCLC cells A427 and A549 [133]. EGCG repressed c-myc expression via upregulation of tumor suppressors miR-let-7a-1 and miR-let-7g in lung cancer cells [134,135]. Quercetin displayed anti-cancer properties by opposing cell survival and enhancing apoptosis in

NSCLC cells by increased miR-34a-5p and downregulation of a long noncoding RNA small nucleolar RNA host gene 7 (SNHG7) [136], while in oral squamous cell carcinoma Cal-27 cells quercetin inhibited cell proliferation and metastasis via accumulation of miR-1254 and subsequent downregulation of CD36 [137], and suppressed proliferation and MMP-9 and -2 levels via a miR-16/homeobox A10 (HOXA10) axis increase [138]. In vitro treatment with quercetin promoted apoptosis and repressed metastatic feature in esophageal cancer cells by upregulating miR-1-3p and suppression of Transgelin 2 (TAGNL2) expression [139], while an increase in genistein-induced mir-34a led to production of reactive oxygen species (ROS) and apoptosis in head and neck cancer [140].

3.3.4. Neuroectodermal Cancers

Recent reports described the curcumin-induced miR-222-3p upregulation, thus negatively modulating the expression levels of its target SOX10, causing the inactivation of the SOX10/Notch pathway and limiting proliferation, migration, and invasion of melanoma cells [141]. Similarly, treatment with EGCG upregulated miR-let-7b, thus suppressing growth and development in melanoma cells [142]. Resveratrol induced apoptosis via miR-21 in human glioma cells [143] and genistein inhibited the retinoblastoma cell viability by miR-145 upregulation [144]. The glycoside flavonoid purple sweet potato delphinidin-3-rutin (PSPD3R) suppressed in vitro and in vivo glioma proliferation regulating autophagy by inducing the AKT/cAMP response element-binding protein (CREB)/miR-20b-5p/autophagy related 7 (Atg7) pathway [145].

4. Latest Dietary miRNA-Based Animal Models and Clinical Trials

Most of the evidence on the effects of food-borne bioactive compounds on the regulation of human miRNAs in various diseases comes from preliminary in vitro studies, recently validated in animal models. The antidiabetic effects of quercetin and ECGC were proved in mice fed with an enriched-polyphenol diet (0.05% w/w) ad libitum for 10 weeks [97]. Results revealed the capacity of quercetin and EGCG enrichment to increase miR-27a-3p and miR-96-5p and inhibit gluconeogenesis and FOXO1 pathways, with enhanced effects when combined (Table 1) [97]. BALB/c mice overexpressing or not miR-483-3p were treated for two weeks with ad libitum 0%, 0.1%, or 0.5% EGCG solution, then HepG2 cells were inoculated, and the diet prolonged for two months [112]. Supplementation with EGCG reduced hepatocarcinoma lung metastasis and opposed EMT via miR-483-3p inhibition (Table 1) [112]. Although few clinical trials evaluating the relationship between food-borne miRNAs and human health have been conducted, the number of clinical trials is continuously increasing (www.clinicaltrials.gov) (Table 1). New insights into alterations of skeletal muscle miRNA expression when consuming 1 g/kg/h carbohydrate during the first 3 h of recovery from aerobic exercise (NCT03250234) have been recently described [146]. Authors reported that carbohydrate consumption during an 80 min bout of steady-state treadmill exercise led to increased expression of miR-19b-3p, miR-99a-5p, miR-100-5p, miR-222-3p, miR-324-3p, and miR486-5p immediately following and/or within 3 h from recovery compared with a nutrient-free control, thus resulting in downregulation of breakdown protein gene expression and better muscle recovery (Table 1) [146].

Results from the RESMENA study (NCT01087086) evaluated the effect of the Mediterranean dietary pattern on miRNA levels in white blood cells of 40 patients with metabolic syndrome. Data showed that 8-week hypocaloric diet (30% caloric deficiency) based on Mediterranean diet reduced the expression of miR-155, miR-125, miR-130, miR-132, and miR-422, associated with cancer, atherogenic and adipogenic processes, and other inflammatory conditions (Table 1) [147]. The effects of 60 months with a typical Mediterranean regimen (Med diet) versus a low-fat high complex carbohydrate (LFHCC) diet were correlated to T2DM development and differences in miRNA plasma levels in CORDIOPREV study (NCT00924937) [148]. Following LFHCC consumption, patients with low plasma miR-145 levels showed a higher risk of developing T2DM, as well as the subjects assuming a Med diet with low levels of miR-29a, miR-28-3p, and miR-126 and high miR-150 expression (Table 1) [148]. Current therapeutic options for the treatment of antiphospholipid syndrome showed the efficacy of daily ubiquinol treatment (200 mg for 1 month) in the regulation of a profile of monocyte miRNAs and identified novel and specific miRNA-mRNA regulatory networks associated with atherothrombosis development (NCT02218476) [149]. A completed clinical trial (NCT01634841) provided a systematic investigation of the role of walnuts in preventing or slowing age-related cognitive decline and macular degeneration [150]. Authors screened miRNA profiles in serum samples (before and after intervention) of eight randomly selected participants from the walnut arm, showing 53 miRNAs modulated after one year assuming 15% of daily energy as walnuts, 36 of them being upregulated and 17 downregulated [150]. Compared with participants in the control diet, walnuts consumed for 1 year significantly increased the serum concentration of miR-551 related to the inhibited progression of several cancers [150]. The antineoplastic effects of vitamin D were evaluated in prostate cancer [118]. A cohort of prostate cancer patients was treated with three different vitamin D3 doses (400, 10,000 or 40,000 IU/day) in the time between randomization and prostatectomy (approximately 3–8 weeks). Vitamin D3 assumption determined an increase in tumor suppressors miR-100 and miR-125b in both pathological and healthy prostatic tissue [118]. The HYPODD study correlated the vitamin D supplementation to miR-21 circulating levels in the pathogenesis of cardiometabolic disorders [151]. Hypovitaminosis D correction (50,000 UI/week for 8 weeks and then 50,000 UI/month for 10 months) ameliorated the cardiovascular risk profiles in hypertensive patients without affecting the miR-21 circulating expression (Table 1) [151]. The effects of 4-week time-restricted eating (TRE), a popular form of intermittent fasting, determined downregulation of a miRNA panel (miR-4649-5p, miR-2467-3p, miR-543, miR-301a-3p, miR-3132, miR-19a-5p, miR-495-3p, and miR-4761-3p), which, in turn, could inhibit cell growth pathways while activating cell survival and promoting healthy aging (NCT03590847) [152]. A study conducted on 125 subjects with hypercholesterolemia (ACTRN12619000170123) evaluated the effect of daily assumption of a nutraceutical combination containing 400 mg phytosterols, 100 mg bergamot extract, 20 mg olive extract, and 52 µM vitamin K2 up to 12 weeks of treatment [153]. The evaluated nutraceutical combination did not change the serum lipid profile and inflammation-related miRNAs and biomarkers [153].

Table 1. Dose effect sizes, in vivo models, target miRNAs, and biological relevance to foods, constituents, and dietary regimen or supplementation.

Food, Constituent or Regimen	Dose Effect Size	Model	Target miRNA	Biological Relevance	Refs.
Quercetin	0.05% w/w	Mouse	miR-27a-3p, miR-96-5p	Antidiabetic	[97]
EGCG	0.05% w/w	Mouse	miR-27a-3p, miR-96-5p, miR-483	Antidiabetic	[97]
	0%, 0.1%, 0.5% solution ad libitum	Mouse	miR-483	Anticancer properties in hepatocellular carcinoma	[112]
Walnut	30–60 g/d	Human	miR-551	Anticancer properties	[150]
Vitamin D	400, 10,000 or 40,000 IU/day	Human	miR-100, miR-125b	Anticancer properties in prostate cancer	[118]
	50,000 UI/week for 8 weeks, 50,000 UI/month for 10 months	Human	miR-21	Lower cardiovascular risk in hypertensive patients	[151]

Table 1. *Cont.*

Food, Constituent or Regimen	Dose Effect Size	Model	Target miRNA	Biological Relevance	Refs.
Carbohydrates	1 g/kg/h in 3 h after 2 cycle ergometry glycogen depletion	Human	miR-19b-3p, miR-99a-5p, miR-100-5p, miR-222-3p, miR-324-3p, miR-486-5p	Enhanced recovery after exercise	[146]
Ubiquitinol	200 mg/d	Human	20 different miRNAs	Anti-phospholipids syndrome	[149]
Mediterranean diet	8-week hypocaloric diet	Human	miR-155, miR-125, miR-130, miR-132, miR-422	Anti-inflammatory, anticancer, anti-atherogenic	[147]
	low-fat high complex carbohydrate vs. Mediterranean diet for 60 months	Human	miR-145, miR-29a, miR-28-3p, miR-126, miR-150	Diabetic risk	[148]
Nutraceutical combination	400 mg phytosterols, 100 mg bergamot extract, 20 mg olive extract, 52 µM vitamin K2	Human	miR-21, miR-146a miR-126	No significant effects on lipid and inflammatory profile, as on miRNA levels	[153]

5. Questions Opening on the Potential Impact of Dietary miRNAs on Health and Disease

Increasing evidence highlight the potential of dietary miRNAs to modulate human pathophysiology, suggesting new dietary-based intervention approaches [154]. However, a preventive strategy based on xenomiRNAs denotes multiple limitations, due to their poor bioavailability, the restricted knowledge of the potential side effects related to high consumption, and the appropriate dietary intake according to their stability due to manufacturing processes and food storage [155]. The bioavailability of food-targeted miRNAs after ingestion is still a controversial issue. In vitro and in vivo evidences reported upregulated miR-29b, miR-200c, miR-21-5p, and miR-30a-5p plasma levels after milk consumption, supporting the availability of these molecules [17,156]. On the other hand, given the base sequence complementarity between miR-21-5p and miR-30a-5p in humans and animals, the precise assessment of xenomiRNA uptaken by diet is quite uncertain [157]. Moreover, the increase in miRNA plasmatic concentration could be ascribed to endogenous responses to other milk-derived compounds [158]. Analyses by real time quantitative PCR (RT-qPCR) and RNA-sequencing on human blood did not provide supporting evidences about the absorption of specific bovine miRNAs after milk consumption [159], as well as results on milk-fed mice highlighted the absence of miRNA absorption and revealed their rapid degradation in intestinal fluids [160]. Analyses by RT-qPCR performed on post-prandial plasma of pigtail macaques reported absent or low-levels of nonspecific amplified miRNAs, thus supporting the scarce intestinal absorption of plant xenomiRNAs [161]. Likewise, the plant-derived miR-168 has been detected in feces and gastrointestinal mucosa while being undetectable in blood, confirming that the potential availability of gastrointestinal tract is not accompanied by systemic absorption [162]. On the other hand, the detection of the plant miR-172 in gastrointestinal tract, serum and feces of mice fed with plant RNA extracts, confirmed the possibility of a dietary-derived miRNA amount absorbed by intestinal tract [163]. Growing evidence reported xenomiRNAs as food contaminants, describing some plant-derived miRNAs as a consequence of experimental contamination and artifacts [19,164]. In addition, the biological and functional role of dietary miRNAs from different sources in human health is still controversial. Different milk-derived miRNAs have been reported to modulate oncogenic and adipogenic pathways, promoting the development of B-cell lymphoma, hormone-dependent breast and prostate cancer [43–45,47], as well as the ginger-related miRNA has been associated with colitis development [64] and the pork-derived miRNAs to the development of metabolic disorders in mice [22]. The evaluation of food-derived xenomiRNA effects cannot refrain from considering the co-existence of a great variety of dietary bioactive compounds. In the absence of supplementary intake of dietary exogenous miRNAs, many phytochemicals or animal-based food derivatives may modify the risk of diseases, targeting the reported biological effects [29,165]. Indeed, several food-derived compounds exert their regulatory effects on different diseases either by upregulating or downregulating different signaling pathways, as well as acting on many epigenetic patterns [166]. Dietary constituents are able to affect epigenetic mechanisms, including DNA status modulation, histone methylation, and acetylation, by aiming key epigenetic modulators such as DNA methyltransferases and histone deacetylases, thus resulting in local or global changes in epigenetics and subsequent gene transcription and expression levels [29,165,166]. Attractive strategies from a better knowledge of nutrimiromics are undeniable [167], although further studies are needed to determine the pharmacokinetics and the possible side effects of dietary miRNA-based intervention in human health. Based on current evidence here summarized, it has to take into account both the promising results of food-derived miRNAs and negative effects exerted by the dietary molecules on human health, thus their dual role in chronic diseases still represents an open door in nutrition-based strategies.

6. Conclusions

Herein, we provided an up-to-date comprehensive review of food-derived miRNA activities in human health and disease, reporting both beneficial and controversial issues of dietary miRNAs as regulators of chronic conditions. Recent reports aim to elucidate the association between altered miRNA expression and pathological processes contributing to the onset of several chronic diseases. The crucial roles of different miRNAs in the development of T2DM, insulin resistance and obesity [168–171] have been described, as well as in the progression of other chronic syndromes, such as asthma, allergy, and chronic kidney disease (CKD) [172–176]. This evidence points out nutrient-regulated miRNAs and food-derived miRNAs as intriguing players in food-related health and disease, although the knowledge on miRNA specific role is partially known and still debatable, requiring future studies to broaden knowledge on possible molecular targets and their modulation. In this regard, lifestyle habits, affecting the expression levels of miRNAs, represent a crucial element in the perspective of preventive and personalized medicine. A healthy diet with a personalized choice of nutrients based on individual needs related to age and state of health, i.e., ranging from health to disease or disability/rehabilitative conditions, is essential for maintaining the state of health and to slow down the aging clock. To this end, dietary miRNAs could represent intervention tools in precision nutrition, although with several limitations to overcome, including bioinstability, poor availability, unknown side effects, and multiple molecular targets. Within this framework, future preclinical and clinical studies will benefit from multidisciplinary and translational design taking into consideration some host-related aspects such as microbiome, circadian rhythm and self-susceptibility, and miRNA-derived limitations, as scarce bioavailability and undefined content in body fluids, which undoubtedly add complexity in dissecting the still controversial role of dietary miRNAs in human health and diseases.

Author Contributions: Conceptualization, E.M., N.D. and M.L.B.; methodology, E.M., N.D. and M.L.B.; visualization, A.C. and C.A.; writing- original draft, E.M., N.D. and M.L.B.; supervision, A.B., C.S., R.M., G.C. and M.L.B.; funding acquisition, N.D. and M.L.B. All authors have read and agreed to the published version of the manuscript.

Funding: This research was funded by STUPORANIMA Project, Funder: Italian Ministry of Health-RC, Number: IZS ME 09/22; ENDO-CARE Project, Funder: Ministero dell'Università e della Ricerca,

Next Generation EU Number: P2022SZE5Y; Fuelmilk Project, Funder: Ministero dell'Università e della Ricerca, Number: 2022KH87XS; FORMULAMI Project, Funder: Ministero dello Sviluppo Economico, Number: F/310110/04/X56.

Conflicts of Interest: The authors declare no conflicts of interest.

References

1. Di Renzo, L.; Gualtieri, P.; Romano, L.; Marrone, G.; Noce, A.; Pujia, A.; Perrone, M.A.; Aiello, V.; Colica, C.; De Lorenzo, A. Role of Personalized Nutrition in Chronic-Degenerative Diseases. *Nutrients* **2019**, *11*, 1707. [CrossRef]
2. Shi, Y.; Liu, Z.; Lin, Q.; Luo, Q.; Cen, Y.; Li, J.; Fang, X.; Gong, C. MiRNAs and Cancer: Key Link in Diagnosis and Therapy. *Genes* **2021**, *12*, 1289. [CrossRef]
3. Leitão, A.L.; Enguita, F.J. A Structural View of miRNA Biogenesis and Function. *Noncoding RNA* **2022**, *8*, 10. [CrossRef]
4. Sadri, M.; Shu, J.; Kachman, S.D.; Cui, J.; Zempleni, J. Milk exosomes and miRNA cross the placenta and promote embryo survival in mice. *Reproduction* **2020**, *160*, 501–509. [CrossRef]
5. Mori, M.A.; Ludwig, R.G.; Garcia-Martin, R.; Brandão, B.B.; Kahn, C.R. Extracellular miRNAs: From Biomarkers to Mediators of Physiology and Disease. *Cell Metab.* **2019**, *30*, 656–673. [CrossRef]
6. Kučuk, N.; Primožič, M.; Knez, Ž.; Leitgeb, M. Exosomes Engineering and Their Roles as Therapy Delivery Tools, Therapeutic Targets, and Biomarkers. *Int. J. Mol. Sci.* **2021**, *22*, 9543. [CrossRef]
7. Abozaid, Y.J.; Zhang, X.; Mens, M.M.J.; Ahmadizar, F.; Limpens, M.; Ikram, M.A.; Rivadeneira, F.; Voortman, T.; Kavousi, M.; Ghanbari, M. Plasma circulating microRNAs associated with obesity, body fat distribution, and fat mass: The Rotterdam Study. *Int. J. Obes.* **2022**, *46*, 2137–2144. [CrossRef]
8. McNeill, E.M.; Hirschi, K.D. Roles of Regulatory RNAs in Nutritional Control. *Annu. Rev. Nutr.* **2020**, *40*, 77–104. [CrossRef]
9. Quintanilha, B.J.; Reis, B.Z.; Duarte, G.B.S.; Cozzolino, S.M.F.; Rogero, M.M. Nutrimiromics: Role of microRNAs and Nutrition in Modulating Inflammation and Chronic Diseases. *Nutrients* **2017**, *9*, 1168. [CrossRef]
10. Sanchita; Trivedi, R.; Asif, M.H.; Trivedi, P.K. Dietary plant miRNAs as an augmented therapy: Cross-kingdom gene regulation. *RNA Biol.* **2018**, *15*, 1433–1439. [CrossRef]
11. Lukasik, A.; Brzozowska, I.; Zielenkiewicz, U.; Zielenkiewicz, P. Detection of Plant miRNAs Abundance in Human Breast Milk. *Int. J. Mol. Sci.* **2017**, *19*, 37. [CrossRef]
12. Cannataro, R.; Cione, E. Diet and miRNA: Epigenetic Regulator or a New Class of Supplements? *Microrna* **2022**, *11*, 89–90. [CrossRef]
13. Otsuka, K.; Ochiya, T. Possible connection between diet and microRNA in cancer scenario. *Semin. Cancer Biol.* **2021**, *73*, 4–18. [CrossRef]
14. Rasheed, Z.; Rasheed, N.; Al-Shaya, O. Epigallocatechin-3-O-gallate modulates global microRNA expression in interleukin-1β-stimulated human osteoarthritis chondrocytes: Potential role of EGCG on negative co-regulation of microRNA-140-3p and ADAMTS5. *Eur. J. Nutr.* **2018**, *57*, 917–928. [CrossRef]
15. Preethi, K.A.; Sekar, D. Dietary microRNAs: Current status and perspective in food science. *J. Food Biochem.* **2021**, *45*, e13827. [CrossRef]
16. Fan, Y.; Habib, M.; Xia, J. Xeno-miRNet: A comprehensive database and analytics platform to explore xeno-miRNAs and their potential targets. *PeerJ* **2018**, *6*, e5650. [CrossRef]
17. Baier, S.R.; Nguyen, C.; Xie, F.; Wood, J.R.; Zempleni, J. MicroRNAs are absorbed in biologically meaningful amounts from nutritionally relevant doses of cow milk and affect gene expression in peripheral blood mononuclear cells, HEK-293 kidney cell cultures, and mouse livers. *J. Nutr.* **2014**, *144*, 1495–1500. [CrossRef]
18. Zhang, L.; Chen, T.; Yin, Y.; Zhang, C.Y.; Zhang, Y.L. Dietary microRNA-A Novel Functional Component of Food. *Adv. Nutr.* **2019**, *10*, 711–721. [CrossRef]
19. Fromm, B.; Kang, W.; Rovira, C.; Cayota, A.; Witwer, K.; Friedländer, M.R.; Tosar, J.P. Plant microRNAs in human sera are likely contaminants. *J. Nutr. Biochem.* **2019**, *65*, 139–140. [CrossRef]
20. Wade, B.; Cummins, M.; Keyburn, A.; Crowley, T.M. Isolation and detection of microRNA from the egg of chickens. *BMC Res. Notes* **2016**, *9*, 283. [CrossRef]
21. Fratantonio, D.; Munir, J.; Shu, J.; Howard, K.; Baier, S.R.; Cui, J.; Zempleni, J. The RNA cargo in small extracellular vesicles from chicken eggs is bioactive in C57BL/6 J mice and human peripheral blood mononuclear cells ex vivo. *Front. Nutr.* **2023**, *10*, 1162679. [CrossRef]
22. Shen, L.; Ma, J.; Yang, Y.; Liao, T.; Wang, J.; Chen, L.; Zhang, S.; Zhao, Y.; Niu, L.; Hao, X.; et al. Cooked pork-derived exosome nanovesicles mediate metabolic disorder-microRNA could be the culprit. *J. Nanobiotechnol.* **2023**, *21*, 83. [CrossRef]
23. Pieri, M.; Theori, E.; Dweep, H.; Flourentzou, P.; Kalampalika, F.; Maniori, M.A.; Papagregoriou, G.; Papaneophytou, C.; Felekkis, K. A bovine miRNA, bta-miR-154c, withstands in vitro human digestion but does not affect cell viability of colorectal human cell lines after transfection. *FEBS Open Bio* **2022**, *12*, 925–936. [CrossRef]
24. Servillo, L.; D'Onofrio, N.; Giovane, A.; Casale, R.; Cautela, D.; Castaldo, D.; Iannaccone, F.; Neglia, G.; Campanile, G.; Balestrieri, M.L. Ruminant meat and milk contain δ-valerobetaine, another precursor of trimethylamine N-oxide (TMAO) like γ-butyrobetaine. *Food Chem.* **2018**, *260*, 193–199. [CrossRef]

25. D'Onofrio, N.; Balestrieri, A.; Neglia, G.; Monaco, A.; Tatullo, M.; Casale, R.; Limone, A.; Balestrieri, M.L.; Campanile, G. Antioxidant and Anti-Inflammatory Activities of Buffalo Milk δ-Valerobetaine. *J. Agric. Food Chem.* **2019**, *67*, 1702–1710. [CrossRef]
26. D'Onofrio, N.; Cacciola, N.A.; Martino, E.; Borrelli, F.; Fiorino, F.; Lombardi, A.; Neglia, G.; Balestrieri, M.L.; Campanile, G. ROS-Mediated Apoptotic Cell Death of Human Colon Cancer LoVo Cells by Milk δ-Valerobetaine. *Sci. Rep.* **2020**, *10*, 8978. [CrossRef]
27. D'Onofrio, N.; Mele, L.; Martino, E.; Salzano, A.; Restucci, B.; Cautela, D.; Tatullo, M.; Balestrieri, M.L.; Campanile, G. Synergistic Effect of Dietary Betaines on SIRT1-Mediated Apoptosis in Human Oral Squamous Cell Carcinoma Cal 27. *Cancers* **2020**, *12*, 2468. [CrossRef]
28. D'Onofrio, N.; Martino, E.; Mele, L.; Colloca, A.; Maione, M.; Cautela, D.; Castaldo, D.; Balestrieri, M.L. Colorectal Cancer Apoptosis Induced by Dietary δ-Valerobetaine Involves PINK1/Parkin Dependent-Mitophagy and SIRT3. *Int. J. Mol. Sci.* **2021**, *22*, 8117. [CrossRef]
29. López de Las Hazas, M.C.; Del Pozo-Acebo, L.; Hansen, M.S.; Gil-Zamorano, J.; Mantilla-Escalante, D.C.; Gómez-Coronado, D.; Marín, F.; Garcia-Ruiz, A.; Rasmussen, J.T.; Dávalos, A. Dietary bovine milk miRNAs transported in extracellular vesicles are partially stable during GI digestion, are bioavailable and reach target tissues but need a minimum dose to impact on gene expression. *Eur. J. Nutr.* **2022**, *61*, 1043–1056. [CrossRef]
30. Tong, L.; Hao, H.; Zhang, Z.; Lv, Y.; Liang, X.; Liu, Q.; Liu, T.; Gong, P.; Zhang, L.; Cao, F.; et al. Milk-derived extracellular vesicles alleviate ulcerative colitis by regulating the gut immunity and reshaping the gut microbiota. *Theranostics* **2021**, *11*, 8570–8586. [CrossRef]
31. García-Martínez, J.; Pérez-Castillo, Í.M.; Salto, R.; López-Pedrosa, J.M.; Rueda, R.; Girón, M.D. Beneficial Effects of Bovine Milk Exosomes in Metabolic Interorgan Cross-Talk. *Nutrients* **2022**, *14*, 1442. [CrossRef] [PubMed]
32. Chen, Z.; Xie, Y.; Luo, J.; Chen, T.; Xi, Q.; Zhang, Y.; Sun, J. Milk exosome-derived miRNAs from water buffalo are implicated in immune response and metabolism process. *BMC Vet. Res.* **2020**, *16*, 123. [CrossRef] [PubMed]
33. Melnik, B.C. Milk exosomal miRNAs: Potential drivers of AMPK-to-mTORC1 switching in β-cell de-differentiation of type 2 diabetes mellitus. *Nutr. Metab.* **2019**, *16*, 85. [CrossRef] [PubMed]
34. Melnik, B.C. Synergistic Effects of Milk-Derived Exosomes and Galactose on α-Synuclein Pathology in Parkinson's Disease and Type 2 Diabetes Mellitus. *Int. J. Mol. Sci.* **2021**, *22*, 1059. [CrossRef] [PubMed]
35. Shome, S.; Jernigan, R.L.; Beitz, D.C.; Clark, S.; Testroet, E.D. Non-coding RNA in raw and commercially processed milk and putative targets related to growth and immune-response. *BMC Genom.* **2021**, *22*, 749. [CrossRef] [PubMed]
36. Aarts, J.; Boleij, A.; Pieters, B.C.H.; Feitsma, A.L.; van Neerven, R.J.J.; Ten Klooster, J.P.; M'Rabet, L.; Arntz, O.J.; Koenders, M.I.; van de Loo, F.A.J. Flood Control: How Milk-Derived Extracellular Vesicles Can Help to Improve the Intestinal Barrier Function and Break the Gut-Joint Axis in Rheumatoid Arthritis. *Front. Immunol.* **2021**, *12*, 703277. [CrossRef] [PubMed]
37. Kaur, K.; Vig, S.; Srivastava, R.; Mishra, A.; Singh, V.P.; Srivastava, A.K.; Datta, M. Elevated Hepatic miR-22-3p Expression Impairs Gluconeogenesis by Silencing the Wnt-Responsive Transcription Factor Tcf7. *Diabetes* **2015**, *64*, 3659–3669. [CrossRef] [PubMed]
38. Lönnerdal, B. *Human Milk MicroRNAs/Exosomes: Composition and Biological Effects*; Nestlé Nutrition Institute Workshop Series; Nestlé Nutrition Institute: La Tour-de-Peilz, Switzerland; S. Karger AG: Basel, Switzerland, 2019; Volume 90, pp. 83–92. [CrossRef]
39. Su, Y.; Yuan, J.; Zhang, F.; Lei, Q.; Zhang, T.; Li, K.; Guo, J.; Hong, Y.; Bu, G.; Lv, X.; et al. MicroRNA-181a-5p and microRNA-181a-3p cooperatively restrict vascular inflammation and atherosclerosis. *Cell Death Dis.* **2019**, *10*, 365. [CrossRef]
40. Lin, Y.; Lu, Y.; Huang, Z.; Wang, L.; Song, S.; Luo, Y.; Ren, F.; Guo, H. Milk-Derived Small Extracellular Vesicles Promote Recovery of Intestinal Damage by Accelerating Intestinal Stem Cell-Mediated Epithelial Regeneration. *Mol. Nutr. Food Res.* **2022**, *66*, e2100551. [CrossRef]
41. Yan, C.; Chen, J.; Wang, C.; Yuan, M.; Kang, Y.; Wu, Z.; Li, W.; Zhang, G.; Machens, H.G.; Rinkevich, Y.; et al. Milk exosomes-mediated miR-31-5p delivery accelerates diabetic wound healing through promoting angiogenesis. *Drug Deliv.* **2022**, *29*, 214–228. [CrossRef]
42. Jiang, R.; Lönnerdal, B. Milk-Derived miR-22-3p Promotes Proliferation of Human Intestinal Epithelial Cells (HIECs) by Regulating Gene Expression. *Nutrients* **2022**, *14*, 4901. [CrossRef] [PubMed]
43. Abbas, M.A.; Al-Saigh, N.N.; Saqallah, F.G. Regulation of adipogenesis by exosomal milk miRNA. *Rev. Endocr. Metab. Disord.* **2023**, *24*, 297–316. [CrossRef] [PubMed]
44. Melnik, B.C.; Stadler, R.; Weiskirchen, R.; Leitzmann, C.; Schmitz, G. Potential Pathogenic Impact of Cow's Milk Consumption and Bovine Milk-Derived Exosomal MicroRNAs in Diffuse Large B-Cell Lymphoma. *Int. J. Mol. Sci.* **2023**, *24*, 6102. [CrossRef] [PubMed]
45. Melnik, B.C. Lifetime Impact of Cow's Milk on Overactivation of mTORC1: From Fetal to Childhood Overgrowth, Acne, Diabetes, Cancers, and Neurodegeneration. *Biomolecules* **2021**, *11*, 404. [CrossRef] [PubMed]
46. Melnik, B.C.; Schmitz, G. Exosomes of pasteurized milk: Potential pathogens of Western diseases. *J. Transl. Med.* **2019**, *17*, 3. [CrossRef] [PubMed]
47. Melnik, B.C.; John, S.M.; Carrera-Bastos, P.; Cordain, L.; Leitzmann, C.; Weiskirchen, R.; Schmitz, G. The Role of Cow's Milk Consumption in Breast Cancer Initiation and Progression. *Curr. Nutr. Rep.* **2023**, *12*, 122–140. [CrossRef] [PubMed]
48. Shi, X.B.; Xue, L.; Ma, A.H.; Tepper, C.G.; Kung, H.J.; White, R.W. miR-125b promotes growth of prostate cancer xenograft tumor through targeting pro-apoptotic genes. *Prostate* **2011**, *71*, 538–549. [CrossRef]

49. Zhang, X.; Chen, X.; Xu, Y.; Yang, J.; Du, L.; Li, K.; Zhou, Y. Milk consumption and multiple health outcomes: Umbrella review of systematic reviews and meta-analyses in humans. *Nutr. Metab.* **2021**, *18*, 7. [CrossRef]
50. Martino, E.; Balestrieri, A.; Aragona, F.; Bifulco, G.; Mele, L.; Campanile, G.; Balestrieri, M.L.; D'Onofrio, N. MiR-148a-3p Promotes Colorectal Cancer Cell Ferroptosis by Targeting SLC7A11. *Cancers* **2023**, *15*, 4342. [CrossRef]
51. Martino, E.; Balestrieri, A.; Mele, L.; Sardu, C.; Marfella, R.; D'Onofrio, N.; Campanile, G.; Balestrieri, M.L. Milk Exosomal miR-27b Worsen Endoplasmic Reticulum Stress Mediated Colorectal Cancer Cell Death. *Nutrients* **2022**, *14*, 5081. [CrossRef]
52. Hou, D.; He, F.; Ma, L.; Cao, M.; Zhou, Z.; Wei, Z.; Xue, Y.; Sang, X.; Chong, H.; Tian, C.; et al. The potential atheroprotective role of plant MIR156a as a repressor of monocyte recruitment on inflamed human endothelial cells. *J. Nutr. Biochem.* **2018**, *57*, 197–205. [CrossRef] [PubMed]
53. Li, M.; Chen, T.; He, J.J.; Wu, J.H.; Luo, J.Y.; Ye, R.S.; Xie, M.Y.; Zhang, H.J.; Zeng, B.; Liu, J.; et al. Plant MIR167e-5p Inhibits Enterocyte Proliferation by Targeting β-Catenin. *Cells* **2019**, *8*, 1385. [CrossRef] [PubMed]
54. Alshehri, B. Plant-derived xenomiRs and cancer: Cross-kingdom gene regulation. *Saudi J. Biol. Sci.* **2021**, *28*, 2408–2422. [CrossRef] [PubMed]
55. Chin, A.R.; Fong, M.Y.; Somlo, G.; Wu, J.; Swiderski, P.; Wu, X.; Wang, S.E. Cross-kingdom inhibition of breast cancer growth by plant miR159. *Cell Res.* **2016**, *26*, 217–228. [CrossRef] [PubMed]
56. Xiao, X.; Sticht, C.; Yin, L.; Liu, L.; Karakhanova, S.; Yin, Y.; Georgikou, C.; Gladkich, J.; Gross, W.; Gretz, N.; et al. Novel plant microRNAs from broccoletti sprouts do not show cross-kingdom regulation of pancreatic cancer. *Oncotarget* **2020**, *11*, 1203–1217. [CrossRef] [PubMed]
57. Rakhmetullina, A.; Pyrkova, A.; Aisina, D.; Ivashchenko, A. In silico prediction of human genes as potential targets for rice miRNAs. *Comput. Biol. Chem.* **2020**, *87*, 107305. [CrossRef] [PubMed]
58. Kumazoe, M.; Ogawa, F.; Hikida, A.; Shimada, Y.; Yoshitomi, R.; Watanabe, R.; Onda, H.; Fujimura, Y.; Tachibana, H. Plant miRNA osa-miR172d-5p suppressed lung fibrosis by targeting Tab1. *Sci. Rep.* **2023**, *13*, 2128. [CrossRef]
59. Zhang, L.; Hou, D.; Chen, X.; Li, D.; Zhu, L.; Zhang, Y.; Li, J.; Bian, Z.; Liang, X.; Cai, X.; et al. Exogenous plant MIR168a specifically targets mammalian LDLRAP1: Evidence of cross-kingdom regulation by microRNA. *Cell Res.* **2012**, *22*, 107–126. [CrossRef]
60. Rabuma, T.; Gupta, O.P.; Chhokar, V. Recent advances and potential applications of cross-kingdom movement of miRNAs in modulating plant's disease response. *RNA Biol.* **2022**, *19*, 519–532. [CrossRef]
61. Akao, Y.; Kuranaga, Y.; Heishima, K.; Sugito, N.; Morikawa, K.; Ito, Y.; Soga, T.; Ito, T. Plant hvu-MIR168-3p enhances expression of glucose transporter 1 (SLC2A1) in human cells by silencing genes related to mitochondrial electron transport chain complex I. *J. Nutr. Biochem.* **2022**, *101*, 108922. [CrossRef]
62. Link, J.; Thon, C.; Petkevicius, V.; Steponaitiene, R.; Malfertheiner, P.; Kupcinskas, J.; Link, A. The Translational Impact of Plant-Derived Xeno-miRNA miR-168 in Gastrointestinal Cancers and Preneoplastic Conditions. *Diagnostics* **2023**, *13*, 2701. [CrossRef] [PubMed]
63. Xiao, J.; Feng, S.; Wang, X.; Long, K.; Luo, Y.; Wang, Y.; Ma, J.; Tang, Q.; Jin, L.; Li, X.; et al. Identification of exosome-like nanoparticle-derived microRNAs from 11 edible fruits and vegetables. *PeerJ* **2018**, *6*, e5186. [CrossRef] [PubMed]
64. Manzaneque-López, M.C.; Sánchez-López, C.M.; Pérez-Bermúdez, P.; Soler, C.; Marcilla, A. Dietary-Derived Exosome-like Nanoparticles as Bacterial Modulators: Beyond MicroRNAs. *Nutrients* **2023**, *15*, 1265. [CrossRef] [PubMed]
65. Teng, Y.; Ren, Y.; Sayed, M.; Hu, X.; Lei, C.; Kumar, A.; Hutchins, E.; Mu, J.; Deng, Z.; Luo, C.; et al. Plant-Derived Exosomal MicroRNAs Shape the Gut Microbiota. *Cell Host Microbe* **2018**, *24*, 637–652.e8. [CrossRef] [PubMed]
66. Mlotshwa, S.; Pruss, G.J.; MacArthur, J.L.; Endres, M.W.; Davis, C.; Hofseth, L.J.; Peña, M.M.; Vance, V. A novel chemopreventive strategy based on therapeutic microRNAs produced in plants. *Cell Res.* **2015**, *25*, 521–524. [CrossRef] [PubMed]
67. Liu, J.; Wang, F.; Weng, Z.; Sui, X.; Fang, Y.; Tang, X.; Shen, X. Soybean-derived miRNAs specifically inhibit proliferation and stimulate apoptosis of human colonic Caco-2 cancer cells but not normal mucosal cells in culture. *Genomics* **2020**, *112*, 2949–2958. [CrossRef]
68. Marzano, F.; Caratozzolo, M.F.; Consiglio, A.; Licciulli, F.; Liuni, S.; Sbisà, E.; D'Elia, D.; Tullo, A.; Catalano, D. Plant miRNAs Reduce Cancer Cell Proliferation by Targeting MALAT1 and NEAT1: A Beneficial Cross-Kingdom Interaction. *Front Genet.* **2020**, *11*, 552490. [CrossRef]
69. Yu, W.Y.; Cai, W.; Ying, H.Z.; Zhang, W.Y.; Zhang, H.H.; Yu, C.H. Exogenous Plant gma-miR-159a, Identified by miRNA Library Functional Screening, Ameliorated Hepatic Stellate Cell Activation and Inflammation via Inhibiting GSK-3β-Mediated Pathways. *J. Inflamm. Res.* **2021**, *14*, 2157–2172. [CrossRef]
70. Komori, H.; Fujita, D.; Shirasaki, Y.; Zhu, Q.; Iwamoto, Y.; Nakanishi, T.; Nakajima, M.; Tamai, I. MicroRNAs in Apple-Derived Nanoparticles Modulate Intestinal Expression of Organic Anion-Transporting Peptide 2B1/SLCO2B1 in Caco-2 Cells. *Drug Metab. Dispos.* **2021**, *49*, 803–809. [CrossRef]
71. Javaid, A.; Zahra, D.; Rashid, F.; Mashraqi, M.; Alzamami, A.; Khurshid, M.; Ali Ashfaq, U. Regulation of micro-RNA, epigenetic factor by natural products for the treatment of cancers: Mechanistic insight and translational association. *Saudi J. Biol. Sci.* **2022**, *29*, 103255. [CrossRef]
72. Song, J.; Jun, M.; Ahn, M.R.; Kim, O.Y. Involvement of miR-Let7A in inflammatory response and cell survival/apoptosis regulated by resveratrol in THP-1 macrophage. *Nutr. Res. Pract.* **2016**, *10*, 377–384. [CrossRef] [PubMed]

73. Tili, E.; Michaille, J.J.; Adair, B.; Alder, H.; Limagne, E.; Taccioli, C.; Ferracin, M.; Delmas, D.; Latruffe, N.; Croce, C.M. Resveratrol decreases the levels of miR-155 by upregulating miR-663, a microRNA targeting JunB and JunD. *Carcinogenesis* **2010**, *31*, 1561–1566. [CrossRef] [PubMed]
74. Liang, F.; Xu, X.; Tu, Y. Resveratrol inhibited hepatocyte apoptosis and alleviated liver fibrosis through miR-190a-5p/HGF axis. *Bioorganic Med. Chem.* **2022**, *57*, 116593. [CrossRef] [PubMed]
75. Ma, F.; Liu, F.; Ding, L.; You, M.; Yue, H.; Zhou, Y.; Hou, Y. Anti-inflammatory effects of curcumin are associated with down regulating microRNA-155 in LPS-treated macrophages and mice. *Pharm. Biol.* **2017**, *55*, 1263–1273. [CrossRef] [PubMed]
76. Roessler, C.; Kuhlmann, K.; Hellwing, C.; Leimert, A.; Schumann, J. Impact of Polyunsaturated Fatty Acids on miRNA Profiles of Monocytes/Macrophages and Endothelial Cells-A Pilot Study. *Int. J. Mol. Sci.* **2017**, *18*, 284. [CrossRef] [PubMed]
77. Trentini, M.; Zanotti, F.; Tiengo, E.; Camponogara, F.; Degasperi, M.; Licastro, D.; Lovatti, L.; Zavan, B. An Apple a Day Keeps the Doctor Away: Potential Role of miRNA 146 on Macrophages Treated with Exosomes Derived from Apples. *Biomedicines* **2022**, *10*, 415. [CrossRef] [PubMed]
78. Duchnik, E.; Kruk, J.; Tuchowska, A.; Marchlewicz, M. The Impact of Diet and Physical Activity on Psoriasis: A Narrative Review of the Current Evidence. *Nutrients* **2023**, *15*, 840. [CrossRef]
79. Xu, J.; Tan, Y.L.; Liu, Q.Y.; Huang, Z.C.; Qiao, Z.H.; Li, T.; Hu, Z.Q.; Lei, L. Quercetin regulates fibrogenic responses of endometrial stromal cell by upregulating miR-145 and inhibiting the TGF-β1/Smad2/Smad3 pathway. *Acta Histochem.* **2020**, *122*, 151600. [CrossRef]
80. Park, S.; Lim, W.; Bazer, F.W.; Whang, K.Y.; Song, G. Quercetin inhibits proliferation of endometriosis regulating cyclin D1 and its target microRNAs in vitro and in vivo. *J. Nutr. Biochem.* **2019**, *63*, 87–100. [CrossRef]
81. Benameur, T.; Soleti, R.; Porro, C. The Potential Neuroprotective Role of Free and Encapsulated Quercetin Mediated by miRNA against Neurological Diseases. *Nutrients* **2021**, *13*, 1318. [CrossRef]
82. Abozaid, O.A.R.; Sallam, M.W.; El-Sonbaty, S.; Aziza, S.; Emad, B.; Ahmed, E.S.A. Resveratrol-Selenium Nanoparticles Alleviate Neuroinflammation and Neurotoxicity in a Rat Model of Alzheimer's Disease by Regulating Sirt1/miRNA-134/GSK3β Expression. *Biol. Trace Elem. Res.* **2022**, *200*, 5104–5114. [CrossRef] [PubMed]
83. Cannataro, R.; Carbone, L.; Petro, J.L.; Cione, E.; Vargas, S.; Angulo, H.; Forero, D.A.; Odriozola-Martínez, A.; Kreider, R.B.; Bonilla, D.A. Sarcopenia: Etiology, Nutritional Approaches, and miRNAs. *Int. J. Mol. Sci.* **2021**, *22*, 9724. [CrossRef] [PubMed]
84. El-Sayed, N.S.; Elatrebi, S.; Said, R.; Ibrahim, H.F.; Omar, E.M. Potential mechanisms underlying the association between type II diabetes mellitus and cognitive dysfunction in rats: A link between miRNA-21 and Resveratrol's neuroprotective action. *Metab. Brain Dis.* **2022**, *37*, 2375–2388. [CrossRef] [PubMed]
85. Unger, A.L.; Torres-Gonzalez, M.; Kraft, J. Dairy Fat Consumption and the Risk of Metabolic Syndrome: An Examination of the Saturated Fatty Acids in Dairy. *Nutrients* **2019**, *11*, 2200. [CrossRef] [PubMed]
86. Yang, W.M.; Jeong, H.J.; Park, S.Y.; Lee, W. Induction of miR-29a by saturated fatty acids impairs insulin signaling and glucose uptake through translational repression of IRS-1 in myocytes. *FEBS Lett.* **2014**, *588*, 2170–2176. [CrossRef] [PubMed]
87. Tashiro, E.; Nagasawa, Y.; Itoh, S.; Imoto, M. Involvement of miR-3180-3p and miR-4632-5p in palmitic acid-induced insulin resistance. *Mol. Cell Endocrinol.* **2021**, *534*, 111371. [CrossRef]
88. Takahashi, K.; Sasano, T.; Sugiyama, K.; Kurokawa, J.; Tamura, N.; Soejima, Y.; Sawabe, M.; Isobe, M.; Furukawa, T. High-fat diet increases vulnerability to atrial arrhythmia by conduction disturbance via miR-27b. *J. Mol. Cell Cardiol.* **2016**, *90*, 38–46. [CrossRef]
89. Alisi, A.; Da Sacco, L.; Bruscalupi, G.; Piemonte, F.; Panera, N.; De Vito, R.; Leoni, S.; Bottazzo, G.F.; Masotti, A.; Nobili, V. Mirnome analysis reveals novel molecular determinants in the pathogenesis of diet-induced nonalcoholic fatty liver disease. *Lab Investig.* **2011**, *91*, 283–293. [CrossRef]
90. Deng, P.; Li, M.; Wu, Y. The Predictive Efficacy of Serum Exosomal microRNA-122 and microRNA-148a for Hepatocellular Carcinoma Based on Smart Healthcare. *J. Healthc. Eng.* **2022**, *2022*, 5914541. [CrossRef]
91. Monraz-Méndez, C.A.; Escutia-Gutiérrez, R.; Rodriguez-Sanabria, J.S.; Galicia-Moreno, M.; Monroy-Ramírez, H.C.; Sánchez-Orozco, L.; García-Bañuelos, J.; De la Rosa-Bibiano, R.; Santos, A.; Armendáriz-Borunda, J.; et al. Moringa oleifera Improves MAFLD by Inducing Epigenetic Modifications. *Nutrients* **2022**, *14*, 4225. [CrossRef]
92. Nur, S.M.; Rath, S.; Ahmad, V.; Ahmad, A.; Ateeq, B.; Khan, M.I. Nutritive vitamins as epidrugs. *Crit. Rev. Food Sci. Nutr.* **2021**, *61*, 1–13. [CrossRef] [PubMed]
93. Bae, M.; Kim, M.B.; Lee, J.Y. Astaxanthin Attenuates the Changes in the Expression of MicroRNAs Involved in the Activation of Hepatic Stellate Cells. *Nutrients* **2022**, *14*, 962. [CrossRef] [PubMed]
94. Sharifzadeh, M.; Esmaeili-Bandboni, A.; Emami, M.R.; Naeini, F.; Zarezadeh, M.; Javanbakht, M.H. The effects of all trans retinoic acid, vitamin D3 and their combination on plasma levels of miRNA-125a-5p, miRNA-34a, and miRNA-126 in an experimental model of diabetes. *Avicenna J. Phytomed.* **2022**, *12*, 67–76. [CrossRef] [PubMed]
95. Wan, H.; Wang, Y.; Pan, Q.; Chen, X.; Chen, S.; Li, X.; Yao, W. Quercetin attenuates the proliferation, inflammation, and oxidative stress of high glucose-induced human mesangial cells by regulating the miR-485-5p/YAP1 pathway. *Int. J. Immunopathol. Pharmacol.* **2022**, *36*, 20587384211066440. [CrossRef] [PubMed]
96. Wang, D.; Li, Y.; Zhai, Q.Q.; Zhu, Y.F.; Liu, B.Y.; Xu, Y. Quercetin ameliorates testosterone secretion disorder by inhibiting endoplasmic reticulum stress through the miR-1306-5p/HSD17B7 axis in diabetic rats. *Bosn. J. Basic Med. Sci.* **2022**, *22*, 191–204. [CrossRef] [PubMed]

97. Liu, H.; Guan, H.; Tan, X.; Jiang, Y.; Li, F.; Sun-Waterhouse, D.; Li, D. Enhanced alleviation of insulin resistance via the IRS-1/Akt/FOXO1 pathway by combining quercetin and EGCG and involving miR-27a-3p and miR-96-5p. *Free Radic. Biol. Med.* **2022**, *181*, 105–117. [CrossRef] [PubMed]
98. Chen, W.T.; Yang, M.J.; Tsuei, Y.W.; Su, T.C.; Siao, A.C.; Kuo, Y.C.; Huang, L.R.; Chen, Y.; Chen, S.J.; Chen, P.C.; et al. Green Tea Epigallocatechin Gallate Inhibits Preadipocyte Growth via the microRNA-let-7a/HMGA2 Signaling Pathway. *Mol. Nutr. Food Res.* **2023**, *67*, e2200336. [CrossRef]
99. Chen, C.P.; Su, T.C.; Yang, M.J.; Chen, W.T.; Siao, A.C.; Huang, L.R.; Lin, Y.Y.; Kuo, Y.C.; Chung, J.F.; Cheng, C.F.; et al. Green tea epigallocatechin gallate suppresses 3T3-L1 cell growth via microRNA-143/MAPK7 pathways. *Exp. Biol. Med.* **2022**, *247*, 1670–1679. [CrossRef]
100. Capetini, V.C.; Quintanilha, B.J.; de Oliveira, D.C.; Nishioka, A.H.; de Matos, L.A.; Ferreira, L.R.P.; Ferreira, F.M.; Sampaio, G.R.; Hassimotto, N.M.A.; Lajolo, F.M.; et al. Blood orange juice intake modulates plasma and PBMC microRNA expression in overweight and insulin-resistant women: Impact on MAPK and NFκB signaling pathways. *J. Nutr. Biochem.* **2023**, *112*, 109240. [CrossRef]
101. Gowd, V.; Kanika; Jori, C.; Chaudhary, A.A.; Rudayni, H.A.; Rashid, S.; Khan, R. Resveratrol and resveratrol nano-delivery systems in the treatment of inflammatory bowel disease. *J. Nutr. Biochem.* **2022**, *109*, 109101. [CrossRef]
102. Cadieux, Z.; Lewis, H.; Esquela-Kerscher, A. *Role of Nutrition, the Epigenome, and microRNAs in Cancer Pathogenesis*; The Royal Society of Chemistry: London, UK, 2019; Volume 1, pp. 1–35. [CrossRef]
103. Farooqi, A.A.; Khalid, S.; Ahmad, A. Regulation of Cell Signaling Pathways and miRNAs by Resveratrol in Different Cancers. *Int. J. Mol. Sci.* **2018**, *19*, 652. [CrossRef] [PubMed]
104. Huang, L.; Zhang, S.; Zhou, J.; Li, X. Effect of resveratrol on drug resistance in colon cancer chemotherapy. *RSC Adv.* **2019**, *9*, 2572–2580. [CrossRef] [PubMed]
105. Khan, A.W.; Farooq, M.; Haseeb, M.; Choi, S. Role of Plant-Derived Active Constituents in Cancer Treatment and Their Mechanisms of Action. *Cells* **2022**, *11*, 1326. [CrossRef] [PubMed]
106. Qin, J.; Chen, J.X.; Zhu, Z.; Teng, J.A. Genistein inhibits human colorectal cancer growth and suppresses miR-95, Akt and SGK1. *Cell Physiol. Biochem.* **2015**, *35*, 2069–2077. [CrossRef] [PubMed]
107. Yang, X.; Jiang, W.; Kong, X.; Zhou, X.; Zhu, D.; Kong, L. Genistein Restricts the Epithelial Mesenchymal Transformation (EMT) and Stemness of Hepatocellular Carcinoma via Upregulating miR-1275 to Inhibit the EIF5A2/PI3K/Akt Pathway. *Biology* **2022**, *11*, 1383. [CrossRef]
108. Tsoukas, M.A.; Ko, B.J.; Witte, T.R.; Dincer, F.; Hardman, W.E.; Mantzoros, C.S. Dietary walnut suppression of colorectal cancer in mice: Mediation by miRNA patterns and fatty acid incorporation. *J. Nutr. Biochem.* **2015**, *26*, 776–783. [CrossRef]
109. Tu, M.; Wang, W.; Zhang, G.; Hammock, B.D. ω-3 Polyunsaturated Fatty Acids on Colonic Inflammation and Colon Cancer: Roles of Lipid-Metabolizing Enzymes Involved. *Nutrients* **2020**, *12*, 3301. [CrossRef]
110. Negri, M.; Gentile, A.; de Angelis, C.; Montò, T.; Patalano, R.; Colao, A.; Pivonello, R.; Pivonello, C. Vitamin D-Induced Molecular Mechanisms to Potentiate Cancer Therapy and to Reverse Drug-Resistance in Cancer Cells. *Nutrients* **2020**, *12*, 1798. [CrossRef]
111. Padi, S.K.; Zhang, Q.; Rustum, Y.M.; Morrison, C.; Guo, B. MicroRNA-627 mediates the epigenetic mechanisms of vitamin D to suppress proliferation of human colorectal cancer cells and growth of xenograft tumors in mice. *Gastroenterology* **2013**, *145*, 437–446. [CrossRef]
112. Kang, Q.; Tong, Y.; Gowd, V.; Wang, M.; Chen, F.; Cheng, K.W. Oral administration of EGCG solution equivalent to daily achievable dosages of regular tea drinkers effectively suppresses miR483-3p induced metastasis of hepatocellular carcinoma cells in mice. *Food Funct.* **2021**, *12*, 3381–3392. [CrossRef]
113. Su, N.; Li, L.; Zhou, E.; Li, H.; Wu, S.; Cao, Z. Resveratrol Downregulates miR-155-5p to Block the Malignant Behavior of Gastric Cancer Cells. *BioMed Res. Int.* **2022**, *2022*, 6968641. [CrossRef] [PubMed]
114. Dhar, S.; Hicks, C.; Levenson, A.S. Resveratrol and prostate cancer: Promising role for microRNAs. *Mol. Nutr. Food Res.* **2011**, *55*, 1219–1229. [CrossRef] [PubMed]
115. Maleki Dana, P.; Sadoughi, F.; Asemi, Z.; Yousefi, B. The role of polyphenols in overcoming cancer drug resistance: A comprehensive review. *Cell Mol. Biol. Lett.* **2022**, *27*, 1. [CrossRef] [PubMed]
116. Chiyomaru, T.; Yamamura, S.; Fukuhara, S.; Hidaka, H.; Majid, S.; Saini, S.; Arora, S.; Deng, G.; Shahryari, V.; Chang, I.; et al. Genistein up-regulates tumor suppressor microRNA-574-3p in prostate cancer. *PLoS ONE* **2013**, *8*, e58929. [CrossRef] [PubMed]
117. Ji, X.; Liu, K.; Li, Q.; Shen, Q.; Han, F.; Ye, Q.; Zheng, C. A Mini-Review of Flavone Isomers Apigenin and Genistein in Prostate Cancer Treatment. *Front. Pharmacol.* **2022**, *13*, 851589. [CrossRef] [PubMed]
118. Giangreco, A.A.; Vaishnav, A.; Wagner, D.; Finelli, A.; Fleshner, N.; Van der Kwast, T.; Vieth, R.; Nonn, L. Tumor suppressor microRNAs, miR-100 and -125b, are regulated by 1,25-dihydroxyvitamin D in primary prostate cells and in patient tissue. *Cancer Prev. Res.* **2013**, *6*, 483–494. [CrossRef] [PubMed]
119. Stephan, C.; Ralla, B.; Bonn, F.; Diesner, M.; Lein, M.; Jung, K. Vitamin D Metabolites in Nonmetastatic High-Risk Prostate Cancer Patients with and without Zoledronic Acid Treatment after Prostatectomy. *Cancers* **2022**, *14*, 1560. [CrossRef] [PubMed]
120. Khan, S.; Wall, D.; Curran, C.; Newell, J.; Kerin, M.J.; Dwyer, R.M. MicroRNA-10a is reduced in breast cancer and regulated in part through retinoic acid. *BMC Cancer* **2015**, *15*, 345. [CrossRef]

121. Min, D.; Lv, X.B.; Wang, X.; Zhang, B.; Meng, W.; Yu, F.; Hu, H. Downregulation of miR-302c and miR-520c by 1,25(OH)2D3 treatment enhances the susceptibility of tumour cells to natural killer cell-mediated cytotoxicity. *Br. J. Cancer* **2013**, *109*, 723–730. [CrossRef]
122. Muñoz, A.; Grant, W.B. Vitamin D and Cancer: An Historical Overview of the Epidemiology and Mechanisms. *Nutrients* **2022**, *14*, 1448. [CrossRef]
123. Wang, X.; Hang, Y.; Liu, J.; Hou, Y.; Wang, N.; Wang, M. Anticancer effect of curcumin inhibits cell growth through miR-21/PTEN/Akt pathway in breast cancer cell. *Oncol. Lett.* **2017**, *13*, 4825–4831. [CrossRef] [PubMed]
124. Kronski, E.; Fiori, M.E.; Barbieri, O.; Astigiano, S.; Mirisola, V.; Killian, P.H.; Bruno, A.; Pagani, A.; Rovera, F.; Pfeffer, U.; et al. miR181b is induced by the chemopreventive polyphenol curcumin and inhibits breast cancer metastasis via down-regulation of the inflammatory cytokines CXCL1 and -2. *Mol. Oncol.* **2014**, *8*, 581–595. [CrossRef] [PubMed]
125. Norouzi, S.; Majeed, M.; Pirro, M.; Generali, D.; Sahebkar, A. Curcumin as an Adjunct Therapy and microRNA Modulator in Breast Cancer. *Curr. Pharm. Des.* **2018**, *24*, 171–177. [CrossRef] [PubMed]
126. Al-Ansari, M.M.; Aboussekhra, A. miR-146b-5p mediates p16-dependent repression of IL-6 and suppresses paracrine procarcinogenic effects of breast stromal fibroblasts. *Oncotarget* **2015**, *6*, 30006–30016. [CrossRef] [PubMed]
127. Zan, L.; Chen, Q.; Zhang, L.; Li, X. Epigallocatechin gallate (EGCG) suppresses growth and tumorigenicity in breast cancer cells by downregulation of miR-25. *Bioengineered* **2019**, *10*, 374–382. [CrossRef]
128. de la Parra, C.; Castillo-Pichardo, L.; Cruz-Collazo, A.; Cubano, L.; Redis, R.; Calin, G.A.; Dharmawardhane, S. Soy Isoflavone Genistein-Mediated Downregulation of miR-155 Contributes to the Anticancer Effects of Genistein. *Nutr. Cancer* **2016**, *68*, 154–164. [CrossRef]
129. Javed, Z.; Khan, K.; Herrera-Bravo, J.; Naeem, S.; Iqbal, M.J.; Sadia, H.; Qadri, Q.R.; Raza, S.; Irshad, A.; Akbar, A.; et al. Genistein as a regulator of signaling pathways and microRNAs in different types of cancers. *Cancer Cell Int.* **2021**, *21*, 388. [CrossRef] [PubMed]
130. Esposito, A.; Ferraresi, A.; Salwa, A.; Vidoni, C.; Dhanasekaran, D.N.; Isidoro, C. Resveratrol Contrasts IL-6 Pro-Growth Effects and Promotes Autophagy-Mediated Cancer Cell Dormancy in 3D Ovarian Cancer: Role of miR-1305 and of Its Target ARH-I. *Cancers* **2022**, *14*, 2142. [CrossRef]
131. Wan Mohd Tajuddin, W.N.B.; Lajis, N.H.; Abas, F.; Othman, I.; Naidu, R. Mechanistic Understanding of Curcumin's Therapeutic Effects in Lung Cancer. *Nutrients* **2019**, *11*, 2989. [CrossRef]
132. Wang, N.; Feng, T.; Liu, X.; Liu, Q. Curcumin inhibits migration and invasion of non-small cell lung cancer cells through up-regulation of miR-206 and suppression of PI3K/AKT/mTOR signaling pathway. *Acta Pharm.* **2020**, *70*, 399–409. [CrossRef]
133. Pan, Y.; Sun, Y.; Liu, Z.; Zhang, C. miR-192-5p upregulation mediates the suppression of curcumin in human NSCLC cell proliferation, migration and invasion by targeting c-Myc and inactivating the Wnt/β-catenin signaling pathway. *Mol. Med. Rep.* **2020**, *22*, 1594–1604. [CrossRef] [PubMed]
134. Zhong, Z.; Dong, Z.; Yang, L.; Chen, X.; Gong, Z. Inhibition of proliferation of human lung cancer cells by green tea catechins is mediated by upregulation of let-7. *Exp. Ther. Med.* **2012**, *4*, 267–272. [CrossRef] [PubMed]
135. Qamar, M.; Akhtar, S.; Ismail, T.; Wahid, M.; Barnard, R.T.; Esatbeyoglu, T.; Ziora, Z.M. The Chemical Composition and Health-Promoting Effects of the Grewia Species—A Systematic Review and Meta-Analysis. *Nutrients* **2021**, *13*, 4565. [CrossRef] [PubMed]
136. Chai, R.; Xu, C.; Lu, L.; Liu, X.; Ma, Z. Quercetin inhibits proliferation of and induces apoptosis in non-small-cell lung carcinoma via the lncRNA SNHG7/miR-34a-5p pathway. *Immunopharmacol. Immunotoxicol.* **2021**, *43*, 693–703. [CrossRef] [PubMed]
137. Chen, L.; Xia, J.S.; Wu, J.H.; Chen, Y.G.; Qiu, C.J. Quercetin suppresses cell survival and invasion in oral squamous cell carcinoma via the miR-1254/CD36 cascade in vitro. *Hum. Exp. Toxicol.* **2021**, *40*, 1413–1421. [CrossRef] [PubMed]
138. Zhao, J.; Fang, Z.; Zha, Z.; Sun, Q.; Wang, H.; Sun, M.; Qiao, B. Quercetin inhibits cell viability, migration and invasion by regulating miR-16/HOXA10 axis in oral cancer. *Eur. J. Pharmacol.* **2019**, *847*, 11–18. [CrossRef] [PubMed]
139. Wang, Y.; Chen, X.; Li, J.; Xia, C. Quercetin Antagonizes Esophagus Cancer by Modulating miR-1-3p/TAGLN2 Pathway-Dependent Growth and Metastasis. *Nutr. Cancer* **2022**, *74*, 1872–1881. [CrossRef] [PubMed]
140. Hsieh, P.L.; Liao, Y.W.; Hsieh, C.W.; Chen, P.N.; Yu, C.C. Soy Isoflavone Genistein Impedes Cancer Stemness and Mesenchymal Transition in Head and Neck Cancer through Activating miR-34a/RTCB Axis. *Nutrients* **2020**, *12*, 1924. [CrossRef]
141. Tang, Y.; Cao, Y. Curcumin Inhibits the Growth and Metastasis of Melanoma via miR-222-3p/SOX10/Notch Axis. *Dis. Markers* **2022**, *2022*, 3129781. [CrossRef]
142. Yamada, S.; Tsukamoto, S.; Huang, Y.; Makio, A.; Kumazoe, M.; Yamashita, S.; Tachibana, H. Epigallocatechin-3-O-gallate up-regulates microRNA-let-7b expression by activating 67-kDa laminin receptor signaling in melanoma cells. *Sci. Rep.* **2016**, *6*, 19225. [CrossRef]
143. Li, H.; Jia, Z.; Li, A.; Jenkins, G.; Yang, X.; Hu, J.; Guo, W. Resveratrol repressed viability of U251 cells by miR-21 inhibiting of NF-κB pathway. *Mol. Cell Biochem.* **2013**, *382*, 137–143. [CrossRef]
144. Wei, D.; Yang, L.; Lv, B.; Chen, L. Genistein suppresses retinoblastoma cell viability and growth and induces apoptosis by upregulating miR-145 and inhibiting its target ABCE1. *Mol. Vis.* **2017**, *23*, 385–394.
145. Wang, M.; Liu, K.; Bu, H.; Cong, H.; Dong, G.; Xu, N.; Li, C.; Zhao, Y.; Jiang, F.; Zhang, Y.; et al. Purple sweet potato delphinidin-3-rutin represses glioma proliferation by inducing miR-20b-5p/Atg7-dependent cytostatic autophagy. *Mol. Ther. Oncolytics* **2022**, *26*, 314–329. [CrossRef]

146. Margolis, L.M.; Carrigan, C.T.; Murphy, N.E.; DiBella, M.N.; Wilson, M.A.; Whitney, C.C.; Howard, E.E.; Pasiakos, S.M.; Rivas, D.A. Carbohydrate intake in recovery from aerobic exercise differentiates skeletal muscle microRNA expression. *Am. J. Physiol Endocrinol. Metab.* **2022**, *323*, E435–E447. [CrossRef]
147. Marques-Rocha, J.L.; Milagro, F.I.; Mansego, M.L.; Zulet, M.A.; Bressan, J.; Martínez, J.A. Expression of inflammation-related miRNAs in white blood cells from subjects with metabolic syndrome after 8 wk of following a Mediterranean diet-based weight loss program. *Nutrition* **2016**, *32*, 48–55. [CrossRef]
148. Jimenez-Lucena, R.; Alcala-Diaz, J.F.; Roncero-Ramos, I.; Lopez-Moreno, J.; Camargo, A.; Gomez-Delgado, F.; Quintana-Navarro, G.M.; Vals-Delgado, C.; Rodriguez-Cantalejo, F.; Luque, R.M.; et al. MiRNAs profile as biomarkers of nutritional therapy for the prevention of type 2 diabetes mellitus: From the CORDIOPREV study. *Clin. Nutr.* **2021**, *40*, 1028–1038. [CrossRef]
149. Pérez-Sánchez, C.; Aguirre, M.Á.; Ruiz-Limón, P.; Ábalos-Aguilera, M.C.; Jiménez-Gómez, Y.; Arias-de la Rosa, I.; Rodriguez-Ariza, A.; Fernández-Del Río, L.; González-Reyes, J.A.; Segui, P.; et al. Ubiquinol Effects on Antiphospholipid Syndrome Prothrombotic Profile: A Randomized, Placebo-Controlled Trial. *Arter. Thromb. Vasc. Biol.* **2017**, *37*, 1923–1932. [CrossRef]
150. Gil-Zamorano, J.; Cofán, M.; López de Las Hazas, M.C.; García-Blanco, T.; García-Ruiz, A.; Doménech, M.; Serra-Mir, M.; Roth, I.; Valls-Pedret, C.; Rajaram, S.; et al. Interplay of Walnut Consumption, Changes in Circulating miRNAs and Reduction in LDL-Cholesterol in Elders. *Nutrients* **2022**, *14*, 1473. [CrossRef] [PubMed]
151. Rendina, D.; D Elia, L.; Abate, V.; Rebellato, A.; Buondonno, I.; Succoio, M.; Martinelli, F.; Muscariello, R.; De Filippo, G.; D Amelio, P.; et al. Vitamin D Status, Cardiovascular Risk Profile, and miRNA-21 Levels in Hypertensive Patients: Results of the HYPODD Study. *Nutrients* **2022**, *14*, 2683. [CrossRef] [PubMed]
152. Saini, S.K.; Singh, A.; Saini, M.; Gonzalez-Freire, M.; Leeuwenburgh, C.; Anton, S.D. Time-Restricted Eating Regimen Differentially Affects Circulatory miRNA Expression in Older Overweight Adults. *Nutrients* **2022**, *14*, 1843. [CrossRef] [PubMed]
153. Protic, O.; Di Pillo, R.; Montesanto, A.; Galeazzi, R.; Matacchione, G.; Giuliani, A.; Sabbatinelli, J.; Gurău, F.; Silvestrini, A.; Olivieri, F.; et al. Randomized, Double-Blind, Placebo-Controlled Trial to Test the Effects of a Nutraceutical Combination Monacolin K-Free on the Lipid and Inflammatory Profile of Subjects with Hypercholesterolemia. *Nutrients* **2022**, *14*, 2812. [CrossRef]
154. Li, Y.; Teng, Z.; Zhao, D. Plant-derived cross-kingdom gene regulation benefits human health. *Trends Plant Sci.* **2023**, *28*, 626–629. [CrossRef]
155. Mar-Aguilar, F.; Arreola-Triana, A.; Mata-Cardona, D.; Gonzalez-Villasana, V.; Rodríguez-Padilla, C.; Reséndez-Pérez, D. Evidence of transfer of miRNAs from the diet to the blood still inconclusive. *PeerJ* **2020**, *8*, e9567. [CrossRef]
156. Wang, L.; Sadri, M.; Giraud, D.; Zempleni, J. RNase H2-Dependent Polymerase Chain Reaction and Elimination of Confounders in Sample Collection, Storage, and Analysis Strengthen Evidence That microRNAs in Bovine Milk Are Bioavailable in Humans. *J. Nutr.* **2018**, *148*, 153–159. [CrossRef]
157. Fromm, B.; Tosar, J.P.; Lu, Y.; Halushka, M.K.; Witwer, K.W. Human and Cow Have Identical miR-21-5p and miR-30a-5p Sequences, Which Are Likely Unsuited to Study Dietary Uptake from Cow Milk. *J. Nutr.* **2018**, *148*, 1506–1507. [CrossRef]
158. Witwer, K.W. Diet-responsive mammalian miRNAs are likely endogenous. *J. Nutr.* **2014**, *144*, 1880–1881. [CrossRef]
159. Auerbach, A.; Vyas, G.; Li, A.; Halushka, M.; Witwer, K. Uptake of dietary milk miRNAs by adult humans: A validation study. *F1000Res* **2016**, *5*, 721. [CrossRef]
160. Title, A.C.; Denzler, R.; Stoffel, M. Uptake and Function Studies of Maternal Milk-derived MicroRNAs. *J. Biol. Chem.* **2015**, *290*, 23680–23691. [CrossRef]
161. Witwer, K.W.; McAlexander, M.A.; Queen, S.E.; Adams, R.J. Real-time quantitative PCR and droplet digital PCR for plant miRNAs in mammalian blood provide little evidence for general uptake of dietary miRNAs: Limited evidence for general uptake of dietary plant xenomiRs. *RNA Biol.* **2013**, *10*, 1080–1086. [CrossRef] [PubMed]
162. Link, J.; Thon, C.; Schanze, D.; Steponaitiene, R.; Kupcinskas, J.; Zenker, M.; Canbay, A.; Malfertheiner, P.; Link, A. Food-Derived Xeno-microRNAs: Influence of Diet and Detectability in Gastrointestinal Tract-Proof-of-Principle Study. *Mol. Nutr. Food Res.* **2019**, *63*, e1800076. [CrossRef] [PubMed]
163. Liang, G.; Zhu, Y.; Sun, B.; Shao, Y.; Jing, A.; Wang, J.; Xiao, Z. Assessing the survival of exogenous plant microRNA in mice. *Food Sci. Nutr.* **2014**, *2*, 380–388. [CrossRef]
164. Witwer, K.W. Alternative miRNAs? Human sequences misidentified as plant miRNAs in plant studies and in human plasma. *F1000Research* **2018**, *7*, 244. [CrossRef]
165. Jia, M.; He, J.; Bai, W.; Lin, Q.; Deng, J.; Li, W.; Bai, J.; Fu, D.; Ma, Y.; Ren, J.; et al. Cross-kingdom regulation by dietary plant miRNAs: An evidence-based review with recent updates. *Food Funct.* **2021**, *12*, 9549–9562. [CrossRef]
166. Agrawal, P.; Kaur, J.; Singh, J.; Rasane, P.; Sharma, K.; Bhadariya, V.; Kaur, S.; Kumar, V. Genetics, Nutrition, and Health: A New Frontier in Disease Prevention. *J. Am. Nutr. Assoc.* **2023**, *28*, 1–13. [CrossRef]
167. Otsuka, K.; Yamamoto, Y.; Matsuoka, R.; Ochiya, T. Maintaining good miRNAs in the body keeps the doctor away?: Perspectives on the relationship between food-derived natural products and microRNAs in relation to exosomes/extracellular vesicles. *Mol. Nutr. Food Res.* **2018**, *62*, 1700080. [CrossRef]
168. Dalgaard, L.T.; Sørensen, A.E.; Hardikar, A.A.; Joglekar, M.V. The microRNA-29 family: Role in metabolism and metabolic disease. *Am. J. Physiol. Cell Physiol.* **2022**, *323*, C367–C377. [CrossRef]
169. Hung, Y.H.; Kanke, M.; Kurtz, C.L.; Cubitt, R.; Bunaciu, R.P.; Miao, J.; Zhou, L.; Graham, J.L.; Hussain, M.M.; Havel, P.; et al. Acute suppression of insulin resistance-associated hepatic miR-29 in vivo improves glycemic control in adult mice. *Physiol. Genom.* **2019**, *51*, 379–389. [CrossRef]

170. Ma, E.; Fu, Y.; Garvey, W.T. Relationship of Circulating miRNAs with Insulin Sensitivity and Associated Metabolic Risk Factors in Humans. *Metab. Syndr. Relat. Disord.* **2018**, *16*, 82–89. [CrossRef] [PubMed]
171. Pordzik, J.; Eyileten-Postuła, C.; Jakubik, D.; Czajka, P.; Nowak, A.; De Rosa, S.; Gąsecka, A.; Cieślicka-Kapłon, A.; Sulikowski, P.; Filipiak, K.J.; et al. MiR-126 Is an Independent Predictor of Long-Term All-Cause Mortality in Patients with Type 2 Diabetes Mellitus. *J. Clin. Med.* **2021**, *10*, 2371. [CrossRef] [PubMed]
172. Fourdinier, O.; Schepers, E.; Metzinger-Le Meuth, V.; Glorieux, G.; Liabeuf, S.; Verbeke, F.; Vanholder, R.; Brigant, B.; Pletinck, A.; Diouf, M.; et al. Serum levels of miR-126 and miR-223 and outcomes in chronic kidney disease patients. *Sci. Rep.* **2019**, *9*, 4477. [CrossRef] [PubMed]
173. Franczyk, B.; Gluba-Brzózka, A.; Olszewski, R.; Parolczyk, M.; Rysz-Górzyńska, M.; Rysz, J. miRNA biomarkers in renal disease. *Int. Urol. Nephrol.* **2022**, *54*, 575–588. [CrossRef] [PubMed]
174. Kim, J.Y.; Stevens, P.; Karpurapu, M.; Lee, H.; Englert, J.A.; Yan, P.; Lee, T.J.; Pabla, N.; Pietrzak, M.; Park, G.Y.; et al. Targeting ETosis by miR-155 inhibition mitigates mixed granulocytic asthmatic lung inflammation. *Front. Immunol.* **2022**, *13*, 943554. [CrossRef]
175. Weidner, J.; Bartel, S.; Kılıç, A.; Zissler, U.M.; Renz, H.; Schwarze, J.; Schmidt-Weber, C.B.; Maes, T.; Rebane, A.; Krauss-Etschmann, S.; et al. Spotlight on microRNAs in allergy and asthma. *Allergy* **2021**, *76*, 1661–1678. [CrossRef]
176. Zhang, K.; Liang, Y.; Feng, Y.; Wu, W.; Zhang, H.; He, J.; Hu, Q.; Zhao, J.; Xu, Y.; Liu, Z.; et al. Decreased epithelial and sputum miR-221-3p associates with airway eosinophilic inflammation and CXCL17 expression in asthma. *Am. J. Physiol. Lung Cell Mol. Physiol.* **2018**, *315*, L253–L264. [CrossRef]

Disclaimer/Publisher's Note: The statements, opinions and data contained in all publications are solely those of the individual author(s) and contributor(s) and not of MDPI and/or the editor(s). MDPI and/or the editor(s) disclaim responsibility for any injury to people or property resulting from any ideas, methods, instructions or products referred to in the content.

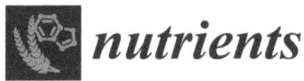

Review

Systematic Review of Management of Moderate Wasting in Children over 6 Months of Age

Zahra A. Padhani [1,2,*], Bernardette Cichon [3,*], Jai K. Das [2,4], Rehana A. Salam [5], Heather C. Stobaugh [6,7], Muzna Mughal [3], Alexandra Rutishauser-Perera [3], Robert E. Black [8] and Zulfiqar A. Bhutta [2,4,9]

1. Robinson Research Institute, Adelaide Medical School, University of Adelaide, Adelaide, SA 5000, Australia
2. Institute for Global Health and Development, Aga Khan University, Karachi 74800, Pakistan; jai.das@aku.edu (J.K.D.); zulfiqar.bhutta@aku.edu or zulfiqar.bhutta@sickkids.ca (Z.A.B.)
3. Action against Hunger UK, London SE10 0ER, UK; muznamughal15@gmail.com (M.M.); a.rutishauserperera@actionagainsthunger.org.uk (A.R.-P.)
4. Division of Women and Child Health, Aga Khan University, Karachi 74800, Pakistan
5. Centre of Research Excellence, Melanoma Institute Australia, University of Sydney, Sydney, NSW 2006, Australia; asalam.rehana@gmail.com
6. Action against Hunger USA, Technical Services and Innovation Department, Washington, DC 20463, USA; hstobaugh@actionagainsthunger.org or heather.stobaugh@tufts.edu
7. Friedman School of Nutrition Science and Policy, Tufts University, Boston, MA 02111, USA
8. Bloomberg School of Public Health, Johns Hopkins University, Baltimore, MD 21205, USA; rblack1@jhu.edu
9. Centre for Global Child Health, Hospital for Sick Children, Toronto, ON M5G 0A4, Canada
* Correspondence: zahraali.padhani@adelaide.edu.au (Z.A.P.); b.cichon@actionagainsthunger.org.uk (B.C.)

Abstract: The effective management of the 33 million children with moderate acute malnutrition (MAM) is key to reducing childhood morbidity and mortality. In this review, we aim to evaluate the effectiveness of specially formulated foods (SFFs) compared to non-food-based approaches to manage MAM in children >6 months old. We conducted a search on ten databases until 23 August 2021 and included five studies, covering 3387 participants. Meta-analysis of four studies comparing SFFs to counselling or standard of care showed that SFFs likely increase recovery rate, reduce non-response, and may improve weight-for-height z-score, weight-for-age z-score and time to recovery, but have little or no effect on MUAC gain. One study on a multicomponent intervention (SFFs, antibiotics and counselling provided to high-risk MAM) compared to counselling only was reported narratively. The intervention may increase weight gain after 24 weeks but may have little or no effect on weight gain after 12 weeks and on non-response and mortality after 12 and 24 weeks of enrollment. The effect of this intervention on recovery was uncertain. In conclusion, SFFs may be beneficial for children with moderate wasting in humanitarian contexts. Programmatic recommendations should consider context and cost-effectiveness.

Keywords: moderate wasting; moderate acute malnutrition; specialized formulated foods; fortified-blended foods (FBF); ready-to use supplementary foods (RUSF); nutrition counselling

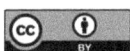

1. Introduction

Children who suffer from moderate wasting (also referred to as moderate acute malnutrition (MAM), which is characterized as a weight-for-height z-score (WHZ) < −2 and ≥ −3 or a mid-upper arm circumference (MUAC) < 125 mm and ≥115 mm in children 6–59 months), face a threefold higher risk of mortality as compared to adequately nourished children [1].

If not treated, the condition can easily lead to severe acute malnutrition (SAM), which entails an even more pronounced risk of near-term mortality [1]. Those that survive experience adverse health effects and negative developmental outcomes. Recent prevalence estimates suggest that in 2020, nearly 31 million children <5 years of age had moderate wasting [2]. The actual number of children impacted by MAM every year is likely much larger than this estimate because many factors, such as the incidence of moderate wasting and MUAC-based case definitions, are not considered in this figure [3–5].

The effective management of children with MAM is therefore key to reducing childhood morbidity and mortality, and to reaching the World Health Assembly (WHA) targets of lowering wasting prevalence to below five percent by 2025 and less than three percent by 2030 [6]. Until very recently, the World Health Organization (WHO) had no guidelines for the management of MAM, but the Essential Nutrition Actions encompassed some guidance based on breastfeeding promotion and support and nutrition education or counselling. Furthermore, in humanitarian emergencies where the increased nutrient and energy requirements for moderately wasted children cannot be met through locally available foods, specially formulated foods can be provided. Such foods typically take the form of fortified blended foods (FBFs) or ready-to-use supplementary foods (RUSFs) that are provided as part of outpatient-based, supplementary feeding programs [7–9].

Overall, the practice for managing MAM differs by location, national-level guidance, and implementing organization. More recently, innovations and adaptations in the management of acute malnutrition, including MAM, have been implemented with aims to improve efficiency in operations, maximize coverage and reduce overall costs. The types of program adaptations vary, but many include reducing the frequency of clinic-based follow-up visits, training caregivers to identify acute malnutrition in their own children, treating children closer to the communities through community health workers, simplifying admission criteria, and/or combining the treatment of SAM and MAM in one program [10–12].

In 2020, WHO initiated the development of a comprehensive guideline focused on the prevention and management of acute malnutrition in infants and children. This guideline now incorporates recommendations for the treatment of MAM for the first time. As part of this, the WHO commissioned two systematic reviews on the management of moderate wasting. The first review explored the effectiveness of different types, quantities and durations of dietary management with specially formulated foods (SFFs) and has recently been published [13]. The aim of this subsequent review was to evaluate the effectiveness of food-based approaches compared to other interventions with or without non-specially formulated food to manage MAM in infants and children over six months of age. Furthermore, an aim was to identify which subgroups of children are most likely to benefit from SFFs.

2. Materials and Methods

2.1. Inclusion and Exclusion Criteria

The inclusion and exclusion criteria have been briefly outlined in Table 1 using the Participant, Intervention, Comparators, Outcomes and Study Design (PICOS) criteria.

Table 1. Eligibility criteria.

Criteria	Details
Study Participants	Children aged over six months with MAM, defined as WHZ ≥ -3 and <-2 and/or a MUAC of ≥ 11.5 cm and <12.5 cm or a WHZ between $>70\%$ and $<80\%$ of the median and without any oedema, treated either as inpatients or outpatients.
Intervention	Food-based approaches for the treatment of MAM with or without SFFs, including multicomponent interventions.
Comparison	Intervention with non-specially formulated foods, non-food based interventions, standard of care or none.
Outcomes	Anthropometric recovery, anthropometric outcomes (such as WHZ, weight for age z-score (WAZ), MUAC, weight and height gain), non-response, sustained recovery, recovery time, deterioration to SAM, and mortality.
Type of Study	Included: Experimental studies (Randomized controlled trials (RCTs) both individual and cluster randomised and quasi experimental/non-RCTs).Excluded: Observational studies, animal studies, grey literature, reviews, conference abstracts, and studies with external comparison groups.

The review included studies evaluating the impact of food-based approaches to manage MAM. Studies including wider definitions of undernutrition were only included if the results were presented separately for moderately wasted children based on at least one of the criteria, either MUAC or WHZ. Specifically, studies assessing the following comparisons were included:

Comparison 1: All food-based vs. non-food-based approaches or none.
Comparison 2: Specially formulated foods vs. non-food-based approaches or none.
Comparison 3: Specially formulated foods vs. non-specially formulated foods.
Comparison 4. Multicomponent interventions vs. standard of care or none.

The intervention categories (Figure 1) are based on the inputs involved in each approach. All food-based approaches include the provision of any type of food, regardless of its composition or originally intended use. Non-food-based approaches include any inputs other than direct food distribution, such as cash or counselling. While counselling often includes instructions for caregivers to provide additional foods and specific types of foods to their malnourished children, the food itself is not directly provided as an input of the program or health service. Therefore, counselling is considered a non-food-based approach. No intervention (labelled as "none" above) is defined as providing either inputs, assistance, or services of any kind.

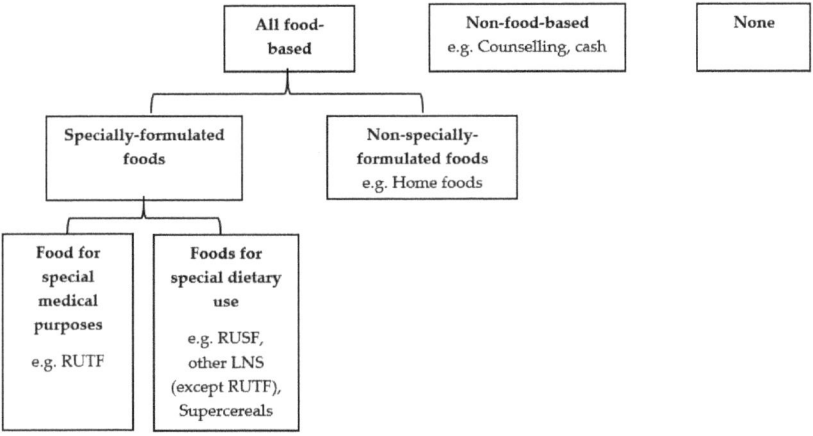

Figure 1. Flow chart of intervention categories.

SFFs for the treatment of MAM are characterized as foods designed, produced, distributed, and utilized in at least one of two distinct ways: (1) foods tailored for specific dietary requirements; or (2) foods intended for particular medical purposes as outlined by the Codex Alimentarius for International Foods [14,15]. In this review, foods classified as "for special dietary uses" pertain to those that can be widely distributed without the need for medical supervision, e.g., RUSF, FBFs, or other diverse forms of lipid-based supplements (LNS). These foods are also frequently used in the management of MAM, but may also have other uses. Foods "for special medical purposes" are intended to be distributed with medical oversight, e.g., ready-to-use-therapeutic food (RUTF). Non-specially formulated foods, often called "local foods" or "home foods", refer to the foods that are commonly consumed by the population without being specifically designed to address malnutrition. This may include imported foods, foods grown locally, or provision of food by development partners or humanitarian organizations in response to food scarcity. Multicomponent interventions are defined as those including any combination of the above categories. Such interventions were included, but analyzed separately.

2.2. Search Strategy and Study Selection

An extensive search was conducted by formulating a search using the PICO criteria as described in Table 1, and the full search strategy can be found in Supporting Table S1. Search was conducted on 10 electronic databases including Medline/PubMed, Embase, Web of Science Index Medicus, CINAHL, Lilacs, the Cochrane Central Register of Controlled Trials (CENTRAL), and eLENA (WHO), Index Medicus for the WHO Eastern Mediterranean Region, and African Index Medicus. No restriction was applied on language or date. The date of the final search was 23 August 2021. We cross-referenced the bibliographies of all included studies, relevant systematic reviews and scoping review on MAM conducted for WHO by this research group in November 2020, to identify studies that may have been missed in the initial search.

Studies identified through database search were exported into EndNote and underwent deduplication. The records were then uploaded into Covidence [16] software for title/abstract and full-text screening. Two reviewers independently screened papers, at both the title/abstract and full-text screening stage, to determine relevance based on the aforementioned selection criteria. Discrepancies were resolved through discussion or by contacting a third reviewer who was a subject expert.

2.3. Data Extraction

Data were extracted from the included studies by two independent reviewers into an Excel spreadsheet. Discrepancies were resolved through discussion or by consulting a third reviewer if consensus was not achieved. Data were extracted on the following: study setting and methods, participants characteristics, inclusion/exclusion criteria, intervention/comparison characteristics, outcomes of interest (at baseline and endline), follow-up details, and additional information such as study limitations, funding, and conflict of interest.

2.4. Risk of Bias (ROB) Assessment

Two authors conducted individual assessments of the quality of all eligible studies using the updated Cochrane risks of bias tool, ROB-2 [17]. Any differences in evaluations were resolved through consensus or by consulting a third author.

2.5. Data Analysis

Analysis was conducted on Review Manager (RevMan) 5.4 software [18]. All the estimates were verified by a second author. Dichotomous outcomes are presented as risk ratios (RR), while the continuous outcomes are presented as mean difference (MD) or standardized mean difference (SMD) along with 95% confidence intervals (CI). Data were analyzed separately for the four comparisons, as mentioned above.

In the comparison of SFFs versus non-food-based or none (Comparison 2), the non-food-based category encompassed a diverse range of intervention types. Nevertheless, a meta-analysis was conducted as the studies fit into this comparison. A separate analysis was conducted for single and multicomponent interventions. All cRCTs were adjusted for clustering so no further adjustment of clusters was deemed necessary during the analysis.

We considered creating funnel plots to investigate potential biases related to small studies and publication biases. However, this was not possible due to the limited number of studies available under each outcome.

2.6. Subgroup and Sensitivity Analysis

Subgroup analyses based on study context, age group, duration of intervention, type of dietary intervention or comparison group, type and dosage of specially formulated food, facility vs. community-based approaches, HIV status and morbidity, concurrent stunting, breastfeeding status, household socio-economic status as well as means of identification (routine screening vs. presentation to a facility) were planned. We were able to perform subgroup analysis based on the type of comparison group for SFFs comparison only; however, we were unable to perform subgroup analysis based on other criteria because of very few studies being included in the review and due to insufficient information being available. We performed sensitivity analysis on the outcomes to assess the impact of high/unclear risk of bias relating to sequence generation and allocation concealment.

Furthermore, a subgroup analysis was planned to identify which children require SFFs, across settings and contexts, but unfortunately this was not possible given the small number of studies identified.

2.7. Evidence Profiles

We constructed GRADE evidence profiles for primary outcomes, summarizing the quality of evidence in accordance to the Grading of Recommendations, Assessment, Development, and Evaluation (GRADE) criteria [19]. It encompasses evaluating factors including within-study risk of bias, indirectness, inconsistency, imprecision, and risk of publication bias. The certainty of evidence for each outcome was rated as "very low" "low", "moderate" or "high".

Preferred Reporting Items for Systematic reviews and Meta-Analyses (PRISMA) guideline was followed for reporting (See Supporting Table S2). The review protocol was registered with the International Prospective Register of Systematic Reviews (PROSPERO: CRD42021273394).

3. Results

3.1. Search Results

We identified a total of 32,180 records for screening. After de-duplication, 23,462 records underwent title and abstract, followed by full-text screening. A total of five papers was included for data extraction and analysis (Figure 2).

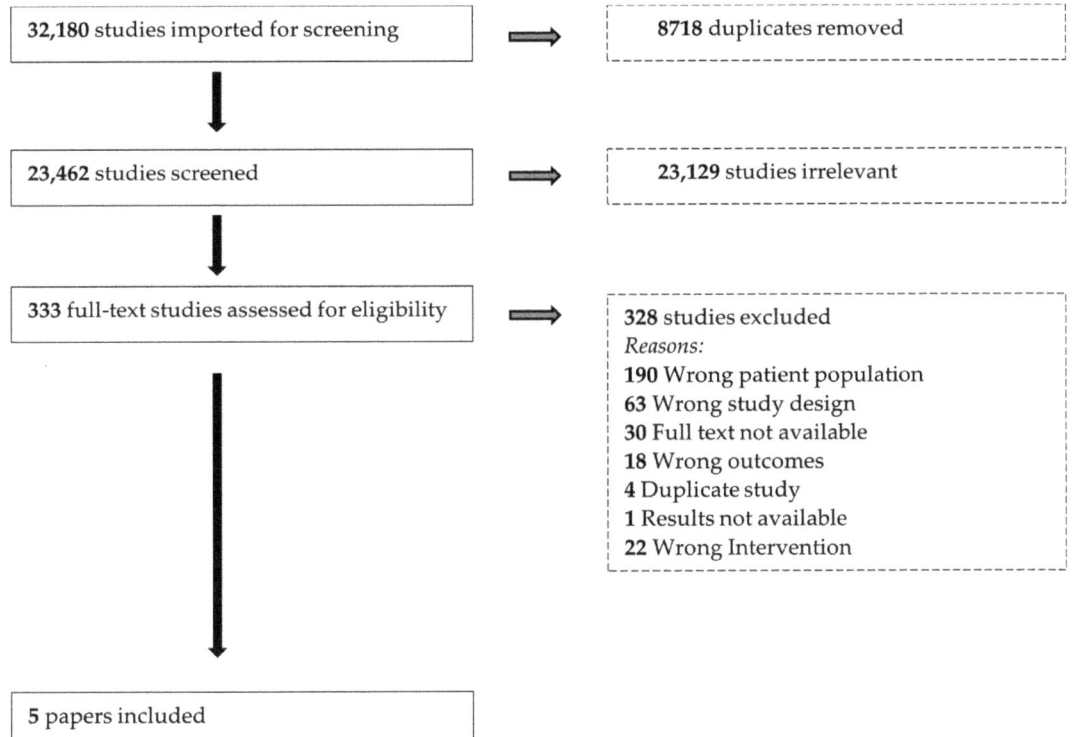

Figure 2. PRISMA flow diagram.

Figure 3 outlines the number of studies included by comparison group. Four studies fit into the first two comparisons. Specially-formulated foods is a subgroup of all food-based approaches, therefore any studies fitting into comparison 2 were also included in comparison 1 (Figure 1). All four studies identified for these two comparisons included interventions using SFFs, including either foods for special medical purposes or special dietary uses. We did not identify any study that looked at non-specially formulated foods only. Therefore, there were no differences in the number of studies between comparison 1 and comparison 2. Going forward in this paper, we will refer to comparison 2 for these included studies.

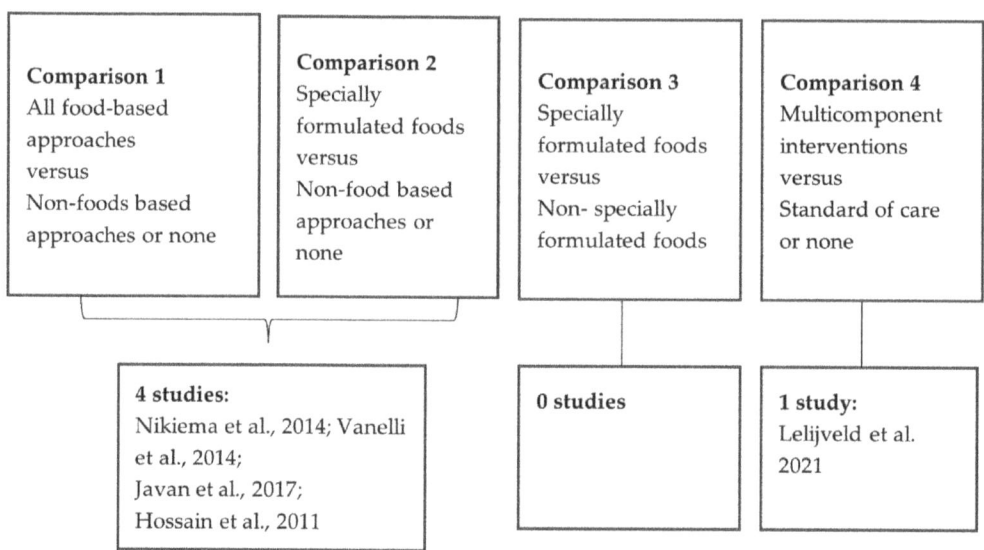

Figure 3. Studies identified by comparison group [20–24].

3.2. Characteristics of Included Studies

Five studies, including 3387 participants, were included in this review [20–24]. Studies were conducted between 2011 and 2021 in Burkina Faso [22], Sierra Leone [23], Malawi [21], Iran [20] and Bangladesh [24]. Out of the five studies, three were individually randomized RCTs [20,23,24] and two were cluster randomized RCTs [21,22].

3.2.1. Comparison 2: Specially-Formulated Foods vs. Non-Food-Based or None

A total of four studies fit into comparison 2, namely the studies by Hossain et al., 2011 [24], Nikièma et al., 2014 [22], Javan et al., 2017 [20] and Vanelli et al. [23]. Table 2 provides a description of these four studies. The studies differed greatly in terms of study design, types of interventions, admission and discharge criteria for treatment, types of SFFs, and dosing of those formulated foods also differed greatly (Table 2). One study used a dose of 150 kcal/day for children < 12 months and 300 kcal/day for children 12–24 months [24], two studies used a dose of approximately 250 kcal/day [20,22], one study used a much higher dose of 200 kcal/kg/day in addition to a food ration providing 1000–1200 kcal/child/day [23].

Table 2. Characteristics of the included studies.

Author, Year	Study Design and Setting	Participants, Admission and Recovery Criteria	Description of Intervention and Control Groups	Outcomes
Hossain et al., 2011 [24]	RCT	507 participants of which 301 had a WHZ < −2 and ≥ −3. In this review we included data only from the subsample of 301 children who met the wasting criteria. Dhaka Hospital and four community clinics in police Districts of Demra, Gulshan, Sabujbagh, and Mirpur.	• Hospital Control (H-C): Fortnightly follow-up care at the International Center for Diarrheal Disease Research, Bangladesh Hospital, including growth monitoring, health education, and micronutrient supplementation. • Community control (C-C): Fortnightly follow-up at community clinics, using the same treatment regimen as group H-C. • Supplementary food group (C-SF): Community-based follow-up as per group C-C plus cereal-based supplementary food (SF). • Psychosocial stimulation: Follow-up as per group C-C plus psychosocial stimulation (PS). • Multicomponent intervention (C-SF+PS): Follow-up as per group C-C plus both SF and PS. Duration: 12 weeks.	Weight-for-age (WAZ), weight-for-length (WHZ), height-for-age (HAZ), weight
Nikièma et al., 2014 [22]	cRCT Rural health centres in Hounde, Burkina Faso	1974 children aged 6–24 months with a WHZ < −2 and ≥ −3 Recovery was defined as a WHZ ≥ −2 at the end of a 12\week period	• Group 1: Child-centered nutrition counselling (CCC) only (n = 605). • Group 2: 273 kcal/day of corn soy blend ++ (CSB++) (n = 675). • Group 3: 258 kcal/day of a locally produced peanut and soy-based ready-to-use supplementary food (RUSF) (n = 694). Duration: 12 weeks.	Number of children recovered, died, or dropped out, attendance, time to recovery, weight, length, and daily mid upper arm circumference (MUAC) gains
Javan et al., 2017 [20]	Randomised investigator blinded (single blind) controlled trial 17 Health centers in Urban areas of Sabzevar, Iran	70 children aged 9–24 months with MAM defined as WHZ < −2 and ≥ −3. Recovery was defined as WHZ > −2 at the end of intervention period	• Intervention group: 273 kcal/day of a blended supplementary food consisting of chickpea, barley, wheat rice and sugar. This food was not fortified and was provided in addition to multivitamins/mineral supplement and nutritional counselling. • Control group: Multivitamins/mineral supplement and nutritional counselling. Duration: 12 weeks.	Rate of weight gain, length gain and Z-score WHZ gain, recovery proportion and adverse events.
Lelijveld 2021 [21]	cRCT 22 community nutrition clinics in Pujehun District, Sierra Leone	1322 children aged 6–59 months with MAM, defined as MUAC ≥ 11.5 and <12.5 cm without oedema or clinical complications. Only 710 of these were in the High-risk group which met inclusion criteriaRecovery was defined as MUAC > 12.5 cm two consecutive visits	• Intervention group: high-reisk MAM children were given 1 sachet of RUTF (92 g, 520 kcal) and a seven-day course of amoxicillin (40–45 mg/kg per dose twice daily) along with standard nutrition counselling. Children with low-risk MAM received standard nutrition counselling only. • Control group: 6 weeks of nutrition counselling alone (delivered via biweekly mother support groups led by a respected community elder). Duration: 2–12 weeks.	MUAC, WAZ, HAZ, WHZ, weight gain Kg, Subscapular skinfold thickness for age, triceps skinfold thickness for age, skinfold thickness ratio, recovered, died, deteriorate to SAM, Remained with MAM, recent illness

Table 2. *Cont.*

Author, Year	Study Design and Setting	Participants, Admission and Recovery Criteria	Description of Intervention and Control Groups	Outcomes
Vanelli et al., 2014 [23]	RCT Outpatient clinics in Makeni, Northern region, Sierra Leone	332 children aged 6–60 months with a WHZ < −2 and ≥ −3. Recovery was defined as achieving a WHZ-score > −2.	• Group 1: World Food Programme Feeding Program supplementations ($n = 177$). These consisted of corn flour, palm oil, dried fishes, and milk powder. The ration for one child provided a maximum of 1000 to 1200 kcal/person/day and 10–12% of energy from protein. • Group 2: In addition to the above-mentioned food ration, children received a locally produced lipid-based paste called "Parma pap" based on the standard RUTF recipe provided in a dose of 200 kcal/kg/day ($n = 159$). Duration: 12 weeks.	Weight, length, WHZ

3.2.2. Comparison 4: Multicomponent Intervention versus Non-Food-Based or None

One study [21] was a multicomponent intervention. In this study by Lelijveld et al., children identified as high-risk MAM received a combination of 520 kcal/day of RUTF, amoxicillin, and nutrition counselling in the intervention group, while low risk MAM children received counselling only.

In the control group, both high-risk and low-risk MAM children received counselling only. In this review, we included only the high-risk subsample given that the low-risk group received counselling in each group and therefore did not meet the PICOS criteria. High-risk MAM children were those with at least one of the following characteristics: MUAC < 11.9, weight for age z-score (WAZ) < -3.5, primary caregiver is not the mother, and non-breastfed if the child is under 2 years. These characteristics have been associated with failure to recover in some Targeted Supplementary Feeding Program (TSFP) in Sierra Leone; thus, "high-risk" equates to failing to respond to the treatment provided in a TSFP.

3.3. Quality of Included Studies

Out of five studies, four had some methodological concerns related to the randomization process, deviation from the intended interventions, and selection of the reported result and one study was judged to be at high risk of bias (Supporting Figure S1).

3.4. Effects of Intervention

Four out of the five studies fit into comparison 1 and 2 with 2677 participants; and one study fit into comparison 4 (multicomponent intervention vs. standard of care) including 710 children. The same four studies were identified for comparison 1 and comparison 2 as all included interventions using SFFs and specially-formulated foods is a subgroup of all food-based approaches (Figure 1). No additional studies were identified that fit only the broader definition of interventions in comparison 1's "all food-based approaches" category.

The results in terms of effect of intervention in comparison 1 and 2 and comparison 4 are presented below. One of the main objectives of this review was to carry out a subgroup analysis to determine which children might need supplementary foods; unfortunately, due to the limited data available, this was not possible.

3.4.1. Comparisons 1 and 2: Specially Formulated Foods versus Non-Food-Based or None

Analysis of the four studies included in this comparison category [20,22–24] suggests that SFFs, when compared to non-food-based interventions or none, likely increase the recovery rate (RR: 1.29; 95% CI: 1.19 to 1.40; n = 2348; three studies; moderate certainty evidence; Figure 4) and have little or no effect on deterioration to severe wasting (RR: 0.78; 95% CI: 0.59 to 1.03; n = 1974; one study; moderate certainty evidence). SFFs may increase WHZ (MD: 0.32; 95% CI: 0.18 to 0.45; n = 365; two studies; low certainty evidence), WAZ (MD: 0.26; 95% CI: 0.14 to 0.38; n = 365; two studies; low certainty evidence), MUAC gain (MD: 0.25 cm; 95% CI: 0.09 to 0.41; n = 301; one study; low certainty evidence), and weight gain (MD 0.26 g/kg/day; 95%CI: 0.11 g/kg/day to 0.41 g/kg/day; n = 64; low certainty evidence), but may have little or no effect on the height for age z-score (HAZ) (MD: 0.10; 95% CI: 0.00 to 0.19; n = 365; two studies; low certainty evidence). SFFs likely reduce non-response by 52% (RR: 0.48; 95% CI: 0.39 to 0.60; n = 1974; one study; moderate certainty evidence) and may decrease the time to recovery (MD: -1.12 weeks; 95% CI: -2.10 to -0.14; n = 1368; one study). The impact on height gain and mortality was uncertain. The effect on sustained recovery was not reported. Forest plots for all the outcomes are shown in Supporting Figures S2–S12 and the full evidence profile can be found in Supporting Table S3.

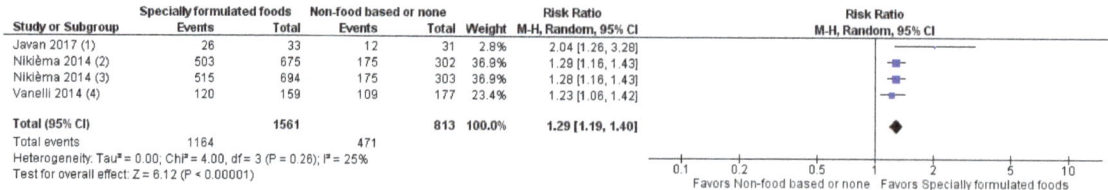

Figure 4. Forest plot of specially formulated foods compared to non-food-based approaches or none. Outcome: anthropometric recovery rate [20,22,23].

Subgroup analysis by a comparison group (i.e., by standard or care group or by counselling) suggests an increase in the recovery rate (RR: 1.29; 95% CI: 1.19 to 1.39; one study) when SFFs were compared with counselling (Supporting Figure S13). However, there was an uncertain effect of specially formulated food on mortality when compared with the standard of care or counselling only (Supporting Figure S14).

Sensitivity analysis was performed for the comparison specially formulated food vs. other or none by excluding studies with unclear risk of bias for both sequence generation and allocation concealment. Notably, the removal of the study by Javan et al., 2017, did not show a significant change in the recovery rate, WHZ, WAZ and HAZ [20].

3.4.2. Comparison 4: Multicomponent Intervention versus Non-Food-Based or None

The findings from one study [21] found an uncertain effect of a multicomponent intervention provided to high-risk MAM children only, on recovery rate after 12 and 24 weeks of enrolment when compared to standard of care. The multicomponent intervention may decrease deterioration to severe wasting by 23% (RR 0.77; 95% CI: 0.6 to 0.98; one study; n = 710; Figure 5) after 12 weeks of intervention, but it may have little or no effect on deterioration to severe wasting after 24 weeks of enrollment. The multicomponent intervention may also have little or no effect on WHZ, WAZ, HAZ, MUAC gain after 12 and 24 weeks of enrollment. It may increase weight by 0.12 g/kg/day (MD 0.02 g/kg/day; 95% CI: 0.22 to 0.22; one study; n = 710) after 24 weeks of enrollment but may have little or no effect on weight gain after 12 weeks of enrollment and on non-response and mortality after 12 and 24 weeks of enrollment. The study did not report on height gain, sustained recovery, and on time to recovery. Forest plots for all the outcomes are shown in Supporting Figures S15–S23 and the full evidence profile can be found in Supporting Table S4.

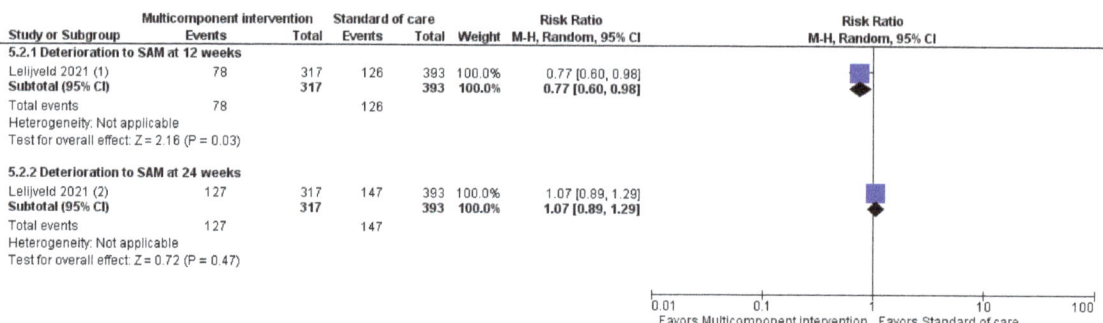

Figure 5. Forest plot of multicomponent intervention compared to non−food−based or none. Outcome: deterioration to SAM [21].

4. Discussion

4.1. Summary of Results

This systematic review summarizes findings from five studies, all of which are RCTs. Evidence indicates that providing SFFs, regardless of formulation or dosing, to children with MAM likely increases recovery, decreases non-response with no effect on deterioration to SAM when compared to other approaches (i.e., counselling) or no intervention. There is low certainty evidence that interventions with SFFs may reduce time to recovery and may increase total weight gain, WHZ, WAZ and MUAC. The intervention may not have an effect on height and HAZ gain. The certainty of evidence relating to mortality was judged to be very low, as none of the studies were sufficiently powered to assess it. Death as an outcome tends to be a rare event in MAM treatment programs. Thus, studies would need to include an extremely large sample size in order to achieve sufficient statistical power to include mortality as a primary outcome, which is often impractical.

The evidence of the multicomponent intervention with RUTF and antibiotics compared to counselling in high-risk MAM children only indicates that it may have little or no effect on recovery, WHZ, WAZ, HAZ and non-response after 12 weeks of intervention, that the multicomponent intervention may decrease deterioration to severe wasting after 12 weeks of intervention and likely has little or no effect on MUAC and weight gain. However, this study was not powered for subgroup analysis of high-risk MAM children.

We did not find any study reporting on comparison 3, i.e., specially formulated foods vs. non-specially formulated foods

4.2. Overall Completeness and Applicability

The existing body of evidence is quite small given only five studies were identified to fit the inclusion criteria for this analysis. Furthermore, these studies only addressed three of the four different comparisons that we sought to conduct. In these studies, the "other approaches" included nutrition counselling alone or standard of care, which was either nutrition counselling with a vitamin mineral supplement and/or a general food ration for malnourished children and/or growth monitoring. Despite differences in interventions in the control group, results and direction of effect remained consistent. While studies were few and specific to the certain contexts in which they were implemented, results may be applicable to other contexts, since nutrition counselling and general food rations are common alternatives to MAM treatment. It is however important to note that both nutrition counselling and general food rations can vary significantly across programs and contexts, which could influence the results of further comparisons.

No studies were identified to assess the effectiveness of SFFs compared to non-specially formulated foods, nor were any identified regarding a comparison between non-SFFs versus other interventions.

Given the small number of studies, we were not able to carry out subgroup analyses to determine which categories of MAM children require SFFs. Nonetheless, the Lelijveld et al. (2021) study [21], by design, aimed to investigate an intervention based on risk stratification within MAM children. While the study was designed to provide a package of interventions to children deemed "high-risk", the authors noted that the criteria for identifying risk may not have been completely appropriate as two criteria ("Mother not the primary caregiver" and "less than 2 years and not breastfeeding") were identified as not being correlated with an increased risk of deterioration. Rather, having a low MUAC for children under 12 months, history of SAM and being a twin were found to be significant risk factors for deterioration among control group children [21]. Two observational studies from Ethiopia not included in this systematic review identified similar risk factors as those noted by the authors in the Lelijveld et al. (2021) study. The first includes a prospective study that followed MAM children without treatment for seven months and found 54% of children recovered, 32.5% remained MAM, and 9.3% encountered a single episode of SAM. Risk factors of poor outcomes, including no recovery from MAM over the seven month period and/or deterioration to SAM, consisted of having a low MUAC and/or low WHZ at baseline, poor child feeding practices, and household food insecurity [25]. A second prospective cohort study in Ethiopia found that without treatment, approximately two-thirds of children from food-insecure and one-third from food-secure households, did not experience recovery from MAM. Dietary diversity and maternal factors, and maternal MUAC demonstrated to be associated with adverse health outcomes [26]. Worse anthropometric measurements upon admission and discharge as well as household food insecurity were cited as factors associated with poor post-discharge outcomes as well in two longitudinal studies investigating relapse in Malawi [27,28]. These studies indicate that moderately wasted children from vulnerable households and those with lower anthropometry status could be at greater risk for poor outcomes and may benefit from more targeted treatment strategies. Other indicators, such as multiple anthropometric deficits, captured by low WAZ, have been shown to be associated with high risk of mortality [29]. A study by Myatt et al. (2019) using data from Senegal found that low WAZ and MUAC were independently associated with near-term mortality [30]. The study also established that a combination of MUAC and WAZ successfully identified all near-term deaths associated with severe anthropometric deficits, encompassing concurrent wasting and stunting [30]. Consistent with these findings, authors of the Lelijveld et al. (2021) study found that a combination of three risk factors: MUAC < 12.0 cm, WAZ < −3, and declining anthropometry during treatment for MAM can effectively predict 90% of cases leading to deterioration into SAM with a specificity rate of 67% in context of Sierra Leone [21]. Further trials are required to confirm the efficacy and cost-effectiveness of prioritizing treatment to children with such risks.

As there were too few studies in this review to allow for subgroup analysis to answer the question of whom should be prioritized for treatment, the WHO commissioned a prognostic factor systematic review as part of the guideline development process to explore the question of who might most benefit from supplementary foods separately [31]. Through this process a series on individual child factors and social factors were identified, namely, which are in line with the above-mentioned studies. These include a MUAC between 115–119 mm, WAZ < −3 SD, age < 24 months, failing to recover from moderate wasting after receiving other interventions (e.g., counselling alone), having relapsed to moderate wasting, history of severe wasting, co-morbidity and personal circumstances such as mother died or poor maternal health and well-being [31].

4.3. Agreements and Disagreements with Other Studies or Reviews

The findings of this systematic review are consistent with previously published systematic reviews on the topic. A recent systematic review conducted in 2020 explored effectiveness of food interventions versus no treatment or nutrition counselling in the management of moderate wasting [32]. Of the included studies, seven concluded that food products demonstrated better anthropometric outcomes in comparison to counseling and/or micronutrient supplementation. Conversely, two studies did not identify a significant advantage of food product interventions, and an additional two studies yielded inconclusive results. The inclusion criteria used in this systematic review were less strict than the ones used in the current analysis, therefore additional studies were identified and included, i.e., studies that did not disaggregate by MAM status as well as studies that only had a small proportion of MAM children were included. It is also worth noting that the studies that did not find an effect only included a small proportion of MAM children and did not disaggregate results by MAM status. In line with our findings, the authors concluded that evidence suggests that supplementary foods indeed contribute to recovery and exhibit to be more effective than counselling; however, the specific type and duration of the supplementary food provided are crucial factors to be considered. Furthermore, the authors highlighted the potential to enhance the effectiveness by focusing on improving the quality and adherence to counseling interventions. A more recent systematic review by Gluning et al. (2021) also found that children had a greater likelihood of recovery if they received a specially formulated food than if they did not [33].

4.4. Implications for Practice

The findings of this systematic review indicate that SFFs are likely beneficial for children with moderate wasting in terms of recovery and other anthropometric outcomes. While the primary aim of wasting interventions is to save lives, any specific recommendations for the use of SFFs in the treatment of MAM may also want to consider potential impacts on other outcome indicators, such as body composition and functional outcomes. Concerns have been raised regarding a potential impact of routinely providing specially formulated lipid-based products (e.g., RUSF and RUTF) to children with MAM on increasing obesity rates, given the escalating challenge of the double burden of malnutrition, whereby populations are experiencing both high rates of undernutrition and also growing rates of overweight. While this review was limited to outcomes in anthropometry and mortality, to our knowledge there is no evidence supporting concerns that treatment of moderately wasted children would contribute to an increase in population-wide rates of overweight and obesity. The study by Lelijveld et al. (2021) did not find any evidence indicating excessive or unhealthy weight gain (based on skinfold thickness) in individuals, in those who received RUTF compared with those who did not receive it [21]. The mean z-scores for skinfold thickness in both groups remained below the global average [21]. This was similar to findings of a study in Kenya, which found that children undergoing treatment for MAM with RUTF exhibited comparable body composition to those treated with RUSF and neither group revealed excessive adiposity [34]. Furthermore, two RCTs comparing fortified blended foods to lipid-based products for treatment also indicated the absence of any adverse effects on body composition [35,36].

Cost-effectiveness is also a practically relevant outcome of interest given many resource constraints in areas where prevalence of child moderate wasting is high. Unfortunately, information to date on cost and cost-effectiveness of acute malnutrition treatment is limited [37]. Among the studies included in this review, only Lelijveld et al. (2021) mentioned costs, and even so, such data were limited to RUTF costs only. Nonetheless, the study found similar RUTF costs per child treated (USD13 and USD19) and recovered (USD27 and USD23) at the intervention and control sites, respectively. Other studies testing a range of supplements for treatment of MAM found supplements costs ranged from USD5 to USD17 per child [38–40], while total program costs ranged from USD28-USD112 per child treated [39,41], where a large variation in costs can be explained by contexts as well as which costs are included in the overall estimate. One study found the treatment of MAM with RUSF to be cost-effective [39].

4.5. Implications for Further Research

The available evidence to answer the research questions included in this review is very limited, leaving obvious gaps in the evidence-base that require further research. Specifically, studies are needed that compare non-specially formulated foods/dietary approaches to other approaches (including counselling or cash) and that compare SFFs to non-specially formulated foods. Formulations and dosing of supplements provided in the intervention groups of the four studies differed significantly. Additional research is required to ascertain the optimal type, composition, and dosage of supplements in terms of both effectiveness and cost-effectiveness.

Only one of the studies in this review [23] achieved a recovery rate > 75%, meeting the Sphere minimum standard for recovery in MAM programs [42]. Nikièma et al. found recovery rates of 74.5% and 74.2% in the CSB++ and RUSF arms, respectively. In the intervention groups of the studies by Javan et al. (2017) and Lelijveld et al. (2021), 68% and 48% recovered, respectively [20,21]. In the control groups recovery rates ranged from 31.6% to 61.6% [20–23]. Further research is needed to determine what programmatic, contextual, or other barriers exist for programs to reach overall higher recovery rates and whether the definition of recovery is appropriate and achievable in all populations.

This review incorporated three studies that included a counseling intervention as part of their research design. In two studies, program attendance and protocol adherence were lower in the counselling arms than in the arms that provided the SFFs [21,22]. In an explorative restricted analysis on non-defaulter children, Nikièma et al. stated that when analyses were adjusted for attendance, the differences between food-supplementation groups and the child-centered counselling groups diminished. Interviews with a subset of women who were less adherent or had dropped out from the program revealed that many did not perceive the advice as useful and encountered difficulty in cooking recommended recipes, given their dependence on their husbands to buy the ingredients. Additionally, the extended waiting time at the healthcare center on the day of counselling was identified as a demotivating factor [22]. Further research is essential to gain a more comprehensive understanding of the impact pathway of counselling and if effectiveness could be improved either through provision of incentives to increase adherence or by better adapting the content or modality of counselling to local causes of malnutrition and dynamics within households. It would also be worth exploring whether a more holistic package of interventions with more focus on morbidity as a cause could improve outcomes of MAM programs. Very high rates of morbidity and inflammation have been found in children with MAM [38,43], but that to date limited attention is placed on the detection and management of illness in children with MAM beyond routine medication which usually includes deworming, vitamin-A, and iron and folic acid supplementation.

Given the large number of children affected by MAM every year, the likely heterogeneity of this population, and the cost of treatment, prioritization of treatment may be needed in some contexts. As mentioned above, this review was not able to conclusively answer the question of whom should be prioritized for treatment. Therefore, a separate prognostic review was commissioned by the WHO, which identified a number of individual and social factors to help determine which MAM children should be prioritized for use of supplementation with specifically formulated foods [31], but noted that research is needed to evaluate the response to interventions in MAM children who have identified prognostic factors and that the prognostic factor review was limited to findings primarily from African contexts [31]. Research should also be conducted to determine the cost-effectiveness of a risk stratification approach in various contexts, which will likely differ across contexts. Cost-effectiveness studies should cost longer term programs, include wider health system costs as well as those for treatment of complicated and uncomplicated SAM, given the impact that treating MAM early can have on the prevention of SAM and duration of treatment.

5. Conclusions

Although data are limited, our results suggest that the provision of specially formulated food may be beneficial for children with MAM. We were not able to answer the question of who should be prioritized for treatment as part of this review due to the paucity of data. The findings of this review contributed to the WHO guideline formulation pertaining to the prevention and management of wasting and nutritional oedema in infants and children, which now recommends that in humanitarian crisis or high-risk contexts all children should be considered for a supplementary food in addition to counseling and the provision of home foods. The guideline also highlights a number of individual and social factors that can aid in prioritizing children for treatment, but acknowledged the need for further research.

Supplementary Materials: The following supporting information can be downloaded at: https://www.mdpi.com/article/10.3390/nu15173781/s1, Supporting Table S1. Search Strategy; Supporting Table S2. PRISMA Checklist; Supporting Table S3. Evidence profile for comparison 2 (Specially formulated foods compared to non-food-based approaches or none); Supporting Table S4. Evidence profile for comparison 4 (multicomponent intervention versus non-food-based or none); Supporting Figure S1a. Quality of included studies—Cluster randomized trials, Supporting Figure S1b. Quality of included studies—Individually randomized trials; Supporting Figure S2. Forest plot of specially formulated foods compared to non-food-based approaches or none. Outcome: Weight-for-height z-score; Supporting Figure S3. Forest plot of specially formulated foods compared to non-food-based approaches or none. Outcome: Deterioration to SAM; Supporting Figure S4. Forest plot of specially formulated foods compared to non-food-based approaches or none. Outcome: Weight-for-height z-score; Supporting Figure S5. Forest plot of specially formulated foods compared to non-food-based approaches or none. Outcome: Weight-for-age z-score; Supporting Figure S6. Forest plot of specially formulated foods compared to non-food-based approaches or none. Outcome: Height-for-age z-score; Supporting Figure S7. Forest plot of specially formulated foods compared to non-food-based approaches or none. Outcome: MUAC gain; Supporting Figure S8. Forest plot of specially formulated foods compared to non-food-based approaches or none. Outcome: Weight gain; Supporting Figure S9. Forest plot of specially formulated foods compared to non-food-based approaches or none. Outcome: Height gain; Supporting Figure S10. Forest plot of specially formulated foods compared to non-food-based approaches or none. Outcome: Non-response; Supporting Figure S11. Forest plot of specially formulated foods compared to non-food-based approaches or none. Outcome: Time to recovery; Supporting Figure S12. Forest plot of specially formulated foods compared to non-food-based approaches or none. Outcome: Mortality; Supporting Figure S13. Forest plot of specially formulated foods compared to non-food-based approaches or none. Outcome: Recovery rate (subgroup analysis based on type of comparison group); Supporting Figure S14. Forest plot of specially formulated foods compared to non-food-based approaches or none. Outcome: Mortality (subgroup analysis based on type of comparison group); Supporting Figure S15: Forest plot of multicomponent intervention compared to non-food-based or none. Outcome: Recovery rate; Supporting Figure S16: Forest plot of multicomponent intervention compared to non-food-based or none. Outcome: Deterioration to SAM; Supporting Figure S17: Forest plot of multicomponent intervention compared to non-food-based or none. Outcome: Weight for height z-score; Supporting Figure S18: Forest plot of multicomponent intervention compared to non-food-based or none. Outcome: Weight for age z-score; Supporting Figure S19: Forest plot of multicomponent intervention compared to non-food-based or none. Outcome: Height for age z-score; Supporting Figure S20: Forest plot of multicomponent intervention compared to non-food-based or none. Outcome: MUAC gain; Supporting Figure S21: Forest plot of multicomponent intervention compared to non-food-based or none. Outcome: Weight gain; Supporting Figure S22: Forest plot of multicomponent intervention compared to non-food-based or none. Outcome: Non-response; Supporting Figure S23: Forest plot of multicomponent intervention compared to non-food-based or none. Outcome: Mortality.

Author Contributions: The initial draft of the methodology was written by J.K.D., Z.A.P., R.A.S. and B.C.; H.C.S., M.M., A.R.-P., Z.A.B. and R.E.B. reviewed the methodology, contributing to its refinement and providing their endorsement; R.A.S., M.M. and B.C. conducted the title and abstract and full-text screening. Data were extracted by J.K.D., Z.A.P., R.A.S. and B.C., risk of bias assessment was performed by Z.A.P., R.A.S., J.K.D. and B.C.; while all authors collectively participated in shaping the manuscript structure and interpreting the data. Z.A.P., B.C., J.K.D., R.A.S. and H.C.S. wrote the first draft of the manuscript. The final draft was revised by M.M., A.R.-P., Z.A.B. and R.E.B., B.C., J.K.D., R.A.S., Z.A.P., H.C.S., M.M., A.R.-P., Z.A.B. and R.E.B. approved the final version of the manuscript. All authors have read and agreed to the published version of the manuscript.

Funding: This review was supported by the WHO as an integral component of the guideline development process for the updated guidelines on the prevention and management of wasting and/or nutritional oedema (acute malnutrition).

Institutional Review Board Statement: This is a systematic review, so ethical approval was exempted.

Informed Consent Statement: Not applicable.

Data Availability Statement: The data presented in this study are available in Supplementary Documents.

Acknowledgments: The PICO question that served as the foundation for this systematic review was formulated by WHO in collaboration with the Guideline Development Group (GDG) for the revision of the guidelines on the prevention and management of wasting and/or nutritional oedema (acute malnutrition). The authors extend their gratitude to Alison Daniel, Kirrily de Polnay, Jaden Bendabenda, Zita Weise Prinzo, Celeste Naude, and Michael McCaul for their invaluable insights throughout the systematic review process. Their contributions were especially instrumental in determining comparison groups and guiding the GRADE assessment.

Conflicts of Interest: The authors declare no conflict of interest.

References

1. Olofin, I.; McDonald, C.; Ezzati, M.; Flaxman, S.; Black, R.; Fawzi, W.; Caulfield, L.; Danaei, G. Associations of Suboptimal Growth with All-Cause and Cause-Specific Mortality in Children under Five Years: A Pooled Analysis of Ten Prospective Studies. *PLoS ONE* **2013**, *8*, e64636. [CrossRef] [PubMed]
2. United Nations Children's Fund (UNICEF); World Health Organization; International Bank for Reconstruction and Development/The World Bank. *Levels and Trends in Child Malnutrition: Key Findings of the 2021 Edition of the Joint Child Malnutrition Estimates*; World Health Organization: Geneva, Switzerlands, 2021. Available online: https://apps.who.int/iris/handle/10665/341135 (accessed on 1 April 2022).
3. Food an Agricultural Organisation (FAO); Tufts University. *Twin Peaks: The Seasonality of Acute Malnutrition, Conflict and Environmental Factors—Chad, South Sudan and the Sudan*; FAO: Rome, Italy, 2019.
4. Grellety, E.; Golden, M.H. Weight-for-Height and Mid-Upper-Arm Circumference Should Be Used Independently to Diagnose Acute Malnutrition: Policy Implications. *BMC Nutr.* **2016**, *2*, 10. [CrossRef]
5. Myatt, M. How Do We Estimate a Caseload of SAM/MAM in a Given Time Period. 2012. Available online: https://www.ennonline.net/attachments/3133/MAM-and-SAM-caseload-calculations.pdf (accessed on 21 March 2022).
6. World Health Organization (WHO); United Nations Children's Fund (UNICEF). Discussion Paper: The Extension of the 2025 Maternal, Infant and Young Child Nutrition Targets to 2030. 2021. Available online: https://data.unicef.org/resources/who-unicef-discussion-paper-nutrition-targets/ (accessed on 21 March 2022).
7. Global Nutrition Cluster (GNC). Moderate Acute Malnutrition: A Decision Tool for Emergencies. 2017. Available online: https://reliefweb.int/report/world/moderate-acute-malnutrition-decision-tool-emergencies (accessed on 30 April 2022).
8. World Health Organization. *Essential Nutrition Actions: Improving Maternal, Newborn, Infant and Young Child Health and Nutrition*; World Health Organization: Geneva, Switzerland, 2013. Available online: https://www.ncbi.nlm.nih.gov/books/NBK258736/ (accessed on 30 April 2022).
9. Golden, M.H.; Grellety, E. Integrated Management of Acute Malnutrition (IMAM) Generic Protocol; English Version 6.6.2. 2011. Available online: https://www.researchgate.net/publication/292131715_Golden_MH_Grellety_Y_Integrated_Management_of_Acute_Malnutrition_IMAM_Generic_Protocol_ENGLISH_version_662 (accessed on 5 August 2023).
10. United Nations Children's Fund (UNICEF); International Rescue Committee (IRC). *Toolkit for CHW Community-Based Treatment of Uncomplicated Wasting for Children 6–59 Months in the Context of COVID-19*; Version 1.0; UNICEF: New York, NY, USA, 2020. Available online: www.ennonline.net/toolkitforchwinthecontextofcovid19 (accessed on 1 May 2022).
11. United Nations Children's Fund (UNICEF); World Health Organization. *Prevention, Early Detection and Treatment of Wasting in Children 0–59 Months through National Health Systems in the Context of COVID-19*; UNICEF: New York, NY, USA, 2020.
12. World Food Programme. *WFP's Additional Recommendations for the Management of Maternal and Child Malnutrition Prevention and Treatment in the Context of COVID 19*; World Food Programme: Rome, Italy, 2020.
13. Cichon, B.; Das, J.K.; Salam, R.A.; Padhani, Z.A.; Stobaugh, H.C.; Mughal, M.; Pajak, P.; Rutishauser-Perera, A.; Bhutta, Z.A.; Black, R.E. Effectiveness of Dietary Management for Moderate Wasting among Children >6 Months of Age—A Systematic Review and Meta-Analysis Exploring Different Types, Quantities, and Durations. *Nutrients* **2023**, *15*, 1076. [CrossRef]
14. *Codex STAN 180-1991*; Standard for Labelling of and Claims for Foods for Special Medical Purposes. Codex Alimentarius Commission: Atlanta, GA, USA; Brussels, Belgium, 1991.
15. *Codex STAN 146-1985*; General Standard for the Labelling of and Claims for Prepackaged Foods for Special Dietary Uses. Codex Alimentarius Commission: Atlanta, GA, USA; Brussels, Belgium, 2009.
16. Covidence Systematic Review Software, Veritas Health Innovation, Melbourne, Australia. Available online: www.covidence.org (accessed on 5 August 2023).
17. Sterne, J.A.C.; Savovic, J.; Page, M.J.; Elbers, R.G.; Blencowe, N.S.; Boutron, I.; Cates, C.J.; Cheng, H.; Corbett, M.S.; Eldridge, S.M.; et al. RoB 2: A Revised Tool for Assessing Risk of Bias in Randomised Trials. *Br. Med. J.* **2019**, *366*, l4898. [CrossRef]
18. The Cochrane Collaboration. *Review Manager (RevMan) [Computer Program]*, Version 5.4.; The Cochrane Collaboration: London, UK, 2020.
19. Guyatt, G.H.; Oxman, A.D.; Vist, G.E.; Kunz, R.; Falck-Ytter, Y.; Alonso-Coello, P.; Schünemann, H.J. GRADE: An Emerging Consensus on Rating Quality of Evidence and Strength of Recommendations. *Br. Med. J.* **2008**, *336*, 924. [CrossRef] [PubMed]

20. Javan, R.; Kooshki, A.; Afzalaghaee, M.; Aldaghi, M.; Yousefi, M. Effectiveness of Supplementary Blended Flour Based on Chickpea and Cereals for the Treatment of Infants with Moderate Acute Malnutrition in Iran: A Randomized Clinical Trial. *Electron. Physician* **2017**, *9*, 6078–6086. [CrossRef]
21. Lelijveld, N.; Godbout, C.; Krietemeyer, D.; Los, A.; Wegner, D.; Hendrixson, D.T.; Bandsma, R.; Koroma, A.; Manary, M. Treating High-Risk Moderate Acute Malnutrition Using Therapeutic Food Compared with Nutrition Counseling (Hi-MAM Study): A Cluster-Randomized Controlled Trial. *Am. J. Clin. Nutr.* **2021**, *114*, 955–964. [CrossRef]
22. Nikièma, L.; Huybregts, L.; Kolsteren, P.; Lanou, H.; Tiendrebeogo, S.; Bouckaert, K.; Kouanda, S.; Sondo, B.; Roberfroid, D. Treating Moderate Acute Malnutrition in First-Line Health Services: An Effectiveness Cluster-Randomized Trial in Burkina Faso. *Am. J. Clin. Nutr.* **2014**, *100*, 241–249. [CrossRef]
23. Vanelli, M.; Virdis, R.; Contini, S.; Corradi, M.; Cremonini, G.; Marchesi, M.; Mele, A.; Monti, F.; Pagano, B.; Proietti, I.; et al. A Hand-Made Supplementary Food for Malnourished Children. *Acta Biomed.* **2014**, *85*, 236–242.
24. Hossain, M.I.; Nahar, B.; Hamadani, J.D.; Ahmed, T.; Brown, K.H. Effects of Community-Based Follow-up Care in Managing Severely Underweight Children. *J. Pediatr. Gastroenterol. Nutr.* **2011**, *53*, 310–319. [CrossRef]
25. James, P.; Sadler, K.; Wondafrash, M.; Argaw, A.; Luo, H.; Geleta, B.; Kedir, K.; Getnet, Y.; Belchew, T.; Bahwere, P. Children with Moderate Acute Malnutrition with No Access to Supplementary Feeding Programmes Experience High Rates of Deterioration and No Improvement: Results from a Prospective Cohort Study in Rural Ethiopia. *PLoS ONE* **2016**, *11*, e0153530. [CrossRef]
26. Adamu, W.; Jara, D.; Alemayehu, M.; Burrowes, S. Risk Factors Associated with Poor Health Outcomes for Children under the Age of 5 with Moderate Acute Malnutrition in Rural Fagita Lekoma District, Awi Zone, Amhara, Ethiopia, 2016. *BMC Nutr.* **2017**, *3*, 88. [CrossRef]
27. Chang, C.Y.; Trehan, I.; Wang, R.J.; Thakwalakwa, C.; Maleta, K.; Deitchler, M.; Manary, M.J. Children Successfully Treated for Moderate Acute Malnutrition Remain at Risk for Malnutrition and Death in the Subsequent Year after Recovery. *J. Nutr.* **2013**, *143*, 215–220. [CrossRef]
28. Stobaugh, H.C.; Ryan, K.N.; Kennedy, J.A.; Grise, J.B.; Crocker, A.H.; Thakwalakwa, C.; Litkowski, P.E.; Maleta, K.M.; Manary, M.J.; Trehan, I. Including Whey Protein and Whey Permeate in Ready-to-Use Supplementary Food Improves Recovery Rates in Children with Moderate Acute Malnutrition: A Randomized, Double-Blind Clinical Trial. *Am. J. Clin. Nutr.* **2016**, *103*, 926–933. [CrossRef]
29. McDonald, C.; Olofin, I.; Flaxman, S.; Fawzi, W.; Spiegelman, D.; Caulfield, L.; Black, R.; Ezzati, M.; Danaei, G. The Effect of Multiple Anthropometric Deficits on Child Mortality: Meta-Analysis of Individual Data in 10 Propective Studies from Developing Countries. *Am. J. Clin. Nutr.* **2013**, *97*, 896–901. [CrossRef] [PubMed]
30. Myatt, M.; Khara, T.; Dolan, C.; Garenne, M.; Briend, A. Improving Screening for Malnourished Children at High Risk of Death: A Study of Children Aged 6-59 Months in Rural Senegal—ERRATUM. *Public Health Nutr.* **2019**, *22*, 872–873. [CrossRef]
31. World Health Organization. *WHO Guideline on the Prevention and Management of Wasting and Nutritional Oedema (Acute Malnutrition) in Infants under 5 Years (Version 1.1)*; WHO: Geneva, Switzerland, 2023. Available online: https://www.childwasting.org/normative-guidance (accessed on 5 August 2023).
32. Lelijveld, N.; Beedle, A.; Farhikhtah, A.; Elrayah, E.E.; Bourdaire, J.; Aburto, N. Systematic Review of the Treatment of Moderate Acute Malnutrition Using Food Products. *Matern. Child. Nutr.* **2020**, *16*, e12898. [CrossRef]
33. Gluning, I.; Kerac, M.; Bailey, J.; Bander, A.; Opondo, C. The Management of Moderate Acute Malnutrition in Children Aged 6-59 Months in Low- and Middle-Income Countries: A Systematic Review and Meta-Analysis. *Trans. R. Soc. Trop. Med. Hyg.* **2021**, *115*, 1317–1329. [CrossRef] [PubMed]
34. Lelijveld, N.; Musyoki, E.; Adongo, S.W.; Mayberry, A.; Wells, J.C.; Opondo, C.; Kerac, M.; Bailey, J. Relapse and Post-Discharge Body Composition of Children Treated for Acute Malnutrition Using a Simplified, Combined Protocol: A Nested Cohort from the ComPAS RCT. *PLoS ONE* **2021**, *16*, e0245477. [CrossRef] [PubMed]
35. Fabiansen, C.; Yaméogo, C.W.; Iuel-Brockdorf, A.-S.; Cichon, B.; Rytter, M.J.H.; Kurpad, A.; Wells, J.C.; Ritz, C.; Ashorn, P.; Filteau, S.; et al. Effectiveness of Food Supplements in Increasing Fat-Free Tissue Accretion in Children with Moderate Acute Malnutrition: A Randomised 2 × 2 × 3 Factorial Trial in Burkina Faso. *PLoS Med.* **2017**, *14*, e1002387. [CrossRef]
36. McDonald, C.M.; Ackatia-Armah, R.S.; Doumbia, S.; Kupka, R.; Duggan, C.P.; Brown, K.H. Percent Fat Mass Increases with Recovery, But Does Not Vary According to Dietary Therapy in Young Malian Children Treated for Moderate Acute Malnutrition. *J. Nutr.* **2019**, *149*, 1089–1096. [CrossRef] [PubMed]
37. Chui, J.; Donnelly, A.; Cichon, B.; Mayberry, A.; Keane, E. *The Cost-Efficiency and Cost-Effectiveness of Management of Wasting in Children: A Review of the Evidence, Approaches and Lessons*; AAH (Action Against Hunger): New York, NY, USA; Save the Children UK: London, UK, 2020. Available online: https://resourcecentre.savethechildren.net/document/cost-efficiency-and-cost-effectiveness-management-wasting-children-review-evidence/ (accessed on 1 May 2022).
38. Ackatia-Armah, R.; McDonald, C.; Doumbia, S.; Erhardt, J.; Hamer, D.; Brown, K. Malian Children with Moderate Acute Malnutrition Who Are Treated with Lipid-Based Dietary Supplements Have Greater Weight Gains and Recovery Rates than Those Treated with Locally Produced Cereal-Legume Products: A Community-Based, Cluster-Randomized Trial. *Am. J. Clin. Nutr.* **2015**, *101*, 632–645. [CrossRef]
39. Isanaka, S.; Barnhart, D.A.; McDonald, C.; Ackatia-Armah, R.; Kupka, R.; Seydou, D.; Brown, K.; Menzies, N.A. Cost-Effectiveness of Community-Based Screening and Treatment of Moderate Acute Malnutrition in Mali. *BMJ Glob. Health* **2019**, *4*, e001227. [CrossRef]

40. LaGrone, L.; Trehan, I.; Meuli, G.; Wang, R.; Thakwalakwa, C.; Maleta, K.; Manary, M. A Novel Fortified Blended Flour, Corn-Soy Blend "plus-plus," Is Not Inferior to Lipid-Based Ready-to-Use Supplementary Foods for the Treatment of Moderate Acute Malnutrition in Malawian Children. *Am. J. Clin. Nutr.* **2012**, *95*, 212–219. [CrossRef] [PubMed]
41. Griswold, S.P.; Langlois, B.K.; Shen, Y.; Cliffer, I.R.; Suri, D.J.; Walton, S.; Chui, K.; Rosenberg, I.H.; Koroma, A.S.; Wegner, D.; et al. Effectiveness and Cost-Effectiveness of 4 Supplementary Foods for Treating Moderate Acute Malnutrition: Results from a Cluster-Randomized Intervention Trial in Sierra Leone. *Am. J. Clin. Nutr.* **2021**, *114*, 973–985. [CrossRef]
42. Sphere Association. *The Sphere Handbook: Humanitarian Charter and Minimum Standards in Humanitarian Response*, 4th ed.; Sphere Association: Geneva, Switzerland, 2018. Available online: www.spherestandards.org/handbook (accessed on 5 August 2023).
43. Cichon, B.; Fabiansen, C.; Yaméogo, C.W.; Rytter, M.J.H.; Ritz, C.; Briend, A.; Christensen, V.B.; Michaelsen, K.F.; Oummani, R.; Filteau, S.; et al. Children with Moderate Acute Malnutrition Have Inflammation Not Explained by Maternal Reports of Illness and Clinical Symptoms: A Cross-Sectional Study in Burkina Faso. *BMC Nutr.* **2016**, *2*, 57. [CrossRef]

Disclaimer/Publisher's Note: The statements, opinions and data contained in all publications are solely those of the individual author(s) and contributor(s) and not of MDPI and/or the editor(s). MDPI and/or the editor(s) disclaim responsibility for any injury to people or property resulting from any ideas, methods, instructions or products referred to in the content.

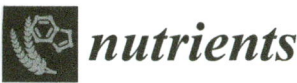

Review

Effects of Unconventional Work and Shift Work on the Human Gut Microbiota and the Potential of Probiotics to Restore Dysbiosis

Aroa Lopez-Santamarina [1], Alicia del Carmen Mondragon [1], Alejandra Cardelle-Cobas [1], Eva Maria Santos [2], Jose Julio Porto-Arias [1], Alberto Cepeda [1,*] and Jose Manuel Miranda [1]

[1] Laboratorio de Higiene Inspección y Control de Alimentos, Departamento de Química Analítica, Nutrición y Bromatología, Campus Terra, Universidade de Santiago de Compostela, 27002 Lugo, Spain; aroa.lopez.santamarina@usc.es (A.L.-S.); alicia.mondragon@usc.es (A.d.C.M.); alejandra.cardelle@usc.es (A.C.-C.); josejulio.porto@usc.gal (J.J.P.-A.); josemanuel.miranda@usc.es (J.M.M.)

[2] Área Académica de Química, Universidad Autónoma del Estado de Hidalgo, Carretera Pachuca-Tulancingo km. 4.5, Pachuca 42076, Hidalgo, Mexico; emsantos@uaeh.edu.mx

* Correspondence: alberto.cepeda@usc.es; Tel.: +34-982-252-231 (ext. 22406)

Abstract: The work environment is a factor that can significantly influence the composition and functionality of the gut microbiota of workers, in many cases leading to gut dysbiosis that will result in serious health problems. The aim of this paper was to provide a compilation of the different studies that have examined the influence of jobs with unconventional work schedules and environments on the gut microbiota of workers performing such work. As a possible solution, probiotic supplements, via modulation of the gut microbiota, can moderate the effects of sleep disturbance on the immune system, as well as restore the dysbiosis produced. Rotating shift work has been found to be associated with an increase in the risk of various metabolic diseases, such as obesity, metabolic syndrome, and type 2 diabetes. Sleep disturbance or lack of sleep due to night work is also associated with metabolic diseases. In addition, sleep disturbance induces a stress response, both physiologically and psychologically, and disrupts the healthy functioning of the gut microbiota, thus triggering an inflammatory state. Other workers, including military, healthcare, or metallurgy workers, as well as livestock farmers or long-travel seamen, work in environments and schedules that can significantly affect their gut microbiota.

Keywords: workers; gut microbiota; military; seafarers; healthcare; farmers; probiotics

1. Introduction

The work pressure and stressful conditions to which workers are exposed in certain jobs can affect their health and safety [1]. Currently, it is estimated that 33% of employees work outside of their country's regular working hours. In fact, according to the US Bureau of Labor Statistics, there are approximately 15 million Americans who work late afternoons, evenings, rotating shifts, or other irregular hours [2]. In Europe, almost one in four workers work night shifts [3]. These work schedules affect the social lives of workers, causing frequent changes in their schedules and lifestyle habits, including changes in sleep patterns and eating habits. Moreover, these unconventional schedules are associated with increased morbidity among workers [4].

In terms of dietary behavior, it was reported that the total energy intake, either on average or in kcal or kcal/week, of workers on a rotating shift schedule does not differ significantly from those working on a conventional schedule [5]. However, there are significant differences in the distribution of caloric intake in the different meals of the day, as well as in the type of food intake [5]. In fact, shift workers have been found to have lower intakes of dietary fiber (because of lower fruit and vegetable intake). This has been linked to excessive energy intake and the

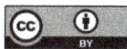

development of overweight and obesity, as foods containing higher amounts of dietary fiber prevent overweight and obesity by avoiding excessive calorie intake through satiety-based signaling [6]. In addition, workers tend to compromise on variety in their diet, often eating on a prearranged schedule that is out of sync with the individual's circadian rhythms. For example, they substitute individual foods for mixed meals and opt for fast or simple meals that are often characterized by a low nutritional value, high-calorie density, high sodium content, and excessive consumption of sugary drinks [7]. In fact, on average, during the first year of employment, new shift workers tend to increase their body mass index (BMI) by about one point, which is attributable to a combination of factors, such as higher-calorie food choices during the working day, lower diet quality, and reduced time spent on leisure activities [8].

In addition, it is known that working hours, the type of work, or even the job position are factors that can affect the gut microbiota (GM) of workers. These alterations may increase the likelihood of developing various metabolic and inflammatory diseases, such as obesity, diabetes, inflammatory bowel diseases, and asthma [9]. In addition, they may also increase the risk of neurological disorders, such as depression, anxiety, and Parkinson's disease [10,11]. It has been shown that an altered feeding rhythm can alter the GM, leading to dysbiosis [12]. Recent research has indicated the existence of a "circadian clock-gut microbiota axis" in which the GM regulates the circadian clock regulation, with evidence of bidirectional communication between them [13–16]. Currently, studies on changes in the GM due to shift work and jet lag focus mainly on the disruption or interruption of this axis [17]. Several recent studies have also shown that GM is crucial for the pathogenesis of stress-related diseases and neurodevelopmental disorders, in addition to the development of brain function [18]. Indeed, it has been shown that even short-term exposure to stress can alter the relative proportions of key human GM phyla [19]. Similarly, experimental modifications of the human genome influence the stress response, anxiety, and hypothalamic-pituitary-adrenal neuroendocrine stress axis [18]. In addition, recent studies suggest that the GM may change depending on the type of work performed, for example, when exposed to chemicals, metals, and particulate matter, and that the GM may modulate the effect of these exposures [12].

The aim of this review is to gather information on how unconventional work affects the health and the GM of workers, as well as the effect of using probiotics to modulate the GM, restore dysbiosis, and improve the quality of life of these workers.

2. Effects of Work in Unconventional Schedules on Human Health

Shift work refers to work activities that take place at times other than traditional daytime hours. While it is true that alternative working hours are often necessary and can facilitate productivity, it is also important to recognize that these unconventional working hours can have an adverse impact on our health and well-being [20]. Several observational studies have shown that shift workers face an increased risk of developing obesity, type 2 diabetes mellitus (DM2), and metabolic syndrome compared to those working equivalent daytime hours [3]. In addition, as the years of shift work accumulate, the risk increases. This phenomenon applies to both night work and rotating shifts [3].

Unconventional shift work, especially at night, is associated with an increased risk of cardiovascular disease, cancer, diabetes, hypertension, chronic fatigue, sleep disorders, increased body weight, and therefore, a higher mortality rate [20–22]. Workers on rotating shifts have a higher prevalence of irritable bowel syndrome, abdominal pain, constipation, and diarrhea than workers on conventional schedules [23–26]. It has been suggested that inadequate nutrition, irregular meal timing, and psychological disorders may contribute to this high prevalence [5]. On the other hand, workers with unconventional work schedules are more likely to suffer from anxiety symptoms due to work schedule problems and disturbed sleep patterns, triggering increased anxiety levels [27].

2.1. Changes in Dietary Pattern

Most workplaces have shifted to less physically demanding tasks (for example, automation), while portability and the availability of dense, high-energy "snacks" have increased in the workplace. This may also be due to an increase in the intake of foods with excess fats, oils, and refined flour, such as junk food. In addition, a lack of physical activity is triggered by a lack of time and feeling more tired. For these reasons, the need to implement nutrition education programs combined with physical exercise is the greatest among shift workers.

A meta-analysis of 24 studies [28] that targeted these workers and included measures as simple as offering fruit at reduced prices in vending machines, providing access to professional nutritional advice, or encouraging physical exercise by giving away sports passes or organizing sports competitions among company members achieved an average weight reduction of 1.2 kg and a decrease in BMI of 0.47 kg/m^2 after one year of implementation. At first glance, this decrease may not seem very significant, but considering that most of the population aged 18–49 years gains, on average, between 0.5 and 1 kg per year, it cancels out the average weight gain resulting from the increasing age of the workforce. Shift workers have been found to have a higher BMI, higher cholesterol and triglyceride levels, and a higher risk of high blood pressure than workers on conventional schedules. Therefore, their risk of developing cardiovascular diseases is up to 40% higher than in conventional shift workers [8,29].

In terms of feeding patterns [30], mice exposed to a 4-week schedule were observed to experience changes in their feeding patterns, consuming food irregularly. This altered feeding schedule was significantly associated with a loss of circadian rhythm and changes in the composition of the gut microbiome in mice. In addition, an association was found between an increased F/B ratio and changes in fat mass and inflammation. Based on these findings, it was hypothesized that the changes in the microbiome observed from baseline to the first energy restriction period might be repeated, and possibly more pronounced, in samples collected during the second energy restriction period [30].

2.2. Hormonal Changes

The elevated risk of cardiometabolic problems in shift workers may also be due to hormones involved in metabolism, such as ghrelin (which increases appetite) and leptin (which reduces appetite), which are regulated by transcription factors in the biological clock. These hormones play a key role in controlling appetite and eating behavior by sending stimulatory and inhibitory signals to the central nervous system, in particular the hypothalamus [31]. During the night, especially in the time interval between 9 p.m. and 4 a.m., circulating blood levels of ghrelin remain very high and are accompanied by low circulating levels of leptin [31]. This imbalance in the ghrelin/leptin ratio means that people who are awake at this time of the day have a greater appetite and are therefore more likely to gain weight. Moreover, this imbalance is intensified in people who suffer from sleep deprivation and/or poor sleep quality. Therefore, this imbalance will chronically increase in workers on rotating or night shifts, which partly explains their higher propensity to obesity [31]. Shift work can also lead to increased circulating levels of resistin, an endocrine hormone implicated in the development and progression of insulin resistance, as well as cortisol, a hormone traditionally associated with stress. This is probably related to a lower insulin response at night, which is an important activator of lipoprotein lipase, an enzyme found in the capillary walls that stimulates the hydrolysis and removal of triacylglycerol [31]. A large body of scientific literature published in recent years demonstrate a link between shift and/or night work and insulin resistance, diabetes, dyslipidemia, and metabolic syndrome [32]. The link between shift work and higher insulin resistance is thought to be due to decreased melatonin production. Melatonin is a key factor in insulin synthesis, secretion, and action. In addition, its concentration also regulates the expression of the glucose transporter GLUT 4. Relevant work in this area has shown that shift work leads to increased insulin resistance and an increased inflammatory state [32]. In addition, cortisol levels have been shown to increase in stressful situations and during prolonged low-calorie diets. These two factors are closely related to shift work, so when stress or blood pressure increases, cortisol levels also increase. When cortisol is high, it is very difficult for the body to regulate blood sugar, and it also inhibits the loss of body fat and the gain in muscle mass. The same is true when the duration of sleep is short and cortisol levels rise and exacerbate the above [33].

Currently, chronic low-grade inflammation has been recognized to play an important role as a biological factor in stress-related ill health [34]. Both sleep disturbance and sleep deprivation have been reported to be associated with changes in different immunological parameters that favor a pro-inflammatory state, which may underlie the negative health effects of sleep disturbance. The slightest loss of sleep has negative health consequences, both physiological and mental, as well as negative effects on performance [35]. This evidence suggests that sleep-mediated immune disruption, together with evidence that pathogen-induced immune responses can negatively affect the sleep cycle, demonstrates that there is a bidirectional relationship between sleep and immunity, which may have profound implications in immune-related human diseases [36]. Any disturbance in sleep can affect the physiological systems that govern immune cell distribution and cytokine activity. A normal sleep cycle plays a key role in regulating the hypothalamic-pituitary-adrenal axis, which controls the circadian rhythm. Systemic cytokine levels show an increase in the mid-morning and late afternoon, reflecting glucocorticoid secretion [37].

2.3. Sleep Disruption

Sleep loss and acute circadian disruption, whether due to total sleep deprivation, sleep restriction, or sleep fragmentation, have been found to be physiological stressors. These changes are analyzed in relation to fluctuations in cortisol levels that occur with sleep loss and circadian disruption. Cortisol elevation following sleep loss and acute circadian disruption is thought to reflect activation of the hypothalamic-pituitary-adrenal (HPA) axis [38]. Indeed, cortisol has significant effects on glucose metabolism. It affects the body's glucose balance by stimulating gluconeogenesis (the production of glucose from sources other than glucose) and reducing peripheral glucose utilization, which can lead to an increase in blood glucose levels. In addition, studies investigating sleep duration disruption have found that sleep loss and acute circadian disruption are associated with increased cortisol levels, especially in the afternoon and early evening [38,39]. This suggests that sleep loss may contribute to metabolic dysfunction, at least in part, via the activation of a cortisol-mediated physiological stress response.

Experimental sleep studies suggest that sleep deprivation can increase adrenal gland activity [38]. Consequently, sleep deprivation may generate physiological stress that alters metabolic homeostasis, leading to a series of low-intensity inflammatory processes that contribute to metabolic dysfunction. If true, this could also provide a new theory for the observed relationship between sleep deprivation, circadian dysregulation, and inflammatory markers [40].

It has been hypothesized that sleep restriction may trigger pro-inflammatory changes in the gut microbiome. These changes could drive the metabolic and cognitive effects observed after sleep restriction [41–43]. In a randomized study of healthy Caucasian volunteers who followed regular eating and exercise schedules, participants were subjected to two nights of partial sleep deprivation and two nights of normal sleep. It was observed that in fecal samples taken after two nights of partial sleep deprivation, there was an increase in the abundance of Firmicutes bacteria and a decrease in Bacteroidetes bacteria compared to those taken after two nights of normal sleep [41,42]. These changes in relative bacterial abundance are similar to the patterns observed in fecal samples from obese people, as described in a study by Benedict et al. [44]. Human research has shown that the presence of higher counts of Firmicutes, which are more prevalent in rotating and night shift workers [43], is associated with an increased predisposition to obesity and metabolic diseases [43,44]. Another study [24] reinforces the results obtained above by showing that humans who experienced an 8 h circadian offset due to flights across different time zones showed a change in the composition of the gut microbiome and a pronounced increase in the phylum Firmicutes [24].

Several previous studies, such as that by Zhang et al. [43], have shown that in sleep-restricted rats, an increased Firmicutes/Bacteroidetes (F/B) ratio, which has been associated with changes in fat mass and inflammation, is observed during rest. There is support for the idea that cortisol levels in the afternoon or early evening may be altered by shorter sleep periods or lack of sleep, as well as by acute circadian mismatch. This physiological response to stress triggered by sleep deprivation is likely to be related to changes in GM. The above-mentioned detailed relationship between cortisol and the GM suggests a possible explanation for the connection between stress triggered by sleep disruption or sleep deprivation, circadian disruption, and possible changes in the GM [43].

2.4. Work Environment

As mentioned above, the community composition and diversity of GM microorganisms are susceptible to change and are affected by various factors, such as diet, activity, sleep patterns, genetics, drugs, and environment, including the type of work and shift work (Figure 1) [45,46].

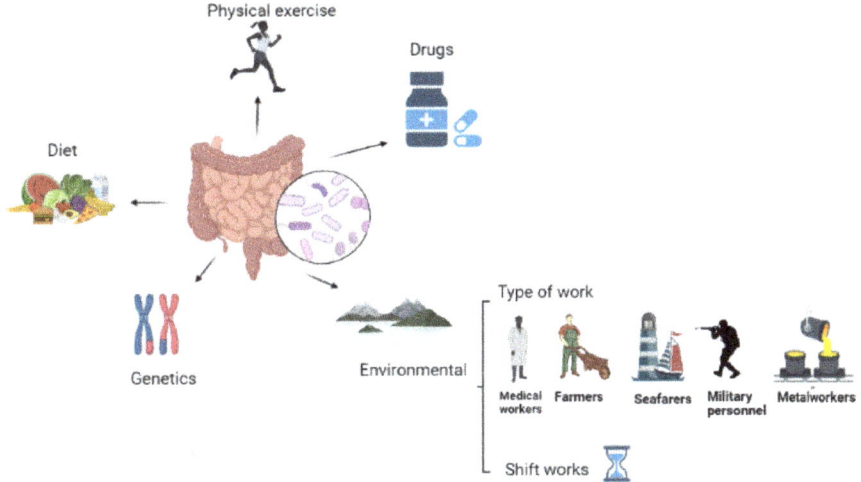

Figure 1. The different factors that can affect the human gut microbiota. Source: own elaboration. (Created in BioRender.com).

Sleep loss and acute circadian disruption are considered physiological stressors that contribute to this susceptibility [46]. For example, in a study by Thaiss et al. [24], jet lag was induced in a group of mice by subjecting them to an 8 h advance in their daily schedule for three days and showed evidence that host circadian misalignment results in microbial dysbiosis, leading to metabolic imbalances.

On the other hand, it is necessary to consider that a specific work environment can also influence the GM and thus the health of workers [47,48]. Table 1 lists the different studies related to the environment of different types of unconventional work and their effects on GM. For example, the chemical and physical conditions present in hospitals give rise to microbial communities that differ widely from those found in the natural external environment [49]. Even within the same workplace, different areas often have their own microecological characteristics. For example, in hospital intensive care units (ICUs), where intensive medical activities are conducted, and frequent exposure to infectious pathogens occurs, microbial communities are particularly hazardous [49–51]. Indeed, the microbiology of the hospital environment has been shown to impact the health of hospital staff [52]. In addition, healthcare workers have been found to have a higher incidence of *Clostridium difficile* infections in their workplaces, suggesting that they may act as potential vectors of infectious diseases [53,54].

Table 1. Effects of work environment on workers' gut microbiota.

Workers	Subjects	Dosage and Time of Exposition	Effects of Gut Microbiota	Other Health Effects	Reference
Tunnel miners	48 healthy men	Before and after 3 weeks of working in a tunnel 8 h/day	Decreased GM diversity; increased Actinobacteria and Bifidobacteriales, Corynebacteriales and Desulfovibrionales; increased Bifidobacterium, Romboutsia, Clostridium, and Leucobacter; decreasing Faecalibacterium and Roseburia	Decreased antioxidant efficacy, digestive and absorptive capacity; increased proinflammatory factors	Lu et al. [1]
Healthcare workers	214 workers	Fecal samples were subjected to an enzyme immunoassay for toxins A and b and for glutamate dehydrogenase	Only 0.8% of healthcare workers were found positive for C. difficile toxins and antigen	The results found did not confirm the hypothesis that a long stay in the hospital is a risk of C. difficile infection	Friedman et al. [53]
Farm workers	6 swine farm workers and 6 local villagers	16S rRNA gene sequencing of fecal samples	Workers had less species diversity compared to the local villagers, as well as higher amounts of Proteobacteria and Clostridiaceae	Analysis of antimicrobial resistance genes did not reveal significant differences among workers and villagers	Sun et al. [48]
Veterinary students in swine farms	14 students who stayed 3 months on swine farms	91 fecal samples investigated by 16S rRNA and whole metagenome shotgun	Moderate decrease in Bacteroidetes and an increase in Proteobacteria phyla	Antibiotic resistance genes were found in similar genetic contexts in student samples and farm environmental samples	Sun et al. [55]
Healthcare workers	71 frontline healthcare workers fighting against COVID-19	A longitudinal investigation at four time points: immediately after they finished treatment and left the isolation wards (Day 0), after a two-week quarantine in a hotel (Day 14), four weeks after their return to normal life (Day 45), and a half year after the frontline work (Day 180)	Microbes associated with mental health were mainly Faecalibacterium spp. and Eubacterium eligens group spp. Of note, the prediction model indicated that a low abundance of Eubacterium hallii group uncultured bacterium and a high abundance of Bacteroides eggerthii immediately after the two-month frontline work were significant determinants of the reappearance of post-traumatic stress symptoms.	Stressful events induced significant depression, anxiety, and stress	Gao et al. [56]

Table 1. *Cont.*

Workers	Subjects	Dosage and Time of Exposition	Effects of Gut Microbiota	Other Health Effects	Reference
Medical workers	175 healthy medical workers	Short-term (1–3 months) workers ($n = 80$) and long-term (>1 year) workers ($n = 95$)	Short-term workers: significantly higher abundances of *Lactobacillus*, *Butyrivibrio*, *Clostridiaceae*, *Clostridium*, *Ruminococcus*, *Dialister*, *Bifidobacterium*, *Odoribacter*, and *Desulfovibrio*, and lower abundances of *Bacteroides* and *Blautia*. Long-term workers: higher abundances of taxa such as *Dialister*, *Veillonella*, *Clostridiaceae*, *Clostridium*, *Bilophila*, *Desulfovibrio*, *Pseudomonas*, and *Akkermansia*, and lower abundances of *Bacteroides* and *Coprococcus*	Not investigated	Zheng et al. [57]
Nurses	51 full-time staff nurses	Worked 12 h day or night shifts	No differences in the richness and diversity of species in samples from nurses working day and night shifts	Not investigated	Rogers et al. [2]
Security officers	10 male security officers working rotational day/night shifts	After working the day shift (7:00 h–15:00 h) for 4 weeks and after working the night shift (23:00 h–7:00 h) for 2 weeks. One-off day per week	The phylum with the highest abundance in the day shift was Firmicutes, followed by Bacteroidetes. In the night shift, the relative abundance of Bacteroidetes decreased; however, Actinobacteria and Firmicutes increased. *Faecalibacterium* was found to be a biomarker of day-shift work.	Not investigated	Mortaş et al. [58]

There is a bidirectional relationship between the GM and circadian rhythm. Thus, the circadian clock influences the composition of the GM; similarly, the GM also regulates the circadian rhythm. Studies are currently focusing on the disruption of this bidirectional axis [12]. Indeed, human GM has been shown to play a key role in the development of brain function, and consequently, in stress-related diseases and neurodevelopmental disorders [12].

3. Effects of Different Types of Unconventional Work on the Human Gut Microbiota

A link between impaired GM and type II diabetes mellitus (DM2), as well as metabolic syndrome, has also been demonstrated [59]. The physiological and psychological stress that occurs during shift work negatively influences intestinal permeability and affects health via impaired GM. In a healthy gut environment, the epithelial barrier is a well-maintained structure designed to restrict the impact of pathogens and promote and support the fight against 'beneficial' inflammatory bacteria [59]. Maintaining an appropriate balance between beneficial and pathogenic bacteria in the mucosa and within the gut is crucial for gut stability. Both the integrity of the epithelial barrier and the protective gut environment can be disrupted by various environmental challenges, including stress [59].

In the human GM, it has been observed that approximately 10–35% of the operational taxonomic units (OTU) show diurnal variations in abundance, according to Bijnens and Depoortere [3]. For example, oscillations in the abundance of *Parabacteroides*, *Lachnospira*, and *Bulleida* have been identified, as mentioned in a study by Thaiss et al. [24]. In addition, short-chain fatty acids (SCFA) show a rhythmic pattern and decrease throughout the day in humans [3]. In vivo studies have shown that oral administration of SCFA induces a phase shift in several peripheral tissues, as observed in a study by Tahara et al. [60]. Importantly, the change in microbiome composition observed in jet-lagged individuals was completely restored after two weeks of recovery from jet lag [24].

3.1. Healthcare Workers

A study by Zheng et al. [57] showed marked differences in the diversity and structure of the GM between healthcare workers and non-healthcare workers. Short-term contract workers were found to have higher microbial diversity than long-term contract workers. Firmicutes, Bacteroidetes, Proteobacteria, and Actinobacteria were found to constitute the majority of the predominant phyla in the GM of all participants. However, the phylum Firmicutes was found to be more abundant in short- and long-term workers than in non-medical individuals. On the other hand, the phylum Bacteroidetes were less abundant among healthcare workers. As for Proteobacteria, they were slightly more abundant in short-term workers, although this difference was not statistically significant [57].

Alterations in the microbiomes of medical workers may have important implications for their health. In this study [57], a deviation in the distribution of medical workers' enterotypes was observed, with an increase in Firmicutes abundance and a decrease in Bacteroides and *Prevotella* levels. It was assessed whether the hospital department (ICU vs. non-ICU) and job position (resident physician vs. nursing staff) of the medical workers had an impact on the composition of the GM. Significant differences in GM composition between individuals belonging to different hospital departments and occupying different job positions were observed in both short- and long-term groups of workers [57]. Significant differences in the composition of the microbiome were observed between ICU and non-ICU workers. Compared to non-ICU workers, it was observed that ICU workers showed a significant increase in the abundance of *Dialister* bacteria, *Enterobacteriaceae*, *Phascolarctobacterium*, *Pseudomonas*, *Veillonella*, and *Streptococcus*, and a marked decrease in *Faecalibacterium*, *Blautia*, and *Coprococcus* bacteria.

It was observed that the GM of ICU workers, who specialize in the treatment of critically ill patients, shows a significant increase in *Enterobacteriaceae*, Pseudomonas, *Veillonella*, and *Streptococcus* bacteria [57]. These findings support the idea that exposure to the hospital environment and interaction with critically ill patients may influence the composition of the microbiome of ICU workers, particularly the abundance of certain bacterial genera. Members of the *Enterobacteriaceae* family are common ICU pathogens. These bacteria are among the pathogens most frequently associated with nosocomial infections in hospital settings, including ICUs [57]. The enrichment of Enterobacteriaceae members in medical workers could be related to exposure to the ICU environment [57].

The risk of colonization by *C. difficile*, a bacterium associated with nosocomial infections, tends to increase steadily during hospitalization. This suggests that there is a cumulative risk of daily exposure to *C. difficile*, possibly in the form of spores, which may persist in the hospital environment for months [53]. These spores could be a potential source of infection and contribute to the transmission of *C. difficile* to the microbiome of exposed medical workers. Colonization with non-toxigenic strains of *C. difficile* may offer some protection against the development of disease caused by toxigenic strains. This means that the presence of non-toxigenic strains in the microbiome may compete with toxigenic strains, thus limiting their growth and pathogenic activity [53].

3.2. Farm Workers

Another worker group studied was farmers. Studies have been conducted on the impact on the microbiota of people working on farms with animals compared to those working in urban environments [55]. Farmers had higher microbial richness and diversity compared to individuals living in urban environments. These results support the hypothesis that residing in urban environments may imply exposure to a less diverse microbial flora, which is associated with an increase in allergic and inflammatory diseases. In addition, they showed a greater similarity to the gut profile of pigs, as evidenced by an increase in bacteria of the genus *Bacteroides* and the family *Clostridiaceae*, as well as a decrease in bacteria of the phylum Firmicutes [55].

Only one study has investigated changes in the oral microbiota associated with exposure to agricultural pesticides. Stanaway et al. [61] found a persistent association across seasons between the detected blood concentration of the insecticide azinphos-methyl and the taxonomic composition of the oral microbiome, specifically a significant reduction in the genus *Streptococcus* [62].

3.3. Military Personnel

Another group in which microbiota-related studies have been conducted is the military personnel. In the study by Walters et al. [63], the relationship between variations in the microbiota of soldiers overseas and the incidence of traveler's diarrhea (TD) infection was investigated. *Ruminococcaceae* was found to be more abundant in soldiers who tested positive for TD, while *Ruminiclostridium* spp. had a higher relative abundance in soldiers who tested negative for TD. In addition, *Haemophilus* spp. and *Turicibacter* spp. were found to be associated with the alleviation of gastrointestinal distress [63].

3.4. Long-Travel Seamen

On the other hand, seafarers also face extreme situations and disruption of conventional patterns [64]. Indeed, the difficult conditions they experience during long sea voyages increase the risk of illness and death compared to workers on land. The ocean environment presents a variety of adverse conditions, such as high humidity, high salinity, intense exposure to sunlight and ultraviolet radiation, heavy waves, monotonous environments, disrupted circadian rhythms, sleep disturbances, and limited access to fresh fruits and vegetables [64,65]. In addition to vitamin deficiency, chronic diseases affecting the immune system and digestive tract have become the main health risk for people working at sea [62]. The human GM plays a key role in the host immune system and is essential for maintaining human health [66]. Recent studies have highlighted the importance of the diversity of gut microbial species and functional genes in the development of various chronic metabolic diseases. Although attention has been paid to the health of seafarers over long voyages, research in this area remains limited [62,67]. In a study by Zhang et al. [68], it was shown that a long sea voyage not only led to changes in the composition of the GM but also reduced the diversity of its functional characteristics. In this study, the microbiome of sailors in the placebo group underwent significant alterations during a long sea voyage, involving changes in key gut bacterial species and a significant reduction in genes for carbohydrate-active enzymes, which are critical for maintaining GM homeostasis and host health [69]. These enzymes help us break down these complex carbohydrates into SCFA, either directly or via a cross-feeding mechanism [70]. This, in turn, promotes gut health and improves fitness. Conversely, the low diversity of gut microbes possessing functional genes represented by these degradative enzymes is closely associated with the growth of pathogens that can trigger chronic diseases [68]. At the same time, during prolonged sea voyages, the limited availability of fresh fruits and vegetables may also be a crucial factor contributing to a decrease in gut microbial diversity [67].

3.5. Metal and Tunnel-Workers

GM and health are also affected in workers exposed daily to dust, metalworking fluids (MWFs), and pesticides. Two studies investigated possible changes in the GM in workers exposed to silica and ceramic dust. A study by Zhou et al. [71] analyzed the characteristics of the GM in patients with early stage pulmonary fibrosis caused by daily exposure to silica in the work environment. It was observed that, at the phylum level, the abundance of Firmicutes and Actinobacteria was lower in patients with silicosis than in healthy control individuals. These findings may be useful for the early diagnosis of silicosis and prevention of pulmonary fibrosis [71]. Furthermore, Ahmed et al. [72] conducted a study on the composition of the nasal microbiota in workers exposed to dust in ceramic factories. It was observed that dust-exposed workers had a significant increase in the relative abundance of the phylum Proteobacteria, specifically *Haemophilus* spp., with a lower presence of Actinobacteria and Bacteroidetes compared to controls [72].

Another study by Wu et al. [73] performed an invasive characterization of the microbiota in lung biopsies obtained from workers exposed to MWFs. Lung biopsies were performed on symptomatic MWF-exposed workers and showed the presence of bacterial species characteristic of MWFs in a new and distinctive MWF-related lung condition. This condition was characterized by lymphocytic bronchiolitis and alveolar ductitis, with B-cell follicle formation and emphysema [74]. Wu et al. [73] also showed the presence of an OTU designated as Pseudomonas in the lung, skin, and nasal samples from exposed workers, as well as in MWFs. Traces of *Pseudomonas pseudoalcaligenes* were found in these samples, and these readings were a close match for the *P. pseudoalcaligenes* readings of the metal working fluid samples, which suggests that the bacterial DNA found in the tissue samples could have originated from the metal working fluid. Interestingly, this OTU was not found to be differentially enriched in the air samples, suggesting that the main mode of transmission of this microorganism is via direct rather than airborne contact [73].

In addition, it is interesting to note that the alterations observed in the GM of the tunnel workers were similar to those found in patients with mental disorders, especially mood disorders [1], and point to the importance of maintaining a proper balance in the GM to promote mental and emotional well-being [1]. Regarding the high abundance of Actinobacteria and *Coriobacteriaceae* in patients with mental disorders, as mentioned in the study by Lu et al. [1], a possible correlation with dyslipidemia has been suggested. This suggests that the composition of the GM may be related to metabolic and cardiovascular health in patients with mental disorders. In addition, the presence of Bifidobacterium bacteria has been found to be significantly higher in patients with major depressive disorder and bipolar disorder with current major depressive episodes. Several studies have found lower levels of *Faecalibacterium* in patients with mental disorders, including bipolar disorder [1]. *Faecalibacterium* is a bacterial genus associated with the production of SCFA, which are important metabolites for gut health. A decrease in SCFA-related bacteria, such as *Faecalibacterium*, could indicate a dysbiosis in anti-inflammatory activities in workers and possibly in patients with mental disorders. SCFA, produced by intestinal bacteria during the fermentation of food substrates, can modulate the immune response and have anti-inflammatory effects. Therefore, a decrease in these bacteria and the corresponding SCFAs could be related to an inflammatory state and dysfunction in microbiota-gut-brain interactions. Furthermore, it has been postulated that SCFA may directly or indirectly mediate GM-brain interactions via various signaling pathways, such as immune, endocrine, neural, and humoral pathways [1].

4. Use of Probiotics to Restore Dysbiosis in Workers

Due to studies showing that both the type of work and unconventional working hours can negatively affect the GM, the use of probiotics has been suggested to alleviate these consequences. Table 2 compiles studies showing the effects of probiotic supplementation on GM and biochemical markers in workers. In fact, they could be used in a personalized way for everyone under the concept of precision probiotics [75].

Probiotics are defined as live microorganisms that, when consumed in adequate amounts, provide health benefits to the host [76]. Commonly, probiotics include bacterial strains of the genera *Lactobacillus* and *Bifidobacterium* [77,78]. To date, most probiotic-related studies have focused on describing variations in the GM and have concluded that limited structural changes in the GM are a common phenomenon following probiotic consumption. These changes are characterized by an increase in the number of beneficial microorganisms and a decrease in pathogens [79,80]. Some clinical studies have investigated the application of probiotics in the treatment of various diseases. For example, their efficacy has been studied in liver disease [81], cardiovascular disease [82], kidney disease [83], irritable bowel syndrome [84], relief of allergy symptoms [85], and against viral infections [82]. Although the results of all these studies were not necessarily positive, probiotics have been found to have common effects on the regulation of GM.

Table 2. Effect of probiotic supplementation of gut microbiota and biochemical markers of workers.

Type of trial	Subjects	Dosage and Time of Exposition	Effects on Gut Microbiota	Other Health Effects	Reference
Double-blind parallel-group trial	94 shift workers	Lactobacillus acidophilus, Bifidobacterium animalis spp. lactis or placebo; 1×10^{10} colony count units (cfu) for 14 days	Not investigated	Probiotic supplementation decreased serum markers such as cortisol, pentraxin, or interleukin-1ra, related to sleep quality.	West et al. [22]
Randomized controlled trial	961 women healthcare workers	1.12×10^9 cfu or more of Lactobacillus bulgaricus OLL1073R-1 and strain of Streptococcus thermophilus daily for 16 weeks	Not investigated	A significant increase in interferon-γ production was found with a daily intake of OLL1073R-1 yogurt.	Kinoshita et al. [86]
A randomized, double-blind, placebo-controlled trial	70 petrochemical workers	100 g/day probiotic yogurt which contained two strains of Lactobacillus acidophilus LA5 and Bifidobacterium lactis BB12 with a total of min 1×10^7 cfu for 6 weeks	Not investigated	The consumption of probiotic yogurt had beneficial effects on mental health parameters in petrochemical workers.	Mohammadi et al. [87]
A double-blind, randomized, placebo-controlled experiment	41 female healthcare workers employed on a rotating shift schedule	4 g/day of freeze-dried powder of the multistrain probiotic mixture (2.5×10^9 cfu/g) for 6 weeks. The prebiotic mixture contained Bifidobacterium bifidum W23, Bifidobacterium lactis W51, Bifidobacterium lactis W52, Lactobacillus acidophilus W37, Lactobacillus brevis W63, Lactobacillus casei W56, Lactobacillus salivarius W24, and Lactococcus lactis (W19 and W58)	Not investigated	Results indicate a potential protective effect of probiotics against fat mass gain. Probiotics may alleviate anxiety and fatigue in shift-working females.	Smith-Ryan et al. [88]
A 30-day longitudinal experiment	82 sailors during a sea voyage	2 g package containing mixed probiotics including 9.70 Log cfu of Lactobacillus casei, 9.70 Log cfu of Lactobacillus plantarum P-8, 9.70 Log^{10} cfu of Lactobacillus rhamnosus M9, 9.88 Log^{10} cfu of Bifidobacterium lactis V9, and 9.88 Log^{10} cfu of Bifidobacterium lactis M8 once daily for 30 days	The compositions of the intestinal microbiota of the two groups (placebo and probiotic) were highly distinct at the end of the sea voyage, which confirmed the positive impacts of the probiotics consumed.	Probiotics maintained intestinal microbiome homeostasis and further prevented anxiety during the long sea voyage.	Zhang et al. [89]

Table 2. Cont.

Type of trial	Subjects	Dosage and Time of Exposition	Effects on Gut Microbiota	Other Health Effects	Reference
A randomized, double-blind placebo-controlled study	262 employees (day workers and three shift workers)	Daily dose of 10^8 cfu of *L. reuteri* for 80 days	Not investigated	Among the 53 shift workers, 33% in the placebo group reported being sick during the study period compared to none in the *L. reuteri* group.	Tubelius et al. [90]
Open-label single-arm study	90 highly stressed information technology specialists	300 mg of lyophilized *L. plantarum* PS128™ powder, which is equivalent to 10 billion cfu for 8 weeks	Not investigated	Significant improvements in self-perceived stress, overall job stress, job burden, cortisol level, general or psychological health, anxiety, depression, sleep disturbances, quality of life, and both positive and negative emotions	Wu et al. [73]
A controlled, parallel, randomized, and double-blind clinical trial	65 military	Symbiotic ice cream containing: 2 × 10^8 cfu/g for *L. acidophilus* LA-5 and 2.7 × 10^9 cfu/g for *B. animalis* BB-12 and 2.3 g of inulin in the 60 g of ice cream for 30 days	No significant differences in α diversity between groups. No significant differences in the proportions of each phyla comparing the two groups.	This supplementation improved tenseness and sleepiness in healthy young military.	Valle et al. [91]

Evidence of the beneficial effects and immune-modulating capacity of probiotics suggests that investigating the use of probiotic supplements to ameliorate sleep disruption-induced changes in night work-associated inflammation is a promising avenue [92]. It is certain that probiotics can transiently colonize the GM [92,93]. It has been postulated that these microorganisms exert beneficial health effects by modifying the immune system.

A study by West et al. [22] investigated the acute effects of two different probiotic strains, *Lactobacillus acidophilus* DDS-1 and *Bifidobacterium animalis* spp. *lactis* UABla-12, on the immune system of night shift workers. These strains, alone or in combination, have previously been shown to reduce the severity of abdominal pain and irritable bowel syndrome symptoms [88,90,93], improve functional constipation [94], provide symptomatic relief in cases of lactose intolerance [94], and show protective effects against atopic dermatitis [95] and respiratory infections [96]. Night shifts are associated with significant changes in the markers of stress and immunity, and probiotic supplementation was found to moderate the severity of these changes. These results suggest that there are wider health implications associated with night work than with circadian disruption [21,97]. They also provide initial evidence for the use of probiotics to attenuate the effects of stress associated with night work.

Another study [27] investigated the acute effects of probiotics on stress indices, acute-phase responses, and inflammation during two nights of night work. It was observed that the most significant changes occurred during the anticipatory stress before the night shift [27]. Anticipatory stress refers to stress associated with upcoming events [90] and is related to illness [98] and dysregulation of the HPA axis and the immune system [99]. The study results provide initial evidence that *L. acidophilus* and *Bifidobacterium lactis* can improve the biological impact of stress and that *B. lactis* can also improve sleep quality. In addition, a high recovery rate of the ingested probiotic species was observed. This study presents a novel approach to understanding the role of probiotic supplementation in inducing stress and immune system alterations. Furthermore, it confirms previous findings that *L. acidophilus* and *B. lactis* can colonize the gut and be detected in feces [94].

On the other hand, there are also studies exploring the possibility that probiotics may play a role in maintaining microbiome homeostasis during long sea voyages. One example is the study by Zhang et al. [68], who investigated the possible effects of probiotics on improving the physical fitness of seafarers. In this study, a questionnaire was designed that included scores related to bowel movement (such as stool consistency and volume; the presence of constipation, diarrhea, and bloody stools; and the frequency of defecation), pain in the stomach, pain in the legs, headache, chest pain, muscle pain, and stress/anxiety at the end of the journey. Following probiotic supplementation, significant differences were found in the reduction in stress and anxiety scores [87,91]. These results indicate that probiotics have the potential to prevent the onset of anxiety during a long sea voyage [72]. Another 30-day longitudinal study on Chinese seafarers revealed that probiotics were able to maintain the homeostasis of the GM during a long sea voyage. The probiotics used in the study included strains such as *Lactobacillus casei*, *Lactobacillus plantarum*, *L. rhamnosus*, and *B. lactis*, which demonstrated excellent probiotic properties in previous studies [68,100].

Another option to reduce anxiety or depression would also be the supplementation of SCFA or dietary fiber intake [41], as recent research indicates that SCFA or the microbiota may influence brain function, such as anxiety or depression [100]. Therefore, it is possible that microbiota-derived metabolites reach the brain, and future studies are required to understand the impact of chronic SCFA administration on the circadian clock system in the brain [41]. The results indicate that bacterial fermentation end products, such as SCFA, show a decrease throughout the day [101]. The two most abundant genera associated with time were *Roseburia* and *Ruminoccocus*, which accounted for 2% and 3% of the bacterial community in our participants, respectively. In addition, both *Roseburia* and *Eubacterium* decreased throughout the day. Both genera are butyrate producers, and a decrease in butyrate concentrations throughout the day was reported [101].

Associations between the time of day and bacterial abundance could be related to specific bacterial characteristics, such as bile resistance. For example, *Oscillospora* and *Bilophila*, which increased during the day, are bile tolerant, which could give them a competitive advantage during waking hours when increased bile secretion occurs due to food intake [101]. Alternatively, these fluctuations could be influenced by factors independent of the presence of food in the gastrointestinal tract. Circadian variations in the murine microbiota are observed even when parenteral nutrition is the only source of food. Other factors may include hormonal signals from the hosts. For example, *Enterobacter aerogenes* may be affected by melatonin, a circadian hormone [101].

A narrative review suggested that probiotics, prebiotics, and postbiotics may improve sleep quality and reduce stress by influencing sleep latency, sleep duration, and cortisol levels. However, it is important to note that stronger evidence and further validation are required to support these findings, as well as to understand the underlying mechanisms in detail. This can be achieved via appropriate methodological adjustments and further research [102].

5. Conclusions

The effects of shift and night work, as well as unconventional work, on human health have various aspects related to both personal characteristics and working and living conditions. Shift work is known to be a risk factor for many health disorders, such as gastrointestinal, psychological, and cardiovascular disorders, but it also disturbs the homeostasis of the sleep/wake cycle and circadian rhythms, as well as hinders family and social life, which triggers other problems. Furthermore, there is a plausible basis for the hypothesis that the suppression of melatonin secretion due to shift or night work may contribute to GM dysbiosis. Furthermore, the work environment or working environment may influence GM, leading to gut dysbiosis in many cases. It has been suggested that the use of probiotics could be a mechanism to restore the intestinal microbiota in workers. The results obtained suggest that probiotic supplementation may be effective in protecting and preserving the diversity and stability of the intestinal microbiota under the special conditions present in various jobs. However, more research is still needed on how the microbiota is affected by probiotics and their use at the individual and personalized level.

Author Contributions: Conceptualization, J.M.M. and A.C.; methodology, J.M.M.; writing—original draft preparation, A.L.-S.; writing—review and editing, J.M.M. and A.C.-C.; visualization, A.d.C.M., E.M.S. and J.J.P.-A.; supervision, J.M.M. All authors have read and agreed to the published version of the manuscript.

Funding: The authors thank the Xunta de Galicia and European Regional Development Funds (FEDER), grant ED431C 2018/05, for covering the cost of this study.

Institutional Review Board Statement: Not applicable.

Informed Consent Statement: Not applicable.

Data Availability Statement: Not applicable.

Acknowledgments: The authors are grateful for the financial support from the European Regional Development Funds (FEDER), grant ED431C 2018/05.

Conflicts of Interest: The authors declare no conflict of interest.

References

1. Lu, Z.H.; Liu, Y.W.; Ji, Z.H.; Fu, T.; Yan, M.; Shao, Z.J.; Lona, Y. Alterations in the intestinal microbiome and mental health status of workers in an underground tunnel environment. *BMC Microbiol.* **2021**, *21*, 7. [CrossRef]
2. Rogers, A.; Hu, Y.-J.; Yue, Y.; Wissel, E.F.; Petit, R.A., III; Jarrett, S.; Christie, J.; Read, T.D. Shiftwork, functional bowel symptoms, and the microbiome. *Peer J.* **2021**, *9*, e11406. [CrossRef]
3. Bijnens, S.; Depoortere, I. Controlled light exposure and intermittent fasting as treatment strategies for metabolic syndrome and gut microbiome dysregulation in night shift works. *Physiol. Behav.* **2023**, *263*, 114103. [CrossRef] [PubMed]

4. Fernández, M.J.; Bello, L.; Sánchez, A.; Serra, L. La turnicidad laboral y su impacto en la alimentación. In *Alimentación y Trabajo*; Editorial Médica Panamericana: Madrid, España, 2012; pp. 53–67.
5. Lowden, A.; Moreno, C.; Holmback, U.; Lennernas, M.; Tucker, P. Eating and shift work—Effects on habits, metabolism and performance. *Scand. J. Work Environ. Health* **2010**, *36*, 150–162. [CrossRef]
6. Parnell, J.A.; Reimer, R.A. Prebiotic fiber modulation of the gut microbiota improves risk factors for obesity and the metabolic syndrome. *Gut Microbes* **2012**, *3*, 29–34. [CrossRef] [PubMed]
7. Tada, Y.; Kawano, Y.; Maeda, I.; Yoshizaki, T.; Sunami, A.; Yokoyama, Y.; Matsumoto, H.; Hida, A.; Komatsu, T.; Togo, F. Association of body mass index with lifestyle and rotating shift working Japanese female nurses. *Obesity* **2014**, *22*, 2489–2493. [CrossRef]
8. Kim, H.I.; Choi, J.Y.; Kim, S.-E.; Jung, H.-K.; Shim, K.-N.; Yoo, K. Impact of shift work on irritable bowel syndrome and functional dyspepsia. *Korean J. Med. Educ.* **2013**, *28*, 431–437.
9. Akere, A.; Akande, K.O. Association between irritable bowel syndrome and shift work: Prevalence and associated factors among nurses. *J. Gastroenterol. Hepatol.* **2014**, *3*, 1328–1331. [CrossRef]
10. Kostic, A.D.; Gevers, D.; Siljander, H.; Vatanen, T.; Hyötyläinen, T.; Hämäläinen, A.-M.; Peet, A.; Tillmann, V.; Pöhö, P.; Mattila, I.; et al. The dynamics of the human infant gut microbiome in development and in progression towards type 1 diabetes. *Cell Host Microbe* **2015**, *17*, 260–273. [CrossRef]
11. Sampson, T.R.; Debelius, J.W.; Thron, T.; Janssen, S.; Shastri, G.G.; Ilhan, Z.E.; Challis, C.; Schretter, C.E.; Rocha, S.; Gradinaru, V.; et al. Gut microbiota regulate motor deficits and neuroinflammation in a model of Parkinson's disease. *Cell* **2016**, *167*, 1469–1480. [CrossRef]
12. Wang, Z.; Wang, Z.; Lu, T.; Chen, W.; Yan, W.; Yuan, K.; Shi, L.; Liu, X.; Zhou, X.; Shi, J.; et al. The microbiota-gut-brain axis in sleep disorders. *Sleep Med. Rev.* **2022**, *65*, 101691. [CrossRef] [PubMed]
13. Han, M.; Yuan, S.; Zhang, J. The interplay between sleep and gut microbiota. *Brain Res. Bull.* **2022**, *180*, 131–146. [CrossRef]
14. Konturek, P.C.; Brzozowski, T.; Konturek, S.J. Gut clock: Implication of circadian rhythms in the gastrointestinal tract. *J. Physiol. Pharmacol.* **2011**, *62*, 139–150. [PubMed]
15. Paulose, J.K.; Wright, J.M.; Patel, A.G.; Cassone, V.M. Human gut bacteria are sensitive to melatonin and express endogenous circadian rhythmicity. *PLoS ONE* **2016**, *11*, e0146643. [CrossRef] [PubMed]
16. Wang, Y.; Kuang, Z.; Yu, X.; Ruhn, K.A.; Kubo, M.; Hooper, L.V. The intestinal microbiota regulates body composition through NFIL3 and the circadian clock. *Science* **2017**, *357*, 912–916. [CrossRef]
17. Tian, Y.; Yang, W.; Chen, G.; Men, C.; Gu, Y.; Song, X.; Zhang, R.; Wang, L.; Zhang, X. An important link between the gut microbiota and the circadian rhythm: Imply for treatments of circadian rhythm sleep disorder. *Food Sci. Biotechnol.* **2022**, *31*, 155–164. [CrossRef]
18. Carabotti, M.; Scirocco, A.; Maselli, M.A.; Severi, C. The gut-brain axis: Interactions between enteric microbiota, central and enteric nervous systems. *Ann. Gastroenterol.* **2015**, *28*, 203–209.
19. Golubeva, A.V.; Crampton, S.; Desbonnet, L.; Edge, D.; O'Sullivan, O.; Lomasney, K.W.; Zhdanov, A.V.; Crispie, F.; Moloney, R.D.; Borre, Y.E.; et al. Prenatal stress-induced alterations in major physiological systems correlate with gut microbiota composition in adulthood. *Psychoneuroendocrinology* **2015**, *60*, 58–74. [CrossRef]
20. Gu, F.; Han, J.; Laden, F.; Pan, A.; Caporaso, N.E.; Stampfer, M.J.; Kawachi, I.; Rexrode, K.M.; Willett, W.C.; Hankinson, S.E.; et al. Total and cause-specific mortality of U.S., nurses working rotating night shifts. *Am. J. Prev. Med.* **2015**, *48*, 241–252. [CrossRef]
21. Myers, J.A.; Haney, M.F.; Griffiths, R.F.; Pierse, N.F.; Powell, D.M.C. Fatigue in air medical clinicians undertaking high-acuity patient transports. *Prehosp. Emerg. Care* **2015**, *19*, 36–43. [CrossRef]
22. West, N.P.; Hughes, L.; Ramsey, R.; Zhang, P.; Martoni, C.J.; Leyer, G.J.; Cripps, A.W.; Cox, A.J. Probiotics, anticipation stress, and the acute immune response to night shift. *Front. Immunol.* **2021**, *11*, 599547. [CrossRef] [PubMed]
23. Wells, M.M.; Roth, L.; Chande, N. Sleep disruption secondary to overnight call shifts is associated with irritable bowel syndrome in residents: A cross sectional study. *Am. J. Gastroenterol.* **2012**, *107*, 1151–1156. [CrossRef] [PubMed]
24. Thaiss, C.A.; Zeevi, D.; Levy, M.; Zilberman-Shapira, G.; Suez, J.; Tengler, A.C.; Abramson, L.; Katz, M.N.; Korem, N.; Kuperman, Y.; et al. Transkingdom control of microbiota diurnal oscillations promotes metabolic homeostais. *Cell* **2014**, *159*, 514–529. [CrossRef]
25. Nojkov, B.; Rubenstein, J.H.; Chey, W.D.; Hoogerwerf, W.A. The impact of rotating shift work on the prevalence of irritable bowel syndrome in nurses. *Am. J. Gastroenterol.* **2010**, *105*, 842–847. [CrossRef] [PubMed]
26. Bhattarai, Y.M.; Pedrogo, D.A.; Kashyap, P.C. Irritable bowel syndrome: A gut microbiota-related disorder. *Am. J. Physiol. Gastrointest. Liver Physiol.* **2017**, *312*, 52–62. [CrossRef]
27. Wang, M.L.; Lin, P.L.; Huang, C.H.; Huang, H.H. Decreased parasympathetic activity of heart rate variability during anticipation of night duty in anesthesiology residents. *Anesth. Analg.* **2018**, *126*, 1013–1018. [CrossRef]
28. Morris, S.B.; Daisley, R.L.; Wheeler, M.; Boyer, P. A meta-analysis of the relationship between individual assessments and job performance. *J. App. Psychol.* **2015**, *100*, 5–20. [CrossRef]
29. Geda, N.R.; Feng, C.X.; Yu, Y. Examining the association between work stress, Life stress and obesity among working adult population in Canada: Findings from a Nationally Representative Data. *Arch. Public Health* **2022**, *80*, 97. [CrossRef]
30. Magnet, F.; Gotteland, M.; Gauthier, L.; Zazueta, A.; Pesoa, S.; Navarrete, P.; Balamurugan, R. The Firmicutes/Bacteroidetes ratio: A relevant marker of gut dysbiosis in obese patients? *Nutrients* **2020**, *12*, 1474. [CrossRef]

31. Briançon-Marjollet, A.; Weiszenstein, M.; Henri, M.; Thomas, A.; Godin-Ribuot, D.; Polak, J. The impact of sleep disorders on glucose metabolism: Endocrine and molecular mechanisms. *Diabetol. Metab. Syndr.* **2015**, *7*, 25. [CrossRef]
32. Young, Y.H.; Kim, H.C.; Lim, H.C.; Park, J.J.; Kim, J.H.; Park, H. Long-term clinical course of post-infectious irritable bowel syndrome after shifellosis: A 10- year follow up study. *J. Neurogastroenterol. Motil.* **2016**, *22*, 490–496. [CrossRef] [PubMed]
33. Burek, K.; Rabstein, S.; Kantermann, T.; Vetter, C.; Rotter, M.; Wang-Sattler, R.; Lehnert, M.; Pallapies, D.; Jöckel, K.-H.; Brüning, T.; et al. Night work, chronotype and cortisol at awakening in female hospital employees. *Sci. Rep.* **2022**, *12*, 6525. [CrossRef] [PubMed]
34. Besedovsky, L.; Lange, T.; Haack, M. The sleep-immune crosstalk in health and disease. *Physiol. Rev.* **2019**, *99*, 1325–1380. [CrossRef] [PubMed]
35. Walker, M.P. A societal sleep prescription. *Neuron* **2019**, *103*, 559–562. [CrossRef] [PubMed]
36. Szentirmai, É.; Kapás, L. Brown adipose tissue plays a central role in systemic inflammation-induced sleep responses. *PLoS ONE* **2018**, *13*, e0197409. [CrossRef]
37. Vgontzas, A.N.; Papanicolaou, D.A.; Bixler, E.O.; Lotsikas, A.; Zachman, K.; Kales, A.; Prolo, P.; Wong, M.L.; Licinio, J.; Gold, P.W.; et al. Circadian interleukin-6 secretion and quantity and depth of sleep. *J. Clin. Endocrinol. Metab.* **1999**, *84*, 2603–2607. [CrossRef] [PubMed]
38. Reynolds, A.C.; Dorrian, J.; Liu, P.Y.; Van Dongen, H.P.; Wittert, G.A.; Harmer, L.J.; Banks, S. Impact of five nights of sleep restriction on glucose metabolism, leptin and testosterone in young adult men. *PLoS ONE* **2012**, *7*, e41218. [CrossRef]
39. Spiegel, K.; Tasali, E.; Penev, P.; Van Cauter, E. Brief communication: Sleep curtailment in healthy young men is associated with decreased leptin levels, elevated ghrelin levels, and increased hunger and appetite. *Ann. Int. Med.* **2004**, *141*, 846–850. [CrossRef]
40. Shearer, W.T.; Reuben, J.M.; Mullington, J.M.; Price, N.J.; Lee, B.N.; Smith, E.O.; Szuba, M.P.; Van Dongen, H.P.; Dinges, D.F. Soluble TNF alpha receptor 1 and IL-6 plasma levels in humans subjected to the sleep deprivation model of spaceflight. *J. Allergy Clin. Immunol.* **2001**, *107*, 165–170. [CrossRef]
41. Litichevskiy, L.; Thaiss, C.A. The Oscillating Gut Microbiome and Its Effects on Host Circadian Biology. *Ann. Rrev. Nutr.* **2022**, *42*, 145–164. [CrossRef]
42. Wollmuth, E.M.; Angert, E.R. Microbial circadian clocks: Host-microbe interplay in diel cycles. *BMC Microbiol.* **2023**, *23*, 124. [CrossRef] [PubMed]
43. Zhang, S.I.; Bai, L.; Goel, N.; Bailey, A.; Jang, C.J.; Bushman, F.D.; Meerlo, P.; Dinges, D.F.; Sehgal, A. Human and rat gut microbiome composition is maintained following sleep restriction. *Proc. Natl. Acad. Sci. USA* **2017**, *114*, E1564–E1571. [CrossRef] [PubMed]
44. Benedict, C.; Vogel, H.; Jonas, W.; Woting, A.; Blaut, M.; Schurmann, A.; Cedernaes, J. Gut microbiota and glucometabolic alterations in response to recurrent particle sleep deprivation in normal-weight young individuals. *Mol. Metab.* **2016**, *5*, 1175–1186. [CrossRef]
45. Voigt, R.M.; Forsyth, C.B.; Green, S.J.; Mutlu, E.; Engen, P.; Vitaterna, M.H.; Turek, F.W.; Keshavarizian, A. Circadian disorganization alters intestinal microbiota. *PLoS ONE* **2014**, *9*, e97500. [CrossRef] [PubMed]
46. Sun, J.; Fang, D.; Wang, Z.; Liu, Y. Sleep Deprivation and Gut Microbiota Dysbiosis: Current Understandings and Implications. *Int. J. Mol. Sci.* **2023**, *24*, 9603. [CrossRef]
47. Rothschild, D.; Weissbrod, O.; Barkan, E.; Kurilshikov, A.; Korem, T.; Zeevi, D.; Costea, P.I.; Godneva, A.; Kalka, I.N.; Bar, N.; et al. Environment dominates over host genetics in shaping human gut microbiota. *Nature* **2018**, *555*, 210–215. [CrossRef] [PubMed]
48. Sun, J.; Liao, X.P.; D'Souza, A.W.; Boolchandani, M.; Li, S.-H.; Cheng, K.; Luis Martínez, J.; Li, L.; Feng, Y.J.; Fang, L.X.; et al. Environmental remodeling of human gut microbiota and antibiotic resistome in livestock farms. *Nat. Commun.* **2020**, *11*, 1427. [CrossRef]
49. Poza, M.; Gayoso, C.; Gómez, M.J.; Rumbo-Feal, S.; Tomás, M.; Aranda, J.; Fernández, A.; Bou, G. Exploring bacterial diversity in hospital environments by GS-FLX Titanium pyrosequencing. *PLoS ONE* **2012**, *7*, e44105. [CrossRef]
50. Chen, C.H.; Tu, C.C.; Kuo, H.Y.; Zeng, R.F.; Yu, C.S.; Lu, H.H.S.; Liou, M.L. Dynamic change of surface microbiota with different environmental cleaning methods between two wards in a hospital. *Appl. Microbiol. Biotechnol.* **2016**, *101*, 771–781. [CrossRef]
51. Brooks, B.; Olm, M.R.; Firek, B.A.; Baker, R.; Thomas, B.C.; Morowitz, M.J.; Banfield, J.F. Strain- resolved analysis of hospital rooms and infants reveals overlap between the human and room microbiome. *Nat. Commun.* **2017**, *8*, 1814. [CrossRef]
52. Lai, P.S.; Allen, J.G.; Hutchinson, D.S.; Ajami, N.J.; Petrosino, J.F.; Winters, T.; Hug, C.; Wartenberg, G.R.; Vallarino, J.; Christiani, D.C. Impact of environmental microbiota on human microbiota of workers in academic mouse research facilities: An observational study. *PLoS ONE* **2017**, *12*, e0180969. [CrossRef] [PubMed]
53. Friedman, N.D.; Pollard, J.; Stupart, D.; Knight, D.R.; Khajehnoori, M.; Davey, E.K.; Parry, L.; Riley, T.V. Prevalence of *Clostridium difficile* colonization among healthcare workers. *BMC Infect. Dis.* **2013**, *13*, 459. [CrossRef] [PubMed]
54. Huttunen, R.; Syrjanen, J. Healthcare workers as vectors of infectious diseases. *Eur. J. Clin. Microbiol. Infect. Dis.* **2014**, *33*, 1477–1488. [CrossRef] [PubMed]
55. Sun, J.; Huang, T.; Chen, C.; Cao, T.T.; Cheng, K.; Liao, X.P.; Liu, Y.H. Comparison of fecal microbial composition and antibiotic resi stance genes from swine, farm workers and the surrounding villagers. *Sci. Rep.* **2017**, *7*, 4965. [CrossRef]
56. Gao, F.; Guo, R.; Ma, Q.; Li, Y.; Wang, W.; Fan, Y.; Ju, Y.; Zhao, B.; Gao, Y.; Qian, L.; et al. Stressful events induce long-term gut microbiota dysbiosis and associated post-traumatic stress symptoms in healthcare workers fighting against COVID-19. *J. Affect. Disord.* **2022**, *303*, 187–195. [CrossRef]

57. Zheng, N.; Li, S.H.; Dong, B.; Sun, W.; Li, H.R.; Zhang, Y.L.; Li, P.; Fang, Z.W.; Chen, C.M.; Han, X.Y.; et al. Comparison of the gut microbiota of short-term and long-term medical workers and non-medical controls: A cross-sectional analysis. *Clin. Microbiol. Infect.* **2021**, *27*, 1285–1292. [CrossRef]
58. Mortaş, H.; Bilici, S.; Karakan, T. The circadian disruption of night work alters gut microbiota consistent with elevated risk for future metabolic and gastrointestinal pathology. *Chronobiol. Internat.* **2020**, *37*, 1067–1081. [CrossRef]
59. Cerf-Bensussan, N.; Gaboriau-Routhiau, V. The immune system and the gut microbiota: Friends or foes? *Nat. Rev. Immunol.* **2010**, *10*, 735–744. [CrossRef]
60. Tahara, Y.; Yamazaki, M.; Sukigara, H.; Motohashi, H.; Sasaki, H.; Miyakawa, H. Gut microbiota-derived short chain fatty acids induce circadian clock entrainment in mouse peripheral tissue. *Sci. Rep.* **2018**, *8*, 1395. [CrossRef]
61. Stanaway, I.B.; Wallace, J.C.; Shojaie, A.; Griffith, W.C.; Hong, S.; Wilder, C.S.; Green, F.H.; Tsai, J.; Knight, M.; Workman, T.; et al. Human oral buccal microbiomes are associated with farmworker status and azinphos-methyl agricultural pesticide exposure. *Appl. Environ. Microbiol.* **2017**, *83*, e02149-16. [CrossRef]
62. Xie, S.; Lin, H.; Meng, Y.; Zhu, J.; Zhang, Y.; Zhang, L.; Li, G. Analysis and determinants of Chinese navy personnel health status: A cross-sectional study. *Health Qual. Life Outcomes* **2018**, *16*, 138. [CrossRef]
63. Walters, W.A.; Reyes, F.; Soto, G.M.; Reynolds, N.D.; Fraser, J.A.; Aviles, R.; Tribble, D.R.; Irvin, A.P.; Kelley-Loughnane, N.; Gutierrez, R.L.; et al. Epidemiology and associated microbiota changes in deployed military personnel at high risk of traveler's Diarrhea. *PLoS ONE* **2020**, *15*, e0236703. [CrossRef] [PubMed]
64. Rydstedt, L.W.; Lundh, M. An ocean of stress? The relationship between psychosocial workload and mental strain among engine officers in the Swedish merchant fleet. *Int. Marit. Health* **2010**, *62*, 168–175. [PubMed]
65. O'Halloran, C.L.; Silver, M.W.; Colford, J.M., Jr. Acute stress symptoms among US ocean lifeguards. *Wilderness Environ. Med.* **2015**, *26*, 442–443. [CrossRef] [PubMed]
66. Lloyd-Price, J.; Mahurkar, A.; Rahnavard, G.; Crabtree, J.; Orvis, J.; Hall, A.B.; Brady, A.; Creasy, H.H.; McCracken, C.; Giglio, M.G.; et al. Strains, functions and dynamics in the expanded Human Microbiome Project. *Nature* **2017**, *550*, 61–66. [CrossRef]
67. Zheng, W.; Zhang, Z.; Liu, C.; Qiao, Y.; Zhou, D.; Qu, J.; An, H.; Xiong, M.; Zhu, Z.; Zhao, X. Metagenomic sequencing reveals altered metabolic pathways in the oral microbiota of sailors during a long sea voyage. *Sci Rep.* **2015**, *5*, 9131. [CrossRef]
68. Zhang, J.; Zhao, J.; Jin, H.; Jin, H.; Lv, R.; Shi, H.; De, G.; Yang, B.; Sun, Z.; Zhang, H. Probiotics maintain the intestinal microbiome homeostasis of the sailors during a long sea voyage. *Gut Microbes* **2020**, *11*, 930–943. [CrossRef]
69. Kriss, M.; Hazleton, K.Z.; Nusbacher, N.M.; Martin, C.G.; Lozupone, C.A. Low diversity gut microbiota dysbiosis: Drivers, functional implications and recovery. *Curr. Opin. Microbiol.* **2018**, *44*, 4–40. [CrossRef]
70. So, D.; Whelan, K.; Rossi, M.; Morrison, M.; Holtmann, G.; Kelly, J.T.; Shanahan, E.R.; Staudacher, H.M.; Campbell, K.L. Dietary fiber intervention on gut microbiota composition in healthy adults: A systematic review and meta-analysis. *Am. J. Clin. Nutr.* **2018**, *107*, 65–983. [CrossRef]
71. Zhou, Y.; Chen, L.; Sun, G.; Li, Y.; Huang, R. Alterations in the gut microbiota of patients with silica-induced pulmonary fibrosis. *J. Occup. Med. Toxicol.* **2019**, *14*, 5. [CrossRef]
72. Ahmed, N.; Mahmoud, N.F.; Solyman, S.; Hanora, A. Human nasal microbiome as characterized by metagenomics differs markedly between rural and industrial communities in Egypt. *Omics J. Integr. Biol.* **2019**, *23*, 573–582. [CrossRef] [PubMed]
73. Wu, B.G.; Kapoor, B.; Cummings, K.J.; Stanton, M.L.; Nett, R.J.; Kreiss, K.; Abraham, J.L.; Colby, T.V.; Franko, A.D.; Green, F.H.; et al. Evidence for environmental–human microbiota transfer at a manufacturing facility with novel work-related respiratory disease. *Am. J. Respir. Crit. Care Med.* **2020**, *202*, 1678–1688. [CrossRef] [PubMed]
74. Cummings, K.J.; Stanton, M.L.; Nett, R.J.; Segal, L.N.; Kreiss, K.; Abraham, J.L.; Colby, T.V.; Franko, A.D.; Green, F.H.Y.; Sanyal, S.; et al. Severe lung disease characterized by lymphocytic bronchiolitis, alveolar ductitis, and emphysema (BADE) in industrial machine-manufacturing workers. *Am. J. Ind. Med.* **2019**, *62*, 927–937. [CrossRef]
75. Le Guern, R.; Stabler, S.; Gosset, P.; Pichavant, M.; Grandjean, T.; Faure, E.; Karaca, Y.; Faure, K.; Kipnis, E.; Dessein, R. Colonization resistance against multi-drug-resistant bacteria: A narrative review. *J. Hosp. Infect.* **2021**, *118*, 48–58. [CrossRef] [PubMed]
76. Hill, C.; Guarner, F.; Reid, G.; Gibson, G.R.; Merenstein, D.J.; Pot, B.; Morelli, L.; Canani, R.B.; Flint, H.J.; Salminen, S.; et al. The international scientific association for probiotics and prebiotics consensus statement on the scope and appropriate use of the term probiotic. *Nat. Rev. Gastroenterol. Hepatol.* **2014**, *11*, 506–514. [CrossRef]
77. Derrien, M.; van Hylckama Vlieg, J.E. Fate, activity, and impact of ingested bacteria within the human gut microbiota. *Trends Microbiol.* **2015**, *23*, 354–366. [CrossRef] [PubMed]
78. Sanchez, B.; Delgado, S.; Blanco-Miguez, A.; Lourenco, A.; Gueimonde, M.; Margolles, A. Probiotics, gut microbiota, and their influence on host health and disease. *Mol. Nutr. Food Res.* **2017**, *61*, 1600240. [CrossRef]
79. Shin, J.H.; Nam, M.H.; Lee, H.; Lee, J.S.; Kim, H.; Chung, M.J.; Seo, J.G. Amelioration of obesity-related characteristics by a probiotic formulation in a high-fat diet-induced obese rat model. *Eur. J. Nutr.* **2017**, *57*, 2081–2090. [CrossRef]
80. Xu, H.; Huang, W.; Hou, Q.; Kwok, L.Y.; Laga, W.; Wang, Y.; Ma, H.; Sun, Z.; Zhang, H. Oral administration of com- pound probiotics improved canine feed intake, weight gain, immunity and intestinal microbiota. *Front Immunol.* **2019**, *10*, 666. [CrossRef]
81. Huang, L.; Yu, Q.; Peng, H.; Zhen, Z. Alterations of gut microbiome and effects of probiotic therapy in patients with liver cirrhosis: A systematic review and meta-analysis. *Medicine* **2022**, *101*, e32335. [CrossRef] [PubMed]

82. Liu, T.X.; Niu, H.T.; Zhang, S.Y. Intestinal microbiota metabolism and atherosclerosis. *Chin. Med. J.* **2015**, *128*, 2805–2811. [CrossRef] [PubMed]
83. Nallu, A.; Sharma, S.; Ramezani, A.; Muralidharan, J.; Raj, D. Gut microbiome in chronic kidney disease: Challenges and opportunities. *Transl. Res.* **2017**, *179*, 24–37. [CrossRef]
84. Wlodarska, M.; Kostic, A.D.; Xavier, R.J. An integrative view of microbiome-host interactions in inflammatory bowel diseases. *Cell Host Microbe* **2015**, *17*, 577–591. [CrossRef]
85. Lopez-Santamarina, A.; Gonzalez, E.G.; Lamas, A.; Mondragon, A.C.; Regal, P.; Miranda, J.M. Probiotics as a possible strategy for the prevention and treatment of allergies. A narrative review. *Foods* **2021**, *10*, 701. [CrossRef] [PubMed]
86. Kinoshita, T.; Maruyama, K.; Suyama, K.; Nishijima, M.; Akamatsu, K.; Jogamoto, A.; Katakami, K.; Saito, I. The effects of OLL1073R-1 yogurt intake on influenza incidence and immunological markers among women healthcare workers: A randomized controlled trial. *Food Funct.* **2019**, *10*, 8129–8136. [CrossRef]
87. Mohammadi, A.A.; Jazayeri, S.; Khosravi-Darani, K.; Solati, Z.; Mohammadpour, N.; Asemi, Z.; Adab, Z.; Djalali, M.; Tehrani-Doost, M.; Hosseini, M.; et al. The effects of probiotics on mental health and hypothalamic–pituitary–adrenal axis: A randomized, double-blind, placebo-controlled trial in petrochemical workers. *Nutr. Neuro* **2015**, *19*, 387–395. [CrossRef] [PubMed]
88. Smith-Ryan, A.E.; Mock, M.G.; Trexler, E.T.; Hirsch, K.R.; Blue, M.N.M. Influence of a multistrain probiotic on body composition and mood in female occupational shift workers. *Appl. Physiol. Nutr. Metab.* **2019**, *44*, 765–773. [CrossRef]
89. Zhang, J.; Sun, Z.; Jiang, S.; Bai, X.; Ma, C.; Peng, Q.; Chen, K.; Chang, H.; Fang, T.; Zhang, H. Probiotic *Bifidobacterium lactis* V9 regulates the secretion of sex hormones in polycystic ovary syndrome patients through the gut-brain axis. *mSystems* **2019**, *4*, e00017-19. [CrossRef]
90. Tubelius, P.; Stan, V.; Zachrisson, A. Increasing work-place healthiness with the probiotic lactobacillus reuteri: A randomised, double-blind placebo-controlled study. *Environm. Health* **2005**, *4*, 25. [CrossRef]
91. Valle, M.C.; Vieira, I.A.; Fino, L.C.; Gallina, D.A.; Esteves, A.M.; da Cunha, D.T.; Cabral, L.; Benatti, F.B.; Marostica, M.R., Jr.; Batista, Â.G.; et al. Immune status, well-being and gut microbiota in military supplemented with synbiotic ice cream and submitted to field training: A randomised clinical trial. *Br. J. Nutr.* **2021**, *126*, 1794–1808. [CrossRef]
92. Vemuri, R.; Shinde, T.; Gundamaraju, R.; Gondalia, S.; Karpe, A.; Beale, D.; Martoni, C.; Eri, R. *Lactobacillus acidophilus* DDS-1 modulates the gut microbiota and improves metabolic profiles in aging mice. *Nutrients* **2018**, *10*, 1255. [CrossRef] [PubMed]
93. Martoni, C.J.; Srivastava, S.; Leyer, G.J. *Lactobacillus acidophilus* DDS-1 and *Bifidobacterium lactis* UABla-12 improve abdominal pain severity and symptomology in irritable bowel syndrome: Randomized controlled trial. *Nutrients* **2020**, *12*, 363. [CrossRef]
94. Gerasimov, S.V.; Vasjuta, V.V.; Myhovych, O.O.; Bondarchuk, L.I. Probiotic supplement reduces atopic dermatitis in preschool children. *Am. J. Clin. Dermatol.* **2010**, *11*, 351–361. [CrossRef]
95. Pakdaman, M.N.; Udani, J.K.; Molina, J.P.; Shahani, M. The effects of the DDS-1 strain of lactobacillus on symptomatic relief for lactose intolerance—A randomized, double-blind, placebo-controlled, crossover clinical trial. *Nutr. J.* **2015**, *15*, 56. [CrossRef] [PubMed]
96. Irwin, C.; McCartney, D.; Desbrow, B.; Khalesi, S. Effects of probiotics and paraprobiotics on subjective and objective sleep metrics: A systematic review and meta-analysis. *Eur. J. Clin. Nutr.* **2020**, *74*, 1536–1549. [CrossRef]
97. Gerasimov, S.V.; Ivantsiv, V.A.; Bobryk, L.M.; Tsitsura, O.O.; Dedyshin, L.P.; Guta, N.V.; Yandyo, B.V. Role of short-term use of *L. acidophilus* DDS-1 and *B. lactis* UABLA-12 in acute respiratory infections in children: A randomized controlled trial. *Eur. J. Clin. Nutr.* **2015**, *70*, 463–469. [CrossRef] [PubMed]
98. Labanki, A.; Langhorst, J.; Engler, H.; Elsenbruch, S. Stress and the brain-gut axis in functional and chronic-inflammatory gastrointestinal diseases: A transdisciplinary challenge. *Psychoneuroendocrinology* **2020**, *111*, 104501. [CrossRef] [PubMed]
99. Casper, A.; Sonnentag, S. Feeling exhausted or vigorous in anticipation of high workload? The role of worry and planning during the evening. *J. Occup. Org. Psychol.* **2020**, *93*, 215–242. [CrossRef]
100. Codoñer-Franch, P.; Gombert, M.; Martínez-Raga, J.; Cenit, M.C. Circadian Disruption and Mental Health: The Chronotherapeutic Potential of Microbiome-Based and Dietary Strategies. *Int. J. Mol. Sci.* **2023**, *24*, 7579. [CrossRef]
101. Kaczmarek, J.L.; Musaad, S.M.; Holster, H.D. Time of day and eating behaviors are associated with the composition and function of the human gastrointestinal microbiota. *Am. J. Clin. Nutr.* **2017**, *106*, 1220–1231. [CrossRef]
102. Haarhuis, J.E.; Kardinaal, A.; Kortman, G.A.M. Probiotics, prebiotics and postbiotics for better sleep quality: A narrative review. *Benef. Microbes* **2022**, *13*, 169–182. [CrossRef] [PubMed]

Disclaimer/Publisher's Note: The statements, opinions and data contained in all publications are solely those of the individual author(s) and contributor(s) and not of MDPI and/or the editor(s). MDPI and/or the editor(s) disclaim responsibility for any injury to people or property resulting from any ideas, methods, instructions or products referred to in the content.

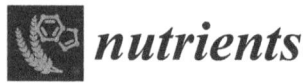

Review

Contextualizing the Neural Vulnerabilities Model of Obesity

Timothy D. Nelson [1,*] and Eric Stice [2]

[1] Department of Psychology, University of Nebraska-Lincoln, Lincoln, NE 68588, USA
[2] Department of Psychiatry and Behavioral Sciences, Stanford University School of Medicine, Stanford, CA 94305, USA; estice@stanford.edu
* Correspondence: tnelson3@unl.edu

Abstract: In recent years, investigators have focused on neural vulnerability factors that increase the risk of unhealthy weight gain, which has provided a useful organizing structure for obesity neuroscience research. However, this framework, and much of the research it has informed, has given limited attention to contextual factors that may interact with key vulnerabilities to impact eating behaviors and weight gain. To fill this gap, we propose a *Contextualized Neural Vulnerabilities Model of Obesity*, extending the existing theory to more intentionally incorporate contextual factors that are hypothesized to interact with neural vulnerabilities in shaping eating behaviors and weight trajectories. We begin by providing an overview of the *Neural Vulnerabilities Model of Obesity*, and briefly review supporting evidence. Next, we suggest opportunities to add contextual considerations to the model, including incorporating environmental and developmental context, emphasizing how contextual factors may interact with neural vulnerabilities to impact eating and weight. We then synthesize earlier models and new extensions to describe a *Contextualized Neural Vulnerabilities Model of Obesity* with three interacting components—food reward sensitivity, top-down regulation, and environmental factors—all within a developmental framework that highlights adolescence as a key period. Finally, we propose critical research questions arising from the framework, as well as opportunities to inform novel interventions.

Keywords: neural vulnerabilities; obesity; context; eating behavior; reward sensitivity; regulation; executive control; inhibitory control; adolescence

Citation: Nelson, T.D.; Stice, E. Contextualizing the Neural Vulnerabilities Model of Obesity. *Nutrients* **2023**, *15*, 2988. https://doi.org/10.3390/nu15132988

Academic Editor: Peter Pribis

Received: 31 May 2023
Revised: 26 June 2023
Accepted: 28 June 2023
Published: 30 June 2023

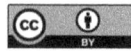

Copyright: © 2023 by the authors. Licensee MDPI, Basel, Switzerland. This article is an open access article distributed under the terms and conditions of the Creative Commons Attribution (CC BY) license (https://creativecommons.org/licenses/by/4.0/).

1. Contextualizing the Neural Vulnerabilities Model of Obesity

In recent years, a framework for conceptualizing obesity risk in the context of specific neural vulnerabilities has emerged [1,2] and provided a useful organizing structure for work in the field of obesity neuroscience. Within this framework, specific individual-level factors, particularly high *reward sensitivity* to high-calorie foods, and low top-down *regulation* abilities (most notably, inhibitory control) are considered critical risk factors for the development of unhealthy eating and, ultimately, obesity. A growing literature documents considerable individual differences in both sensitivity to food rewards and regulation abilities (particularly aspects of executive control, which is also often referred to as executive function), and links these critical neural vulnerability factors to obesogenic eating behaviors and excess weight gain [1,3]. However, the *Neural Vulnerabilities of Obesity* framework, and much of the research informed by this perspective, has given relatively limited attention to contextual factors that may interact with key vulnerabilities to impact eating behaviors and weight gain in important ways. To fill this gap, we propose a *Contextualized Neural Vulnerabilities Model of Obesity*, extending existing theory to more intentionally incorporate the consideration of various contextual factors that are hypothesized to interact with individual reward sensitivity and regulation abilities in shaping eating behaviors and, ultimately, long-term weight trajectories. Our hope is that this extension of the neural vulnerabilities model will provide a useful conceptual framework for increasingly rich and contextualized investigations into the interplay between brain, environment, behavior, and health.

In this paper, we begin by providing an overview of the *Neural Vulnerabilities Model of Obesity* and a brief review of the empirical evidence supporting the model. Next, we suggest opportunities to add contextual considerations to the model, including the incorporation of environmental and developmental context, with an emphasis on how contextual factors may interact with neural vulnerabilities to impact eating and weight trajectories. We then attempt to synthesize earlier models and new extensions to describe a *Contextualized Neural Vulnerabilities Model of Obesity* with three major interacting components – approach factors for unhealthy eating (including food reward sensitivity), top-down regulation abilities (including executive control of attention to food cues, executive control of appetitive response, and emotion regulation), and environmental factors (including availability and cues for unhealthy consumption in the home, neighborhood, family, and peer contexts) – all within a developmental framework highlighting adolescence as a potentially key period. Finally, we propose critical falsifiable research questions arising from the conceptual framework, as well as opportunities to inform novel interventions.

2. The Neural Vulnerabilities Model, Extensions, and Supporting Literature

The *Neural Vulnerabilities Model of Obesity* provides a framework for conceptualizing neural factors that may predispose an individual to the over-consumption of calorically-dense foods and excess weight gain. As reviewed by Stice and Burger [1], the extant literature suggests two specific vulnerabilities with particularly consistent links to obesity: *high reward sensitivity*, as reflected in neural hyper-sensitivity to high-calorie foods; and *regulation deficits*, particularly low inhibitory control. These dual vulnerabilities may also work in tandem, as in an *accelerator/brake* metaphor, with high reward sensitivity creating a strong approach motivation toward unhealthy food (the "accelerator") and regulation serving as a "brake" on excessive consumption. From this perspective, individuals with an overactive accelerator (i.e., too much reward sensitivity), and weak or ineffective brakes (i.e., too little regulation) may be at risk for habitual over-consumption of unhealthy foods. Notably, the factors of reward and regulation—and the idea that they may work in tandem to affect behavior—generally map onto broader neuroscience models of self-regulation failure, such as the *Balance Model of Self-Regulation*, which has also been applied to eating behavior [4,5]. Interestingly, the opposite pattern of low reward responsiveness and very high regulation—not enough accelerator, and too much brake—may characterize individuals at risk of anorexia nervosa (AN). Specifically, women with, or recovered from, AN show a weaker responsivity of the reward and motivational regions (e.g., insula, striatum, anterior cingulate cortex [ACC]) to images and tastes of high-calorie foods versus the healthy controls [6–9]. In addition, women with, or recovered from, AN show greater recruitment of the inhibitory regions (e.g., dorsolateral prefrontal cortex [dlPFC], inferior frontal cortex) in response to high-calorie food images and obesity-related words than do healthy controls [10,11], and they also show less delay discounting for money than do controls, implying elevated self-control [12,13].

Further extending the neural vulnerabilities model, researchers have developed increasingly sophisticated frameworks focusing on how specific regulatory deficits can lead to unhealthy eating patterns and excess weight gain. Hall and Marteau [14] proposed a conceptual model highlighting *executive control* deficits as a key mechanism impacting a wide variety of health behaviors, obesity, and overall health risks in adults. In a developmental extension of this model, Nelson and colleagues [15] detailed how deficits in specific components of executive control (including working memory, inhibitory control, and flexible shifting) in adolescence could contribute to breakdowns of attentional, behavioral, and emotional control, leading to unhealthy eating and weight trajectories. Taken together, these frameworks proposing key roles for a variety of regulatory abilities, particularly those falling under the umbrella of "executive control", extend the neural vulnerabilities model, which has focused primarily on inhibitory control deficits, to include related abilities with a potential relevance to obesity.

A substantial and growing empirical literature supports the role of reward sensitivity and regulation as key neural vulnerability factors for obesity. First, numerous studies have linked a high reward sensitivity with a greater risk for unhealthy food consumption and obesity (see [16] for review). Particularly pertinent to neural vulnerabilities, elevated reward region response to both tastes of high-calorie food and cues for high-calorie food have been associated with overeating and/or obesity in prospective studies. Specifically, elevated responsivity of brain regions implicated in reward valuation (striatum, orbitofrontal cortex) to high-calorie food images and cues has predicted future unhealthy weight gain in longitudinal studies with adolescents and young adults [17–20]. Along these lines, we recently found that elevated activation of reward regions (e.g., caudate and putamen) upon receiving sips of a chocolate milkshake significantly predicted greater weight gain over a one-year period in a large sample drawn from several longitudinal studies of adolescents and adults [21]. Second, a large body of literature has found associations between specific deficits in top-down regulation abilities and dietary and obesity risk. For example, although results have been mixed, studies spanning the developmental spectrum have reported significant correlations between executive control (and related abilities) and unhealthy eating behaviors and/or obesity (see [22,23], for reviews). Moreover, while the majority of this literature has focused narrowly on deficits in inhibitory control (see [1], for review), a growing number of studies have linked other aspects of executive control (such as working memory or flexible shifting; refs. [3,24,25]), or more comprehensive measures incorporating multiple executive control abilities [26,27], to eating and weight outcomes. Third, a more limited set of studies has examined *interactions between reward sensitivity and regulation* in predicting diet and weight trajectories. For example, in a rare study explicitly testing the interaction between the relative reinforcing value of food and inhibitory control, Loch and colleagues [28] reported that this interaction did not significantly predict the change in adiposity over three years in a sample of children and adolescents. However, rigorous large-sample studies, leveraging neural measures to explore interactions between reward sensitivity and regulation in predicting eating behavior and obesity trajectories, are needed.

3. Adding Context to the Neural Vulnerabilities Model

Although the Neural Vulnerabilities of Obesity and related models have guided valuable studies explicating the role of reward sensitivity and top-down regulation in obesity risk, this framework, and much of the research informed by it, gives limited attention to contextual factors. Such factors, including environmental and developmental context, are potentially important in achieving an even more sophisticated understanding of individual risk of unhealthy eating and obesity, which could guide novel interventions. Specifically, as we discuss below, contextual factors may confer risk not only through their direct effects on weight status (which are well-documented in the literature; e.g., refs. [29,30]), but also in how such factors potentially *interact* with neural vulnerabilities of reward sensitivity and top-down regulation to impact weight trajectories. We highlight the particular promise of integrating environmental and developmental contextual factors into the neural vulnerabilities framework.

Environmental Context. Environmental factors could be critical in creating the context in which reward and regulation operate. For example, in highly obesogenic *home and neighborhood environments*—characterized by ubiquitous access to, and cues for, unhealthy consumption—the impact of specific neural vulnerabilities (i.e., high reward, low top-down regulation) could be amplified. Individuals who are highly sensitive to food reward may be especially vulnerable to the consumption cues in such environments, including being drawn to attend to and consume highly appetizing (but nutritionally-poor) foods. Relatedly, individuals with poorer top-down regulation abilities may struggle to direct their attention and behavior in healthy ways when confronted with an obesogenic environment. For example, low executive control of attention may lead to over-attending to food stimuli, making it especially difficult to disengage from tempting stimuli when they are prevalent in the environment [15,31]. Further, deficits in response inhibition may be more likely to lead to impulsive and unhealthy consumption when access to unhealthy foods is easy and immediate. Conversely, in less obesogenic environments, temptation and the need for top-down regulation may be substantially lower, thus moderating the impact of these vulnerabilities. While a large and growing literature has documented the main effects of home, neighborhood, and school environments on diet and weight status, very little research exists exploring *interactions* between individual neural vulnerabilities and the environmental context. Integrating environmental factors into the neural vulnerabilities framework could help guide such research by contextualizing the roles of reward and regulation within the physical environment.

Food insecurity represents a unique environmental factor that may interact with neural vulnerabilities to impact eating and obesity trajectories. The uncertainty that comes with not having reliable access to food could distort reward and regulatory processes, with concerns focusing mostly on consumption whenever food is available, with less attention given to the nutritional quality of the food (see [32] for a review of associations between food insecurity and dietary quality). Further, regulation of portion size may become a less salient goal in the context of food insecurity; rather, such circumstances may encourage overeating whenever food is available, thus enhancing the rewarding value of food while undermining regulation abilities. Such processes may contribute to the paradoxical link between food insecurity and obesity [33] and must be understood as an interaction between context and vulnerability factors.

In addition to the physical environment, the *social or relational environment* in which an individual is embedded creates a critical context for eating and obesity trajectories. Specifically, the behaviors, attitudes, and goals of individuals in close proximity to, and who regularly interact with, the focal person could have a considerable impact in shaping the context in which eating occurs. Families play a critical role in establishing norms around eating. For example, parents who model eating dessert after every meal, and encourage children to do the same, influence the context in which food reward and regulation develop and are deployed. Additionally, friends, partners, and other peers such as roommates or co-workers could be important in supporting or not supporting health goals. For example, having a partner who is supportive of pursuing healthy eating and exercise goals could help mitigate high food reward sensitivity and reduce regulatory demands by helping maintain a home environment that is conducive to these goals. In contrast, living with someone who does not support health goals – for example, by consistently bringing home energy-dense/nutrition-poor foods – may exacerbate neural vulnerabilities by increasing temptation in the home environment. And while the main effects of such social factors on diet and obesity are relatively well-documented (see [34], for review), the ways in which these factors *interact* with individual reward sensitivity and regulation abilities to predict unhealthy weight gain has been largely overlooked and represents an opportunity to integrate the critical context into research guided by the neural vulnerabilities framework.

Just as physical and social environments create the "external context" in which neural vulnerabilities exist, there is also an "internal context" of individual-level characteristics that could interact with reward sensitivity and regulation. Perhaps most notably, *negative affect* could create an internal context in which reward and regulation operate. Depression, anxiety, and loneliness, for example, are prevalent manifestations of negative affect that likely have complex interplays with reward processing, regulation, and eating [4,35]. While the literature surrounding the main effects of negative affect on eating behaviors is considerable (see [36], for review), the interaction between negative affect and neural vulnerabilities in the context of diet and obesity is less frequently studied. The internal context of high negative affect may create conditions that ultimately lead to enhancing the rewarding value of food, both immediately and over time. For example, Wagner and colleagues [35] found that inducing negative affect increased reward region activation in response to appetizing food images compared to a neutral mood control condition. Further, negative affect may create a drive to eat appetizing (yet ultimately unhealthy) foods as a way of combatting negative emotions (a "food as self-medication" hypothesis). In their meta-analysis, Cardi and colleagues [37] reported that experimentally-induced negative mood was associated with greater food consumption. There is also evidence that experimentally-induced stress increases reward region response to milkshake tastes [38]. Because such energy-dense foods are often immediately gratifying, their consumption *in the context of negative affect* could be negatively reinforced through the temporary reduction of unpleasant emotions, thus increasing this behavior when negative emotions are experienced. Along these lines, Ranzenhofer and colleagues [39] assessed negative affect before and after a laboratory meal in a sample of adolescent girls with loss of control eating, and they found that a higher pre-meal negative affect was associated with greater snack and dessert intake, and that there was a significant decrease in negative affect from pre-meal to post-meal.

Relatedly, when negative affect is repeatedly paired with high calorie consumption, the experience of negative affect can theoretically become a cue for eating, even in the absence of hunger, which increases obesity risk. Further, individuals with poor top-down regulation abilities may be especially at risk of falling into these maladaptive processes because they struggle to regulate and respond to negative emotions in healthier ways [15]. Findings from our longitudinal research on developing executive control and obesity risk hint at such a process. We have found that the interaction between negative affect temperament and executive control predicts both unhealthy eating (including high sugar and sugar-sweetened beverage intake [27]) and BMI gain across adolescence [40], with deficits in executive control being particularly predictive in the context of high negative affect. Further, Yang et al. [41] reported an interaction between negative affect and reward region response to appetizing foods, with high negative affect amplifying the association between neural response to food and future weight gain.

Developmental Context. In addition to environmental context, adding *developmental context* to the neural vulnerabilities framework could be valuable. Reward sensitivity, regulation abilities, and eating behaviors all have unique developmental trajectories [42–44], and it is essential to consider the dynamic interplay between these factors at key points in development. Although studies have found associations between neural vulnerabilities and weight from early childhood through adulthood [17,26], we argue that adolescence may be a particularly critical period for consideration within the neural vulnerabilities framework given its importance in the development of eating habits and weight trajectories, as well as it being a time in which the interplay between reward, regulation and the environment may be especially relevant. Adolescence is a unique developmental period characterized by increasing autonomy, which "raises the stakes" for health behaviors and "presses" the adolescent to deploy top-down regulation to direct behavior toward health. Adolescence is also a time of heightened reward sensitivity and emotional reactivity but still-developing regulatory abilities [45], creating a potential developmental imbalance that undermines the top-down control of attention and behavior [46]. Further, adolescents have limited control over their food environments (e.g., they do not typically grocery-shop or decide where they live or go to school), but these environments could be critical in shaping their eating behavior. Because of the combination of increasing health behavior autonomy, heightened reactivity, immature regulation abilities, and vulnerability to environmental context, adolescence represents a unique developmental context in which to understand obesity risk from a contextualized neural vulnerabilities perspective. The importance of this developmental period is further highlighted by the elevated rates of obesity relative to earlier childhood and escalating rates over time [47], as well as generally low dietary quality for adolescents relative to other age groups [44]. Relatedly, adolescence may be an ideal time for intervention to prevent obesity before processes that lead to the habitual overvaluation and overconsumption of energy-dense foods become entrenched. However, much of the extant literature on reward, regulation and obesity has focused on adults, and thus misses critical developmental context.

4. A Contextualized Neural Vulnerabilities Model of Obesity

Integrating the considerations discussed above, we propose a *Contextualized Neural Vulnerabilities Model of Obesity* (see Figure 1). The model is comprised of three major components—reward sensitivity factors, top-down regulation abilities, and environmental factors—all of which are embedded within a developmental context. While each component is expected to have direct effects on eating behaviors and weight trajectories, the novel contribution of this model is in its focus on potential *interactions between components* to create a more contextualized conceptualization of obesity risk that will inform new directions in research, as well as targeted prevention and intervention.

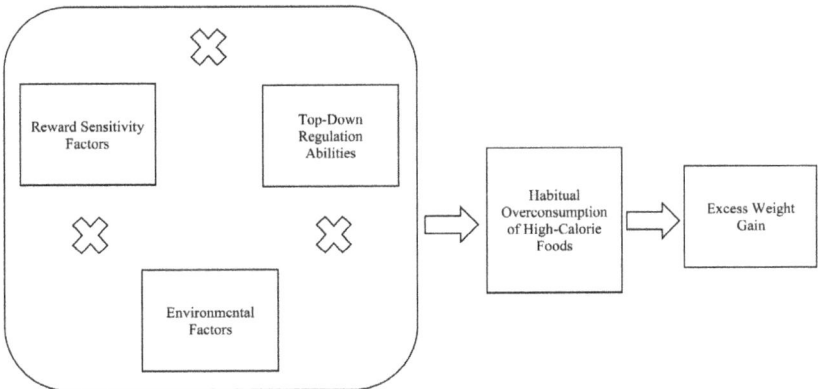

Figure 1. Contextualized Neural Vulnerabilities of Obesity Model.

The three components of the *Contextualized Neural Vulnerabilities Model*, as well as their interactions, are depicted in Figure 1. First, reward sensitivity factors represent individual differences in the reinforcing value of energy-dense/nutrition-poor food, including those high in fat or added sugar, and highly processed foods. It is expected that individuals who are highly sensitive to the rewarding qualities of such foods will be motivated to consume unhealthy foods at a high rate, thus contributing to habitual over-consumption and risk for excess weight gain. An emerging obesity neuroscience literature suggests that elevated reward region response in a variety of situations—including viewing images of high-calorie foods, anticipation of receiving high-calorie food tastes, and actual high-calorie food tastes—may all be relevant in predicting future weight gain [1,21]. Furthermore, it may be useful to distinguish between early-emerging, biologically-determined individual differences in neural responsivity to high-calorie foods and reward region responses to cues that have come to be associated with hedonic pleasure over time. While the former may represent a static individual vulnerability, the latter is conceptualized as more of an *emergent risk factor* that develops through a conditioning *process*. This process may unfold over time with repeated pairing of cues with hedonic pleasure, resulting in an increased attention and reactivity to cues in reward regions, which in turn increases the risk of overeating and weight gain.

Second, regulation factors refer to an individual's ability to exert top-down regulation to direct attention and behavior in intentional ways. Considerable individual differences in such abilities (often conceptualized as executive control or some of its components) have been documented across the developmental spectrum [48–51], and deficits in specific abilities (e.g., inhibitory control, working memory, cognitive flexibility) could impact an individual's ability to achieve health goals (see [14,15], for discussion). By far the most robust literature in this area has focused on low inhibitory control as a risk factor for future weight gain. Inhibitory control deficits in response to high-calorie foods in delay-discounting tasks, which reflect a bias toward immediate rewards, have reliably predicted future weight gain [52–55]. Similar results have emerged from studies using self-report measures of inhibitory control [56–58]. Individuals with inhibitory control deficits also show a poorer response to weight loss treatment and poorer weight loss maintenance [59–61]. Further, individuals who showed less recruitment of inhibitory control regions (dorsolateral prefrontal cortex) during a delay discounting task showed significantly less weight loss in response to weight loss treatment [60] and less weight loss maintenance over a one-year follow-up [61]. Moreover, while the majority of the literature on regulation and obesity has focused on inhibitory control, specifically, other aspects of executive control, particularly working memory and flexible shifting, have begun to receive more attention, both conceptually [14,15] and empirically (see [3,24], for relevant reviews). Therefore, recognizing the potential role of a range of regulatory abilities in eating and obesity, our model includes a broad conceptualization of top-down regulation factors as potentially important neural vulnerabilities for obesity.

One potentially important distinction here is between general top-down regulation (which occurs across a wide variety of stimuli and contexts) and top-down regulation that occurs within the specific context of food. Research rigorously examining the relative impact of these distinct types of regulation is currently lacking, but it is possible that both forms could be relevant for obesity, with general regulation abilities creating a broad foundation for a more food-specific regulation that develops over time. For example, healthy-weight adolescents with versus without a parental history of obesity show greater reward region response to both monetary reward and tastes of high-calorie foods [62,63]. Theoretically, a general deficit in inhibitory control increases the likelihood of beginning to consume high-calorie foods, and the habitual intake of high-calorie foods may create even greater deficits in inhibitory control because it contributes to greater reward region responsivity to cues for high-calorie foods, which is a risk factor for future weight gain [64]. That is, the process of overeating appears to increase a key neural vulnerability factor for future unhealthy weight gain. Research has captured this incentive sensitization conditioning process wherein a previously neutral visual cue acquires motivational significance when it is repeatedly paired with tastes of chocolate milkshake, resulting in an increase in caudate, putamen, and ventral pallidum response to the visual cue [65]. Consistent with expectations, individuals who showed the greatest increase in striatal responsiveness to the cue showed a significantly higher future weight gain [65].

Third, environmental factors include a wide range of contextual considerations that shape diet and weight trajectories. In our conceptualization, these include both "external context" factors and "internal context" factors. External context refers to environments outside the individual such as key physical food environments (e.g., home, neighborhood, school, work) and social or relational systems (e.g., parents, peers, partners), which together comprise the food environment that surrounds the individual on a daily basis [66]. Important aspects of the external food environment include the availability and accessibility of healthy and unhealthy foods (e.g., what foods are easily accessible within the home and community [67]) and environmental cues for consumption (e.g., advertisements for fast food, consumption patterns of others around the individual, social norms around eating [68]). Internal context refers to contextual influences within the individual that can affect dietary behavior, most notably the presence of negative affect (e.g., depression, anxiety, loneliness), which can become a cue for eating high-calorie foods [35]. Broadly speaking, obesogenic environmental contexts—characterized by the high availability of unhealthy foods and various internal and external cues for their consumption—may "set the stage" for habitual unhealthy eating and long-term excess weight gain.

In addition to the main effects of reward sensitivity, regulation abilities, and environment factors, several interactions between these model components are hypothesized to impact dietary and weight outcomes. Existing models have already highlighted some potential roles of reward x regulation interactions, with a greater reward sensitivity expected to create a stronger drive toward overeating, thus requiring stronger regulation abilities to meet dietary goals [4]; however, research rigorously testing such interactions is limited. Our contextualized extension also proposes critical interactions between key neural vulnerabilities (reward sensitivity and regulation abilities) and environmental factors. Individuals with a high food reward sensitivity may be particularly vulnerable to food environments in which highly appetizing foods are readily available and consumption cues are ubiquitous, creating temptation for consumption that may be inconsistent with dietary goals (a reward x environment interaction). Similarly, successfully navigating such challenging environments may require stronger regulation abilities, with obesogenic environments exposing deficits in regulation more than healthy environments which may buffer the risk in individuals with weaker regulation abilities (a regulation x environment interaction). Taken together, these complex interactions suggest that dietary and obesity risk emerge from the *combination* of risk factors in context, with high reward sensitivity creating a motivational approach toward unhealthy foods, the environment creating opportunities for consumption of such foods, and then low regulation resulting in breakdowns in intentional control over eating in the presence of both motivation and opportunity.

Finally, the entire proposed model is further contextualized within a developmental perspective that recognizes that the three model components unfold in unique ways across different developmental periods. Certain regulation abilities, such as executive control, follow an extremely protracted developmental course, with critical growth periods in preschool and adolescence, and maturation continuing into the 20s, before declining later in adulthood [43,69]. Reactivity to rewards may also change across development [42], although normative patterns and individual differences in the trajectories of food reward sensitivity specifically are not well-understood. Similarly, environmental factors must be considered within the developmental context as the centrality of certain relationships (e.g., parents versus peers) and environments (e.g., home versus school, community, or workplace) changes over time. Furthermore, all of these considerations occur against the backdrop of significant shifts in autonomy over health behaviors from childhood to adolescence to adulthood, which may influence the impact of different risk factors. While our contextualized model may be usefully applied to diverse developmental periods, we highlight adolescence as a particularly important time to consider the interactions between reward sensitivity, regulation, and environment. As noted, adolescence is a time when surging reward sensitivity may overwhelm still-developing regulatory abilities, particularly in the context of emerging health behavior autonomy and environmental cues for unhealthy consumption. This combination may make adolescence an especially vulnerable period, particularly for those with deficits in regulation.

5. Pathways to Obesity

One implication of the proposed *Contextualized Neural Vulnerabilities Model* is that there may be diverse pathways to obesity for individuals with different combinations of neural and contextual risk factors. For example, high food reward sensitivity in an environment with easy access to high-calorie foods may overwhelm even relatively strong regulatory abilities, leading to over-consumption. Alternatively, deficits in regulation abilities may combine with cues in the social environment that encourage overeating to increase risk for excess weight gain. However, while we can envision numerous starting points on the path to obesity, we propose that diverse pathways converge on the common process of the habitual over-consumption of high-calorie foods (see Figure 1). Habitual over-consumption, in turn, triggers a conditioning process resulting in the overvaluation of anticipated rewards from high-calorie foods, thus increasing attention and reactivity to these foods and related cues. Once this process of over-consumption and overvaluation begins, it can be difficult to interrupt and reverse, leading to long-term risk of excess weight gain. From this perspective, any factors that lead to the initiation of overeating can kick off a cascade of processes that heighten food rewards, undermine regulation, and entrench overeating patterns. If such a model were supported, the implications for intervention, particularly addressing "upstream" risk factors to prevent initial over-consumption, would be clear.

6. Informing a Contextualized Neural Vulnerabilities Model of Obesity Agenda

The proposed model informs a novel research agenda in contextualized obesity neuroscience, raising key research questions to test and refine components of the model. In addition to exploring the main effects of the three components on eating behavior/weight gain (with innovative research programs in these areas already underway), there is a need for studies incorporating all three components together. Such research could have two purposes. First, because much of the research exploring elements of the neural vulnerabilities model has examined individual components in isolation, studies incorporating multiple elements could help determine which components are the most impactful and, therefore, the most promising targets for intervention. Second, our model points toward explicating the *interactions* between different components and their impact on eating behavior and weight gain. Below, we propose some research questions that could be particularly informative in testing and refining the model, and ultimately informing contextualized approaches to intervention and prevention. For each, we offer specific predictions based on our model. Findings consistent with our predictions would support the model, whereas findings that contradict our hypotheses would suggest the need to revise the model.

Reward x Regulation. Research question: How is the effect of top-down regulation abilities on diet/weight trajectories moderated by individual differences in reward sensitivity? Prediction: We expect a significant reward x food regulation interaction, such that regulation deficits are most predictive of unhealthy dietary and weight trajectories *in the context of high reward sensitivity*. This prediction is based on the idea that strong regulation is needed in the context of high reward sensitivity (which creates a strong approach to unhealthy foods), and that the combination of high reward sensitivity and low regulation is especially conducive to developing unhealthy eating.

Environment x Regulation. Research question: How is the effect of top-down regulation abilities on diet/weight trajectories moderated by individual environmental factors (both "external" and "internal")? Prediction: We expect a significant environment x food regulation interaction, such that regulation deficits are most predictive of unhealthy dietary and weight trajectories *in the context of high obesogenic external environmental factors* (e.g., high availability of unhealthy foods in the home and neighborhood; high parental modeling of the consumption of energy-dense foods; low partner or friend support for health behavior goals). Similarly, we expect a significant environmental x food regulation interaction, such that regulation deficits are most predictive of unhealthy dietary and weight trajectories *in the context of internal factors such as high negative affect* (e.g., high temperamental negative affect; high symptoms of depression, anxiety, and/or loneliness). These predictions are based on the idea that strong regulation is needed in the context of highly obesogenic environments (which creates the opportunity and cues for unhealthy consumption), and that the combination of a highly obesogenic environment and low regulation is especially conducive to developing unhealthy eating.

Reward x Environment. Research Question: Does the combination of high reward sensitivity and an obesogenic environment (external and internal) result in an additive or multiplicative risk of unhealthy dietary and weight trajectories? Prediction: Environmental factors (both external and internal) will moderate the effect of individual differences in reward sensitivity on the prediction of dietary and weight trajectories, such that more obesogenic environments will exacerbate the effect of a high reward sensitivity on eating and weight outcomes. This prediction is based on the idea that high reward sensitivity will create a strong motivation to consume unhealthy foods and that obesogenic environments provide the opportunity for such consumption. We also expect an interplay between food environments and reward sensitivity, such that living in a more obesogenic environment, particularly during critical developmental periods such as adolescence, may condition individuals to overvalue energy-dense foods. This emergent sensitivity to food cues is expected to be a risk factor for future overeating and weight gain.

Food-Specific versus General Regulation. In addition to the proposed interaction analyses, it is also critical to empirically address the relative contributions of food-specific regulation versus general (i.e., non-food) regulation abilities in predicting dietary and weight trajectories. Studies including rigorous measures of both food-specific and general regulation in predicting diet and weight trajectories are currently lacking, leaving a potentially important question regarding optimal intervention targets unanswered. On the one hand, deficits in food-specific inhibitory control are highly correlated with generic inhibitory control ($r = 0.70$) [28], suggesting that the two constructs are highly related, as one would expect. However, there is also evidence that response inhibition training with high-calorie foods produces weight loss compared to a control condition that completed the same response inhibition training with non-food images [70–72]. Future research should further explicate the roles of food- versus non-food regulation to inform targeted treatment approaches.

Developmental Studies. Across the diverse research questions raised, there is a critical need for studies that are informed by a developmental perspective. For example, it would be highly informative to conduct research that charts the developmental trajectories of the contextualized neural vulnerabilities model components over time. We know little about how constructs such as food reward sensitivity and food-specific regulation change across development, and if there are critical periods during which these factors are particularly influential on diet and weight trajectories. These gaps limit our ability to identify key periods when targeted intervention may be most impactful in modifying risk factors and, in turn, changing health trajectories. As noted, we have proposed conceptual reasons for why adolescence might be a particularly important period for observational longitudinal studies (and possibly intervention trials), but rigorous studies of the contextualized model components in this development stage are sparse.

Exploring Differential Risk Pathways to Obesity. It is also important to consider the possibility that individuals may take qualitatively different risk pathways to obesity, rather than all experiencing a single risk pathway. Answering this question may require that we move away from ordinary least squares analyses that seek to fit a single model to the data, and use machine-learning techniques that can detect qualitatively different risk pathways to negative health and mental health outcomes. We have argued that classification tree analyses are particularly well suited to uncovering qualitatively different risk pathways with prospective data [73]. Although a literature search did not identify any prospective study that has used classification tree analyses to predict the future onset of obesity, one study did use it to predict the future onset of binge eating over a two-year follow-up among adolescent girls who initially did not report binge eating [74]. Classification tree analyses select the most potent risk factor and identify the cut-point that shows the greatest potency for differentiating who will, versus will not, experience onset of the outcome (binge eating). Overvaluation of weight/shape for determining self-worth was the first predictor: 20% of girls in the upper 50% of weight/shape overvaluation showed onset of binge eating, whereas only 2% of those in the lower 50% of the distribution showed binge eating onset. The fact that weight/shape overvaluation emerged first signals that it had greater predictive power than all of the other variables included in the model, which included dieting, BMI, body dissatisfaction, pressure for thinness, depressive symptoms, self-esteem, emotional eating, modeling of eating-disordered behaviors, and low social support. Among girls with low weight/shape overvaluation, 9% of those in the upper 25% of depression scores showed binge eating onset, versus 0% for those with lower depression. Among girls with high weight/shape overvaluation, 27% of those with a BMI of 18 or greater showed binge-eating onset, versus 0% for those with a lower BMI. Among girls with a high weight/shape overvaluation and a BMI > 18, 42% showed onset of binge eating if they were in the upper 40% of dieting versus 16% for those with lower dieting. Thus, the results revealed a four-way interaction between weight/shape overvaluation, depression, BMI, and dieting. Findings suggested that an elevated BMI amplified the predictive relation between weight/shape overvaluation and binge eating onset. This amplifying interaction indicates that the attitudinal risk factor of appearance overvaluation only operates among adolescent girls who have an age- and gender-adjusted BMI that places them in the slightly overweight range; thus, for girls who conform to the thin ideal, weight/shape overvaluation was not associated with binge eating onset. The results indicated another amplifying interaction, wherein dieting increased the predictive effects of the combination of weight/shape overvaluation and elevated BMI, with almost half the participants with this triple confluence of risk factors showing binge eating onset. Last, the results suggested an alternative pathway interaction, wherein among adolescent girls with lower weight/shape overvaluation, elevated depression emerged as a risk pathway, theoretically because depression increases the reward value of food or people turn to eating for mood improvement. That is, this classification tree suggested two qualitatively distinct risk pathways to binge eating onset; one involving a combination of weight/shape overvaluation, elevated weight, and dieting, and another involving elevated depression.

It would be useful for future prospective studies to apply classification tree analyses to the prediction of obesity onset over a multi-year follow-up because this might allow us to identify qualitatively different risk pathways to obesity. Results may inform more precision medicine-based prevention programs and treatments.

Randomized Controlled Trials. Finally, there are notable opportunities for research that develops and tests interventions that address key components of the model, particularly during critical developmental periods such as adolescence. Randomized controlled trials, including randomized prevention trials, may be an ideal follow-up for confirming findings from prospective observational risk factor studies (such as those suggested above), and determining the impact of targeted interventions based on a contextualized neural vulnerabilities model framework. Below, we provide a more detailed discussion of potential prevention and intervention implications.

7. Limitations and Opportunities for Further Development

Like all models, the contextualized neural vulnerabilities model described in this paper has limitations that should be acknowledged and considered as opportunities for further model refinement. First, our model does not explicitly focus on the biological foundations of neural vulnerabilities or the biological processes associated with obesity that could exacerbate neural vulnerabilities. For example, inflammatory processes, reduced cerebrovascular function, and disruptions in the gut microbiome could each further compromise cognitive and regulatory processes in ways that create additional risk for unhealthy eating and weight gain over time. Such complex bidirectional effects between neural vulnerabilities and biological processes associated with obesity may be particularly important over the long-term once unhealthy weight gain begins. Research that explicitly explores such processes and integrates the findings into the model would be useful. Second, our model focuses on two specific neural vulnerabilities, high reward sensitivity and regulatory deficits, because these factors have the most research support linking them to obesity risk; however, other neural vulnerabilities may also be relevant. As additional factors are identified in the literature as meaningful neural vulnerabilities for obesity, these factors should be integrated into the contextualized model with a focus on how they interact with key contexts to impact eating and weight trajectories.

8. Implications for Prevention and Intervention

The proposed model, if supported, could inform novel obesity prevention and intervention strategies. Specifically, if the three components are impactful, either via direct effects or through their interactions, this could create multiple points for intervention. We briefly present here some ideas for possible prevention and intervention targets.

If research supports a key role for food reward sensitivity in dietary and obesity risk, interventions could focus on reducing such sensitivity via targeted training. One potential way of reducing elevated reward region response to tastes of high-calorie foods could be to use dietary supplements that block certain taste receptors (e.g., sweet taste receptors), although rigorous trials examining the efficacy of such supplements in preventing weight gain are needed. This review also suggests that reducing the reward region response to cues for high-calorie foods might be useful in preventing future weight gain. Randomized trials have found that computer-training in which participants are cued to make a behavioral response to pictures of fruits and vegetables and to inhibit a behavioral response to high-calorie foods that the participant reports overeating over a 4- to 6-week period significantly reduces reward region response to pictures of high-calorie foods, palatability ratings of and willingness to pay for high-calorie foods, and produces objectively-measured body fat loss that persists through 2-year follow-up [70–72]. Reducing food reward sensitivity may be particularly beneficial for individuals with deficits in regulation because reducing the motivational drive to consume energy-dense foods could lower the demand on regulation abilities.

Enhancing regulation abilities is another possible strategy for prevention and intervention. If food-specific regulation proves particularly important, training could seek to build these specific abilities (rather than more general, non-food regulation) in the context of realistic food stimuli. Training interventions to down-regulate appetitive responses to energy-dense foods could leverage technologies such as virtual reality to create realistic, contextualized opportunities to practice food regulation. Further, interventions focusing on supporting skill *application in context* could provide prompts to remember health goals and direct attention away from tempting but unhealthy cues in the environment to increase the chances of enacting healthy decisions in difficult situations. Relatedly, interventions that focus on developing health goals and enhancing motivation to implement those goals (e.g., by creating cognitive dissonance regarding lifestyle behaviors that contribute to unhealthy weight gain [70–72]), even when confronted with tempting food stimuli, could support efforts to deploy regulation abilities toward health. Alternatively, for individuals with significant deficits in specific regulation abilities, compensatory strategies or "work arounds" might be helpful. For example, for those with poor working memory, targeted messages reminding the individual of their health goals, either periodically or in specific tempting situations, could help to keep such goals top of mind and encourage decisions that are consistent with these goals.

Finally, interventions to modify the external and internal food environment contexts could be useful. A number of interventions already seek to change external contexts such and home, school, work, and neighborhood food environments—with a focus on reducing the availability of and cues for unhealthy foods and increasing the accessibility of healthy alternatives—and have produced positive effects on weight outcomes [75,76]. Such strategies could be especially important for individuals with high food reward sensitivity or regulation deficits that put them at risk for unhealthy consumption, as reducing the opportunities to consume energy-dense foods could help mitigate these risks. Modifying internal contexts by reducing negative affect that can drive emotional eating could also help reduce the demands on food regulation. Alternatively, because environments may not always be modifiable, individuals who encounter particularly challenging food environments may benefit from extra support to enhance food regulation or reduce food reward sensitivity to increase their chances of successfully meeting health goals despite environmental challenges.

To summarize, there is potential for creating novel, comprehensive, multi-component intervention approaches that address all three components of the *Contextualized Neural Vulnerabilities Model of Obesity*. Furthermore, informed by longitudinal observational risk studies with an emphasis on explicating processes and pathways, it may be possible to create targeted screening processes that identify individuals at heightened risk for developing habitual unhealthy eating and obesity. At a minimum, screening could involve assessments of the three model components, and individuals with significant risk in one or more areas could be candidates for targeted prevention efforts. Understanding unique risk pathways may also create opportunities for personalizing prevention efforts by identifying combinations of risk factors and tailoring intervention components to the unique needs of the individual. To facilitate such personalized approaches, it would be necessary to develop a "menu" of effective intervention modules for addressing each of the three main components, and then intervention could be personalized by picking and choosing which intervention strategies best fit a particular case.

Author Contributions: Conceptualization, T.D.N. and E.S.; writing—original draft preparation, T.D.N. and E.S.; writing—review and editing, T.D.N. and E.S. All authors have read and agreed to the published version of the manuscript.

Funding: This work was supported by grants from the National Institute of Diabetes and Digestive and Kidney Diseases (R01DK116693, R01DK125651, R01DK112762), the Eunice Kennedy Shriver National Institute of Child Health and Human Development (R01HD093598), and the National Cancer Institute (R01CA211224) of the National Institutes of Health. The content is solely the responsibility of the authors and does not necessarily represent the official views of the National Institutes of Health.

Institutional Review Board Statement: Not applicable.

Informed Consent Statement: Not applicable.

Data Availability Statement: Not applicable.

Conflicts of Interest: The authors declare no conflict of interest.

References

1. Stice, E.; Burger, K. Neural vulnerability factors for obesity. *Clin. Psychol. Rev.* **2019**, *68*, 38–53. [CrossRef]
2. Stice, E.; Yokum, S. Neural vulnerability factors that increase risk for future weight gain. *Psychol. Bull.* **2016**, *142*, 447–471. [CrossRef]
3. Favieri, F.; Forte, G.; Casagrande, M. The executive functions in overweight and obesity: A systematic review of neuropsychological cross-sectional and longitudinal studies. *Front. Psychol.* **2019**, *10*, 2126. [CrossRef]
4. Heatherton, T.F.; Wagner, D.D. Cognitive neuroscience of self-regulation failure. *Trends Cogn. Sci.* **2011**, *15*, 132–139. [CrossRef]
5. Stoeckel, L.E.; Birch, L.L.; Heatherton, T.; Mann, T.; Hunter, C.; Czajkowski, S.; Onken, L.; Berger, P.K.; Savage, C.R. Psychological and neural contributions to appetite self-regulation. *Obesity* **2017**, *25* (Suppl. 1), S17–S25. [CrossRef]
6. Holsen, L.M.; Lawson, E.A.; Blum, J.; Ko, E.; Makris, N.; Fazeli, P.; Klibanski, A.; Goldstein, J. Food motivation circuitry hypoactivation related to hedonic and nonhedonic aspects of hunger and satiety in women with active anorexia nervosa and weight-restored women with anorexia nervosa. *J. Psychiatry Neurosci.* **2012**, *37*, 322–332. [CrossRef] [PubMed]
7. Oberndorfer, T.A.; Frank, G.K.W.; Simmons, A.N.; Wagner, A.; McCurdy, D.; Fudge, J.L.; Yang, T.T.; Paulus, M.P.; Kaye, W.H. Altered insula response to sweet taste processing after recovery from anorexia and bulimia nervosa. *Am. J. Psychiatry* **2013**, *170*, 1143–1151. [CrossRef] [PubMed]
8. Oberndorfer, T.; Simmons, A.; McCurdy, D.; Strigo, I.; Matthews, S.; Yang, T.; Irvine, Z.; Kaye, W. Greater anterior insula activation during anticipation of food images in women recovered from anorexia nervosa versus controls. *Psychiatry Res. Neuroimaging* **2013**, *214*, 132–141. [CrossRef] [PubMed]
9. Wagner, A.; Aizenstein, H.; Mazurkewicz, L.; Fudge, J.; Frank, G.K.; Putnam, K.; Bailer, U.F.; Fischer, L.; Kaye, W.H. Altered insula response to taste stimuli in individuals recovered from restricting-type anorexia nervosa. *Neuropsychopharmacology* **2008**, *33*, 513–523. [CrossRef]
10. Brooks, S.J.; O'Daly, O.; Uher, R.; Friederich, H.-C.; Giampietro, V.; Brammer, M.; Williams, S.C.R.; Schiöth, H.B.; Treasure, J.; Campbell, I.C. Thinking about eating food activates visual cortex with reduced bilateral cerebellar activation in females with anorexia nervosa: An fMRI study. *PLoS ONE* **2012**, *7*, e34000. [CrossRef]
11. Miyake, Y.; Okamoto, Y.; Onoda, K.; Shirao, N.; Okamoto, Y.; Otagaki, Y.; Yamawaki, S. Neural processing of negative word stimuli concerning body image in patients with eating disorders: An fMRI study. *Neuroimage* **2010**, *50*, 1333–1339. [CrossRef] [PubMed]
12. Steinglass, J.E.; Figner, B.; Berkowitz, S.; Simpson, H.B.; Weber, E.U.; Walsh, B.T. Increased capacity to delay reward in anorexia nervosa. *J. Int. Neuropsychol. Soc.* **2012**, *18*, 773–780. [CrossRef] [PubMed]
13. Steinglass, J.E.; Lempert, K.M.; Choo, T.H.; Kimeldorf, M.B.; Wall, M.; Walsh, B.T.; Fyer, A.J.; Schneier, F.R.; Simpson, H.B. Temporal discounting across three psychiatric disorders: Anorexia nervosa, obsessive compulsive disorder, and social anxiety disorder. *Depress. Anxiety* **2017**, *34*, 463–470. [CrossRef] [PubMed]
14. Hall, P.A.; Marteau, T.M. Executive function in the context of chronic disease prevention: Theory, research and practice. *Prev. Med.* **2014**, *68*, 44–50. [CrossRef]
15. Nelson, T.D.; Nelson, J.M.; Mason, W.A.; Tomaso, C.C.; Kozikowski, C.B.; Espy, K.A. Executive control and adolescent health: Toward A conceptual framework. *Adolesc. Res. Rev.* **2019**, *4*, 31–43. [CrossRef]
16. Sutton, C.A.; L'Insalata, A.M.; Fazzino, T.L. Reward sensitivity, eating behavior, and obesity-related outcomes: A systematic review. *Physiol. Behav.* **2022**, *252*, 113843. [CrossRef]
17. Demos, K.E.; Heatherton, T.F.; Kelley, W.M. Individual differences in nucleus accumbens activity to food and sexual images predict weight gain and sexual behavior. *J. Neurosci.* **2012**, *32*, 5549–5552. [CrossRef]

18. Stice, E.; Burger, K.S.; Yokum, S. Reward region responsivity predicts future weight gain and moderating effects of the TaqIA allele. *J. Neurosci.* **2015**, *35*, 10316–10324. [CrossRef]
19. Yokum, S.; Gearhardt, A.N.; Harris, J.L.; Brownell, K.D.; Stice, E. Individual differences in striatum activity to food commercials predict weight gain in adolescents. *Obesity* **2014**, *22*, 2544–2551. [CrossRef]
20. Yokum, S.; Stice, E. Weight gain is associated with changes in neural response to palatable food tastes varying in sugar and fat and palatable food images: A repeated-measures fMRI study. *Am. J. Clin. Nutr.* **2019**, *110*, 1275–1286. [CrossRef]
21. Nelson, T.D.; Brock, R.L.; Yokum, S.; Tomaso, C.C.; Savage, C.R.; Stice, E. Much Ado About Missingness: A demonstration of full information maximum likelihood estimation to address missingness in functional magnetic resonance imaging data. *Front. Neurosci.* **2021**, *15*, 746424. [CrossRef] [PubMed]
22. Reinert, K.R.S.; Po'e, E.K.; Barkin, S.L. The Relationship between Executive Function and Obesity in Children and Adolescents: A Systematic Literature Review. *J. Obes.* **2013**, *2013*, e820956. [CrossRef] [PubMed]
23. Shields, C.V.; Hultstrand, K.V.; West, C.E.; Gunstad, J.J.; Sato, A.F. Disinhibited eating and executive functioning in children and adolescents: A systematic review and meta-analysis. *Int. J. Environ. Res. Public Health* **2022**, *19*, 13384. [CrossRef] [PubMed]
24. Higgs, S.; Spetter, M.S. Cognitive control of eating: The role of memory in appetite and weight gain. *Curr. Obes. Rep.* **2018**, *7*, 50–59. [CrossRef]
25. Tomaso, C.C.; James, T.; Nelson, J.M.; Espy, K.A.; Nelson, T.D. Longitudinal associations between executive control and body mass index across childhood. *Pediatr. Obes.* **2022**, *17*, e12866. [CrossRef] [PubMed]
26. Nelson, T.D.; James, T.D.; Hankey, M.; Nelson, J.M.; Lundahl, A.; Espy, K.A. Early executive control and risk for overweight and obesity in elementary school. *Child. Neuropsychol.* **2017**, *23*, 994–1002. [CrossRef] [PubMed]
27. Kidwell, K.M.; James, T.D.; Brock, R.L.; Yaroch, A.L.; Hill, J.L.; Nelson, J.M.; Mason, W.A.; Espy, K.A.; Nelson, T.D. Preschool executive control, temperament, and adolescent dietary behaviors. *Ann. Behav. Med.* **2023**, *57*, 260–268. [CrossRef]
28. Loch, L.K.; Tanofsky-Kraff, M.; Parker, M.N.; Haynes, H.E.; Te-Vazquez, J.A.; Bloomer, B.F.; Lazareva, J.; Moursi, N.A.; Nwosu, E.E.; Yang, S.B.; et al. Associations of food reinforcement and food-related inhibitory control with adiposity and weight gain in children and adolescents. *Physiol. Behav.* **2023**, *266*, 114198. [CrossRef] [PubMed]
29. Giskes, K.; van Lenthe, F.; Avendano-Pabon, M.; Brug, J. A systematic review of environmental factors and obesogenic dietary intakes among adults: Are we getting closer to understanding obesogenic environments? *Obes. Rev.* **2011**, *12*, e95–e106. [CrossRef]
30. Saelens, B.E.; Sallis, J.F.; Frank, L.D.; Couch, S.C.; Zhou, C.; Colburn, T.; Cain, K.L.; Chapman, J.; Glanz, K. Obesogenic neighborhood environments, child and parent obesity: The Neighborhood Impact on Kids study. *Am. J. Prev. Med.* **2012**, *42*, e57–e64. [CrossRef]
31. Nelson, T.D.; Kidwell, K.M.; Nelson, J.M.; Tomaso, C.C.; Hankey, M.; Espy, K.A. Preschool executive control and internalizing symptoms in elementary school. *J. Abnorm. Child. Psychol.* **2018**, *46*, 1509–1520. [CrossRef] [PubMed]
32. Morales, M.E.; Berkowitz, S.A. The relationship between food insecurity, dietary patterns, and obesity. *Curr. Nutr. Rep.* **2016**, *5*, 54–60. [CrossRef]
33. Metallinos-Katsaras, E.; Must, A.; Gorman, K. A longitudinal study of food insecurity on obesity in preschool children. *J. Acad. Nutr. Diet.* **2012**, *112*, 1949–1958. [CrossRef]
34. Smith, N.R.; Zivich, P.N.; Frerichs, L. Social influences on obesity: Current knowledge, emerging methods, and directions for future research and practice. *Curr. Nutr. Rep.* **2020**, *9*, 31–41. [CrossRef] [PubMed]
35. Wagner, D.D.; Boswell, R.G.; Kelley, W.M.; Heatherton, T.F. Inducing negative affect increases the reward value of appetizing foods in dieters. *J. Cogn. Neurosci.* **2012**, *24*, 1625–1633. [CrossRef] [PubMed]
36. Devonport, T.J.; Nicholls, W.; Fullerton, C. A systematic review of the association between emotions and eating behaviour in normal and overweight adult populations. *J. Health Psychol.* **2019**, *24*, 3–24. [CrossRef]
37. Cardi, V.; Leppanen, J.; Treasure, J. The effects of negative and positive mood induction on eating behaviour: A meta-analysis of laboratory studies in the healthy population and eating and weight disorders. *Neurosci. Biobehav. Rev.* **2015**, *57*, 299–309. [CrossRef]
38. Rudenga, K.; Sinha, R.; Small, D. Acute stress potentiates brain response to milkshake as a function of body weight and chronic stress. *Int. J. Obes.* **2013**, *37*, 309–316. [CrossRef]
39. Ranzenhofer, L.M.; Hannallah, L.; Field, S.E.; Shomaker, L.B.; Stephens, M.; Sbrocco, T.; Kozlosky, M.; Reynolds, J.; Yanovski, J.A.; Tanofsky-Kraff, M. Pre-meal affective state and laboratory test meal intake in adolescent girls with loss of control eating. *Appetite* **2013**, *68*, 30–37. [CrossRef]
40. Tomaso, C.C.; James, T.D.; Brock, R.L.; Yaroch, A.L.; Hill, J.; Huang, T.T.; Nelson, J.M.; Mason, W.A.; Espy, K.A.; Nelson, T.D. Preschool executive control buffers the relationship between child temperament and adolescent body mass index trajectories. *Pediatric Obesity*. **2023**. under review
41. Yang, X.; Casement, M.; Yokum, S.; Stice, E. Negative affect amplifies the relation between appetitive-food-related neural responses and weight gain over three-year follow-up among adolescents. *Neuroimage Clin.* **2019**, *24*, 102067. [CrossRef] [PubMed]
42. Braams, B.R.; van Duijvenvoorde, A.C.K.; Peper, J.S.; Crone, E.A. Longitudinal changes in adolescent risk-taking: A comprehensive study of neural responses to rewards, pubertal development, and risk-taking behavior. *J. Neurosci.* **2015**, *35*, 7226–7238. [CrossRef] [PubMed]
43. Ferguson, H.J.; Brunsdon, V.E.A.; Bradford, E.E.F. The developmental trajectories of executive function from adolescence to old age. *Sci. Rep.* **2021**, *11*, 1382. [CrossRef]

44. HEI Scores for Americans | Food and Nutrition Service. Available online: https://www.fns.usda.gov/hei-scores-americans (accessed on 23 May 2023).
45. Chung, W.W.; Hudziak, J.J. The transitional age brain: "The best of times and the worst of times". *Child. Adolesc. Psychiatr. Clin. N. Am.* **2017**, *26*, 157–175. [CrossRef] [PubMed]
46. Steinberg, L. Cognitive and affective development in adolescence. *Trends Cogn. Sci.* **2005**, *9*, 69–74. [CrossRef]
47. Fryar, C.D.; Carroll, M.D.; Afful, J. *Prevalence of Overweight, Obesity, and Severe Obesity among Children and Adolescents Aged 2–19 Years: United States, 1963–1965 through 2017–2018*; NCHS Health E-Stats; National Center for Health Statistics: Hyattsville, MD, USA, 2020.
48. Espy, K.A. *The Changing Nature of Executive Control in Preschool*; Monographs of the Society for Research in Child Development; Wiley-Blackwell: Oxford, UK, 2016; p. 81.
49. Lee, K.; Bull, R.; Ho, R.M.H. Developmental changes in executive functioning. *Child. Dev.* **2013**, *84*, 1933–1953. [CrossRef]
50. Nelson, T.D.; James, T.D.; Nelson, J.M.; Tomaso, C.C.; Espy, K.A. Executive control throughout elementary school: Factor structure and associations with early childhood executive control. *Dev. Psychol.* **2022**, *58*, 730–750. [CrossRef]
51. Schmeichel, B.J.; Tang, D. Individual differences in executive functioning and their relationship to emotional processes and responses. *Curr. Dir. Psychol. Sci.* **2015**, *24*, 93–98. [CrossRef]
52. Evans, G.W.; Fuller-Rowell, T.E.; Doan, S.N. Childhood cumulative risk and obesity: The mediating role of self-regulatory ability. *Pediatrics* **2012**, *129*, e68–e73. [CrossRef]
53. Francis, L.A.; Susman, E.J. Self-regulation and rapid weight gain in children from age 3 to 12 years. *Arch. Pediatr. Adolesc. Med.* **2009**, *163*, 297–302. [CrossRef]
54. Schlam, T.R.; Wilson, N.L.; Shoda, Y.; Mischel, W.; Ayduk, O. Preschoolers' delay of gratification predicts their body mass 30 years later. *J. Pediatr.* **2013**, *162*, 90–93. [CrossRef] [PubMed]
55. Seeyave, D.M.; Coleman, S.; Appugliese, D.; Corwyn, R.F.; Bradley, R.H.; Davidson, N.S.; Kaciroti, N.; Lumeng, J.C. Ability to delay gratification at age 4 years and risk of overweight at age 11 years. *Arch. Pediatr. Adolesc. Med.* **2009**, *163*, 303–308. [CrossRef] [PubMed]
56. Anzman, S.L.; Birch, L.L. Low inhibitory control and restrictive feeding practices predict weight outcomes. *J. Pediatr.* **2009**, *155*, 651–656. [CrossRef]
57. Duckworth, A.L.; Tsukayama, E.; Geier, A.B. Self-controlled children stay leaner in the transition to adolescence. *Appetite* **2010**, *54*, 304–308. [CrossRef] [PubMed]
58. Sutin, A.R.; Ferrucci, L.; Zonderman, A.B.; Terracciano, A. Personality and obesity across the adult life span. *J. Pers Soc. Psychol.* **2011**, *101*, 579–592. [CrossRef]
59. Nederkoorn, C.; Jansen, E.; Mulkens, S.; Jansen, A. Impulsivity predicts treatment outcome in obese children. *Behav. Res. Ther.* **2007**, *45*, 1071–1075. [CrossRef] [PubMed]
60. Weygandt, M.; Mai, K.; Dommes, E.; Leupelt, V.; Hackmack, K.; Kahnt, T.; Rothemund, Y.; Spranger, J.; Haynes, J.-D. The role of neural impulse control mechanisms for dietary success in obesity. *Neuroimage* **2013**, *83*, 669–678. [CrossRef]
61. Weygandt, M.; Mai, K.; Dommes, E.; Ritter, K.; Leupelt, V.; Spranger, J.; Haynes, J.-D. Impulse control in the dorsolateral prefrontal cortex counteracts post-diet weight regain in obesity. *Neuroimage* **2015**, *109*, 318–327. [CrossRef]
62. Shearrer, G.E.; Stice, E.; Burger, K.S. Adolescents at high risk of obesity show greater striatal response to increased sugar content in milkshakes. *Am. J. Clin. Nutr.* **2018**, *107*, 859–866. [CrossRef]
63. Stice, E.; Yokum, S.; Burger, K.S.; Epstein, L.H.; Small, D.M. Youth at risk for obesity show greater activation of striatal and somatosensory regions to food. *J. Neurosci.* **2011**, *31*, 4360–4366. [CrossRef]
64. Stice, E.; Yokum, S. Gain in body fat is associated with increased striatal response to palatable food cues, whereas body fat stability is associated with decreased striatal response. *J. Neurosci.* **2016**, *36*, 6949–6956. [CrossRef] [PubMed]
65. Burger, K.S.; Stice, E. Greater striatopallidal adaptive coding during cue-reward learning and food reward habituation predict future weight gain. *Neuroimage* **2014**, *99*, 122–128. [CrossRef] [PubMed]
66. Swinburn, B.; Egger, G.; Raza, F. Dissecting obesogenic environments: The development and application of a framework for identifying and prioritizing environmental interventions for obesity. *Prev. Med.* **1999**, *29*, 563–570. [CrossRef]
67. Kegler, M.C.; Hermstad, A.; Haardörfer, R. Home food environment and associations with weight and diet among U.S. adults: A cross-sectional study. *BMC Public Health* **2021**, *21*, 1032. [CrossRef] [PubMed]
68. Higgs, S. Social norms and their influence on eating behaviours. *Appetite* **2015**, *86*, 38–44. [CrossRef]
69. Korzeniowski, C.; Ison, M.S.; Difabio de Anglat, H. A summary of the developmental trajectory of executive functions from birth to adulthood. In *Psychiatry and Neuroscience Update: From Epistemology to Clinical Psychiatry—Vol. IV*; Gargiulo, P.Á., Arroyo, H.L.M., Eds.; Springer Nature Switzerland AG: Cham, Switzerland, 2021; pp. 459–473. [CrossRef]
70. Stice, E.; Rohde, P.; Butryn, M.L.; Desjardins, C.; Shaw, H. Enhancing efficacy of a brief obesity and eating disorder prevention program: Long-term results from an experimental therapeutics trial. *Nutrients* **2023**, *15*, 1008. [CrossRef]
71. Stice, E.; Rohde, P.; Gau, J.M.; Butryn, M.L.; Shaw, H.; Cloud, K.; D'Adamo, L. Enhancing efficacy of a dissonance-based obesity and eating disorder prevention program: Experimental therapeutics. *J. Consult. Clin. Psychol.* **2021**, *89*, 793–804. [CrossRef]
72. Stice, E.; Yokum, S.; Veling, H.; Kemps, E.; Lawrence, N.S. Pilot test of a novel food response and attention training treatment for obesity: Brain imaging data suggest actions shape valuation. *Behav. Res. Ther.* **2017**, *94*, 60–70. [CrossRef]

73. Stice, E. Interactive and mediational etiologic models of eating disorder onset: Evidence from prospective studies. *Annu. Rev. Clin. Psychol.* **2016**, *12*, 359–381. [CrossRef]
74. Stice, E.; Presnell, K.; Spangler, D. Risk factors for binge eating onset in adolescent girls: A 2-year prospective investigation. *Health Psychol.* **2002**, *21*, 131–138. [CrossRef]
75. Pineda, E.; Bascunan, J.; Sassi, F. Improving the school food environment for the prevention of childhood obesity: What works and what doesn't. *Obes. Rev.* **2021**, *22*, e13176. [CrossRef] [PubMed]
76. Stark, L.J.; Clifford, L.M.; Towner, E.K.; Filigno, S.S.; Zion, C.; Bolling, C.; Rausch, J. A pilot randomized controlled trial of a behavioral family-based intervention with and without home visits to decrease obesity in preschoolers. *J. Pediatr. Psychol.* **2014**, *39*, 1001–1012. [CrossRef] [PubMed]

Disclaimer/Publisher's Note: The statements, opinions and data contained in all publications are solely those of the individual author(s) and contributor(s) and not of MDPI and/or the editor(s). MDPI and/or the editor(s) disclaim responsibility for any injury to people or property resulting from any ideas, methods, instructions or products referred to in the content.

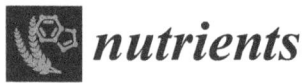

Review

The Human Gut Virome and Its Relationship with Nontransmissible Chronic Diseases

Shahrzad Ezzatpour [1], Alicia del Carmen Mondragon Portocarrero [2], Alejandra Cardelle-Cobas [2], Alexandre Lamas [2], Aroa López-Santamarina [2], José Manuel Miranda [2,*] and Hector C. Aguilar [1]

[1] Department of Microbiology and Immunology, College of Veterinary Medicine, Cornell University, Ithaca, NY 14853, USA
[2] Laboratorio de Higiene, Inspección y Control de Alimentos (LHICA), Departamento de Química Analítica, Nutrición y Bromatología, Universidade de Santiago de Compostela, 27002 Lugo, Spain
* Correspondence: josemanuel.miranda@usc.es; Tel.: +34-982252231 (ext. 22410)

Abstract: The human gastrointestinal tract contains large communities of microorganisms that are in constant interaction with the host, playing an essential role in the regulation of several metabolic processes. Among the gut microbial communities, the gut bacteriome has been most widely studied in recent decades. However, in recent years, there has been increasing interest in studying the influences that other microbial groups can exert on the host. Among them, the gut virome is attracting great interest because viruses can interact with the host immune system and metabolic functions; this is also the case for phages, which interact with the bacterial microbiota. The antecedents of virome-rectification-based therapies among various diseases were also investigated. In the near future, stool metagenomic investigation should include the identification of bacteria and phages, as well as their correlation networks, to better understand gut microbiota activity in metabolic disease progression.

Keywords: Microviridae; Caudovirales; fecal viral transference; virome; obesity; diabetes; inflammatory bowel disease

1. Introduction

The human gut microbiota (GM) is tightly connected to human health through a complex biological system that consists of bacteria, fungi, archaea, and viruses, among other components [1]. The bacterial composition of the GM has been widely investigated in the last two decades in terms of composition, diversity, functionality, and the relationship with human metabolic diseases [2,3]. However, much less attention has been given to other components of the GM, such as viruses. Recent works found that the number of virus-like particles (VLPs) in the gut ranges in a ratio of viruses to bacteria from approximately 0.1 to 10, suggesting that the number of viruses in the human body is close to the number of bacteria [4].

After the colonization of the intestine during birth, the human gut virome (GV) evolves steadily during infancy/childhood, entering a period of major changes during the first 2 years of life, and then stabilizes in later childhood [5,6]. In the first months of life, the GV is dominated by viruses that infect bacteria (phages), whereas eukaryotic viruses increase in both abundance and diversity throughout childhood [6]. In a healthy adult, the human GV comprises phages, viruses that infect other cellular microorganisms, viruses that infect human cells, and viruses derived from food and found in the digestive tract in a transient manner [4,6]. Among eukaryotic viruses, eukaryotic DNA viruses, such as those of the family *Circoviridae*; RNA viruses, such as *Enteroviridae*, *Parechoviridae*, and *Picornaviridae*; and plant viruses, primarily of the family *Vigaviridae*, are frequently found in infants, as are some types of potentially pathogenic viruses, such as those belonging to the genera rotavirus, norovirus, and sapovirus [6].

With respect to phages, at the beginning of infancy, phages of the order *Caudovirales* (tailed phages) predominate, primarily those belonging to the families *Siphoviridae*, *Podoviridae*, and *Myoriviridae*. Subsequently, however, the presence of phages of the order *Caudovirales* decreases as the presence of phages of the family *Microviridae*, order *Petivirales* (icosahedral phages without tails), increases during the first 2 years of life [4,7,8]. Within the order *Caudovirales*, CrAss-type phages, a family of DNA-tailed phages that can infect bacteria of the phylum Bacteroidetes, are currently considered to be the most abundant phages in the adult human GV [5,9,10]. Such CrAss phages are rarely detected in the gastrointestinal tract of infants during the first month of life but subsequently increase in prevalence, accounting for more than 90% of the GV content in an adult human [6,11].

Progressive maturation of the infant GM leads to a reduction in GV abundance and diversity simultaneously compared with those observed for the bacteriome [1]. Subsequently, GV tends to resemble what it will be during the adult stage. Paralleling stability in the cellular microbiome [4], adult GV is usually stable over time, as evident from recent studies showing that >90% of recognizable viral contigs persisted in individuals over one year [1,4].

Most of the viruses included in the human GV are DNA viruses, whereas eukaryotic RNA viruses are rare in healthy individuals, and most of those that meet these characteristics are primarily plant-infecting viruses [4]. However, this lower presence of RNA viruses may not be as real as the background suggests. Thus, it should be noted that, in general, the RNA virome in the human gut is less studied than the DNA virome, as RNA viruses are substantially less stable in samples than DNA viruses, making their identification by metagenomic sequencing difficult [5]. Therefore, it is quite possible that the actual presence of RNA viruses is higher than that published for several environmental niches, including animal feces [5], and that their presence has been systematically underestimated due to technical reasons [4].

The fact that the majority of adult human GV components are phages is an inference because, in most cases, most of the sequences discovered in GV metagenomic sequencing assays do not align with any information present in existing datasets [5]. Therefore, the proportion of GV viruses that can be identified in a completely unambiguous way is extremely low and does not reliably represent all GVs. As the most abundant phage order, *Caudoviridales* includes phages that can infect all major bacterial phyla found in the gut: Firmicutes, Bacteroidetes, Proteobacteria, and Actinobacteria [2].

The human GV, which included both phages and eukaryotic viruses, can be modified in their richness and diversity by factors that depend on the subject's lifestyle [5]. In this regard, different factors, such as geography, diet, genetics, or drugs ingested, can shape the human GV [4] (Table 1). A recent study [12] concluded that geography is the most important contributor to variations in human GV. In addition, other works have shown that diet type can modify GV in adults [4], as well as age [13]. The objectives of this manuscript were therefore to provide and update the state-of-the-art knowledge of the relationship between the GV and nontransmissible chronic diseases. To achieve this goal, a narrative literature search was conducted up to 10 July 2021 for the Web of Science and Scopus databases. The term "human gut virome" was searched in the field "title, abstract and keywords" in the case of Scopus and "topic" in the case of Web of Science. A total of 269 articles were found. The selection of articles will be limited to studies published in English, with no restrictions on the year of publication, although the most prominent articles are those published after 2018. The authors reviewed the titles and the abstracts. If the abstracts reported useful information, full texts were read, and if the pre-established eligibility criteria were met, they were included in the review. After selecting the articles that fell into the selected scope, a total of 87 articles were selected and included in the review.

Table 1. Research works on the metagenomic analysis of the human virome.

Model	Subjects	Determination	Main Findings	References
Humans (twin kids)	12 personal fecal samples (4 twins and his/her mothers)	Metagenomic sequencing of bacterial and viral content from fecal bulk	-The composition of the intestinal phageome has similarities in people from different parts of the world. -Ignorance of sequences in viral metagenomes can lead to errors in determining the diversity of the human virome. -This study identified and validated the genome sequence of CrAssphage.	[11]
Humans (healthy adults)	1986 individuals representing 16 countries	Metagenomic sequencing of the viral content of fecal bulk	-The variability in gut virome (GV) among studies due to technical deficiencies is greater than the effect of any disease. -Gut viral richness increases from birth to median age and declines in elderly individuals.	[13]
Human (1-year-old child)	662 paired samples obtained at 1 year from an unselected childhood cohort	Fecal sample metagenomics and comparison with metaviromics datasets	-An important part of the GV may be lost during the viral enrichment stage or may not be correctly detected as it is in the form of bacteria containing dormant phages (prophages). -Most viral populations in the metavirome were not found in the metagenome datasets.	[1]
Human (healthy children)	60 samples from 18 girls and 12 boys	Isolation and quantification of phages and bacteria from stool, metagenome assembly, and analysis	-Phages can regulate bacterial abundance and composition in an age-specific manner. -Phages could be related to the gut microbiota (GM) changes observed in child stunting.	[14]
Humans (twin kids)	8 infants (4 twin pairs)	Bulk virome characterization	-Both eukaryotic virome and bacterial microbiome expanded from birth to 2 years of age, whereas phageome composition decreased. -The infant microbiome is highly dynamic with respect to bacteria, viruses, and bacteriophages, whereas, in adults, it is more stable.	[7]
Humans (dietary intervention)	Purified virus-like particles from stool samples collected longitudinally from six healthy volunteers	Dietary intervention high-fat/low-fiber diet and comparison of the GV for 8 days	-Viral contigs were rich in functions required in lytic and lysogenic growth, as well as viral CRISPR arrays and genes for antibiotic resistance. -The largest source of variance among GV samples was interpersonal variation. -Dietary intervention caused a change in the GV community, causing convergence of GV in individuals with similar diets.	[15]

Table 1. Cont.

Model	Subjects	Determination	Main Findings	References
Mice (gnotobiotic)	5 Germfree C57BL/6 mice	Gnotobiotic mice subjected to predation by cognate lytic phages	-Shifts in the microbiome caused by phage predation alter the gut metabolome.	[16]
Humans (healthy adults)	10 healthy volunteers	Fecal samples were collected monthly and synchronously over a 12-month period	-Several groups of CrAss-like and *Microviridae* bacteriophages were identified as the most stable colonizers of the human gut. -There are stable, numerically predominant individual-specific persistent viromes typical of each subject.	[10]
Humans (healthy adults)	930 healthy adult subjects	Bulk DNA virome characterization	-Factors associated with urbanization and geography factors were the top covariates of GV variation. -GV showed more heterogeneity than the bacterial microbiome in the investigated samples.	[12]

2. Host-Gut Virome Interactions/Relationships

In general, phages have a narrow activity spectrum, with each phage affecting a small number of closely related bacterial species and, sometimes, only specific serotypes or specific strains within the same species [4]. This fact is important because GV plays a key role in modulating the bacterial populations that are part of the GM. However, since most intestinal phages remain poorly understood, it is often difficult to relate phages to the bacteria that are part of the host GM [17]. Phages exhibit four types of life cycles (including lytic, temperate/lysogenic, pseudolysogenic, and bacterial budding), with lytic and lysogenic life cycles being the two classical forms [5,18] (Figure 1). Another phage cycle is pseudolysogeny, also called the stationary phase of the phage in the host cell [19]. In this phase, there is neither multiplication of the phage genome as in the lytic cycle nor replication synchronized with the cell cycle of the host cell as in the lysogenic cycle [19]. This process usually takes place when the host cell encounters unfavorable conditions such as starvation and ends when the phage enters an actual lysogenic cycle or enters a lytic cycle when bacterial growth conditions improve [20]. This cycle seems to play an important role in phage survival, as bacteria in the natural environment often exhibit very slow growth or starvation [21]. Another cycle of phages is bacterial budding. This cycle is interesting, as phages are released through the bacterial cell membrane without causing lysis of the bacterium by a budding-like process, producing a chronic release of phages [22].

A phage can multiply through the lytic cycle when it kills the bacterium to release progeny phages or as a bacteria containing dormant phages (prophage) when it integrates its DNA into the bacterial chromosome (lysogenic cycle) [4,20]. In a healthy state, the human GV is primarily composed of temperate phages, and its replication switches from temperate to lytic during host inflammation or stress [18]. Because of the predominance of phages over eukaryotic viruses in the GV, as well as their role in regulating bacteriome composition and function, the phageome has been the focus of most human GV research [20].

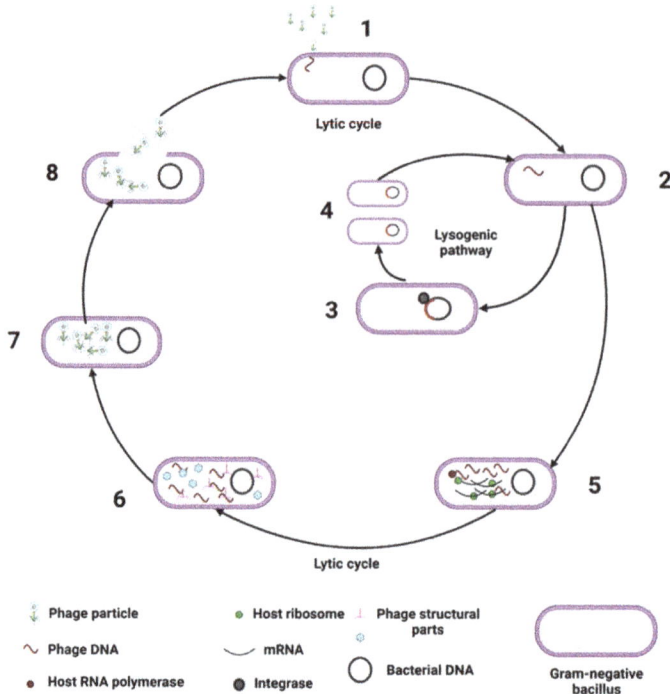

Figure 1. Representation of the main phage infection cycles. (1) Phage interaction with the bacterial surface through specific receptors and injecting its DNA into the host cell cytoplasm; (2) at this point, phages may follow the lysogenic cycle or the lytic cycle; (3) the phage genome integrates into the bacterial host genome using integrases; (4) the resulting bacteria containing dormant phages (prophage) replicate together with the bacterial genome for several generations and can enter the lytic cycle at any moment, e.g., under stress conditions; (5) following the lytic cycle, phages use bacterial molecular tools for protein synthesis and phage DNA polymerase for DNA replication; (6) the structural proteins are expressed; (7) new virions are formed; and (8) phage proteins, such as endoylsins and holins, break the cell membrane and allow the release of new viral particles ready for a new cycle of infections.

In addition to phages, the healthy human intestine often contains low proportions of eukaryotic viruses, which include occasionally detected DNA viral lineages such as *Anelloviridae*, *Geminiviridae*, *Herpesviridae*, *Nanoviridae*, *Papillomaviridae*, *Parvoviridae*, *Polyomaviridae*, *Adenoviridae*, and *Circoviridae* [21]. Eukaryotic RNA viruses primarily comprise multiple plant-related viruses [12], while the most abundant eukaryotic RNA virus infecting animals in the GV belongs to the *Picornaviridae* family [22].

GV plays a highly relevant role in autoimmune and inflammatory intestinal diseases [23]. Therefore, colonization of the intestine by eukaryotic viruses is very important for the maintenance of proper intestinal homeostasis and the development of host immunity. Eukaryotic viruses can increase intestinal inflammation in mice by sensing viral RNA by host Toll-like receptors 3 and 7 and downregulating interferon beta secretion [20], which protects the host from inflammation [23]. Widespread phage predation, lysogeny, and gene transfer also exert an important role in controlling density, diversity, and network interactions within gut-associated symbiotic bacterial communities [8,16]. In addition, phages interact with host innate immunity and cytokine synthesis, and importantly, short-chain fatty acids promote phage production in bacteria [24]. Another important function is providing a direct defense against bacterial invasion in the mucin layer, as well as the interaction with the human immune system to maintain immune homeostasis and reduce the disease process [5]. In addition, several factors encoded by phages may also affect the pathogenicity of intestinal bacteria by promoting their adhesion, invasion, colonization, and toxin production and delivery [5].

3. Gut Virome Determination

Currently, the composition of VLPs is primarily investigated through metagenomics, where high-throughput sequencing is computationally processed to construct genomes of de novo uncultured viruses [5]. The gastrointestinal tract is a habitat with enormous viral colonization, reaching 109 VLPs per g of intestinal content [1].

The assembly of viral genomes is a highly difficult computational task and produces fragmented assemblies and chimeric contigs [1]. However, the identification of viruses without enrichment from bulk metagenomics is increasingly used and overcomes the biases of size filtration steps while allowing the identification of primarily templated but also lytic viruses [1].

Studies on human gut phages are currently limited to relatively low taxonomic levels. Although several human GV databases have been developed in the last 2 years, most bacterial gut viruses (81–93%) are new and cannot be assigned a taxonomic position [8]. Therefore, although these databases have greatly expanded our knowledge of the quality and diversity of human gut viral genomes and provided informative annotation datasets [25], there are still significant barriers that do not allow a complete understanding of human GV composition and dynamics [26]. Unlike bacteria, where 16S rRNA gene sequencing represents a unique tool to identify any bacterial species using a single criterion, DNA viruses have no component that allows similar identification. RNA viruses contain the conserved gene RNA-dependent RNA polymerase (RdRP), which allows broad viral identification [27]. However, the lack of a virome database with comprehensive annotations is a major concern in achieving broad identification of the RNA virome.

Therefore, one of the most critical shortcomings of the metagenomic approach to studying the GV is the large discrepancy between the demonstrable diversity of gut viruses and the number of known human gut-associated bacteriophage genomes, as >80% of viral sequences do not match closed reference databases [8].

4. Relationship between the Gut Virome and Metabolic Pathologies

Although studies of the relationship between the human GM and metabolic diseases have primarily focused on bacteria, in recent years, the relationship between GV and some metabolic diseases has started to be investigated, with increasing emphasis on phages. In this regard, variations in populations of some specific viral families and genera have been shown to be related to the development and progression of some metabolic diseases [28–31]. For example, the high presence of the *Mimiviridae* family in the human gut might be associated with obesity and diabetes [31]. Human adenovirus infection was identified as a significant risk factor for the progression of nonalcoholic fatty liver disease (NAFLD) [32]. Furthermore, in liver cirrhosis, GV alterations correlate with cirrhosis progression [33].

The most widely investigated matter is the relationship between the GM and intestinal diseases, primarily inflammatory bowel disease (IBD) [1,34–42], although there is also a potential relation between GV and type 1 diabetes (T1D) [28,43,44], type 2 diabetes (T2D) [45], obesity [31,46,47], hypertension [48], malnutrition and low growth rate [4,37], metabolic syndrome [49], liver diseases [33,50,51], colorectal cancer (CRC) [52–55], melanoma [56], cognitive maintenance [46], and cerebral ischemia [24] (Table 2).

4.1. Metabolic Syndrome

A variety of conditions that occur simultaneously and increase the risk of heart disease, stroke, and T2D are referred to as metabolic syndrome. These conditions include increased blood pressure, hyperglycemia, excess body fat around the waist, and elevated cholesterol or triglyceride levels [47]. The main factor influencing the development of metabolic syndrome is diet, which has been reported to affect the GM, including the GV [15].

Since the GM is a relevant player in the development of metabolic syndrome, it is reasonable to think that phages infecting these bacteria may also play an important role in metabolic syndrome by regulating such bacterial populations [49]. A recent study has shown that metabolic syndrome is associated with decreases in GV richness and diversity in a manner correlated with bacterial population patterns [49]. Dietary changes that cause a reduction in bacterial diversity have a direct consequence on GV diversity because there are bacterial species that are depleted from the GM and are therefore less accessible for predation by viruses. A recent study found that phages infecting Ruminococcaceae, Clostridiaceae, Bacteroidaceae, and Streptococcaceae predominated in the GV of patients with metabolic syndrome, whereas Bifidobacteriaceae phages were less abundant in patients with metabolic syndrome than in control samples [49]. Such results could reflect unequal predation by phages among the corresponding bacterial families in the gut [49]. This fact is interesting because bacteria of the genus *Bifidobacterium* inhibit the colonization of harmful intestinal bacteria, regulate the immune system, and exhibit anti-obesity and anti-inflammatory activities, thus preventing the progression of metabolic syndrome [57]. The identification of Bifidobacteriaceae species and their phages as more abundant among healthy controls is in line with established studies showing the depletion of these families in metabolic syndrome [58] and disease states associated with metabolic syndrome [59].

Furthermore, viral phages were significantly more prevalent in the GV of controls than in metabolic syndrome patients [49]. This apparent depletion of viral phages in GVs from metabolic syndrome patients may indicate a decrease in their infectivity and could be considered a link between this prominent human gut phage order and a disease state [49]. In contrast to what was reported by [49], the richness and diversity of the GV of children with metabolic syndrome were higher than those of normal-weight children without metabolic syndrome, along with an increased abundance of *Myoviridae* [47].

Table 2. Research works investigating the relationship between the gut virome and metabolic diseases.

Disease/Model	Subjects	Determination	Main Findings	References
Obesity/humans	128 obese subjects and 101 lean subjects	Gut virome (GV), bacteriome, and viral–bacterial correlations	-Obese subjects, especially those with type 2 diabetes (T2D), had a lower gut viral richness and diversity than lean controls. -GV may play an important role in the development of obesity and T2D. -Eleven viruses, including *Escherichia* phage, *Geobacillus* phage, and *Lactobacillus* phage, were higher in obese subjects than in lean controls.	[28]
Inflammatory Bowel disease (IBD)/humans	12 household controls, 18 Crohn's disease patients, and 42 ulcerative colitis patients	Stool samples investigated by virus-like particle enrichment and sequencing as well as bacterial 16S rRNA gene analysis	-Patients with IBD showed a significant increase in *Caudovirales* bacteriophages in their GV. -Changes in the GV may contribute to intestinal inflammation and bacterial dysbiosis.	[33]
Cirrhosis and hepatic encephalopathy/humans	40 controls and 163 cirrhotic patients	Stool metagenomics for bacteria and phages were analyzed in controls versus cirrhosis, within cirrhotic, hospitalized/not, and pre/post rifaximin	-Bacterial α-/β-diversity worsened from controls through cirrhosis patients. Phage α-diversity was similar in both groups. -No changes in α-/β-diversity of phages or bacteria were seen after postrifaximin treatment in cirrhotic patients.	[47]

Table 2. Cont.

Disease/Model	Subjects	Determination	Main Findings	References
Obesity and metabolic syndrome/humans	28 school-aged children (10 with normal weight, 10 obese, and 8 obese + metabolic syndrome)	Characterization of the gut DNA virome using metagenomic sequencing	-Phage richness and diversity of individuals with obese and obese + metabolic syndrome tended to increase with respect to controls. -The abundance of some phages correlated with gut bacterial taxa and with anthropometric and biochemical parameters altered in obese and obese + metabolic syndrome.	[50]
Bile acid metabolism/mice	7 germ-free C57BL/6J mice	Phage-induced repression of a tryptophan-rich sensory protein and repression of bile acid deconjugation	-Phages' presence in the gut can affect the microbial metabolism of bile acids. -Phague BV01 and other phages from the family Salyersviridae are ubiquitous in the human gut, can infect a broad range of Bacteroides hosts, and affect bile acid metabolism.	[24]
Cerebral ischemia/mice	6 adult C57BL/6J mice	Determination of GV composition by shotgun metagenomics in fecal samples	-Following focal ischemia, the abundances of two viral taxa decreased, and those of five viral taxa increased compared with previous cohorts. -Abundances of Clostridia-like phages and Erysipelatoclostridiaceae-like phages were decreased in the stroke compared with previous cohorts	[36]
IBD/humans	40 fecal samples	Stool samples investigated by bioinformatics viral sequencing and bacterial 16S rRNA gene analysis	-Changes in GV and increased numbers of temperate phage sequences were found in individuals with Crohn's disease. -Incorporating both bacteriome and GV composition offered better discrimination power between health and disease.	[49]
Metabolic syndrome/humans	196 participants with metabolic syndrome preceding cardiometabolic disease	Bulk whole genome and virus-like particle communities	-GV from metabolic syndrome patients exhibited low richness and diversity. -Viral clusters revealed that Candidatus Heliusviridae, a highly widespread gut phage, was found in >90% of metabolic syndrome patients.	[37]
Environmental enteric dysfunction and low growth rate/humans	94 children without diarrhea or human immunodeficiency virus	Gut bacterial and GV sequencing and analysis	- Three differentially abundant phages were identified in GV, depending on child growth velocities. -A positive correlation was found between bacteria and bacteriophage richness in children with subsequent adequate/moderate growth.	[35]
IBD/humans	Fecal samples from 24 children, 12 with inflammatory bowel disease and 12 controls	Identification of viral sequences and bacterial microbiota sequencing	-Caudovirales' relative abundance was greater than that of Microviridae in both inflammatory bowel disease patients and healthy controls. -Caudovirales was more abundant in Chron´s disease patients than in ulcerative colitis patients, but not than in control patients. -Pediatric inflammatory bowel disease patients can be distinguished from healthy controls by bacterial community composition.	[34]
Crohn´s disease/mice	12–23 BALB/CYJ mice	Disruption of normal resident microbiota with streptomycin sulphate administration and phage therapy	-A single day of treatment with a phage cocktail significantly decreased the number of adherent invasive Escherichia coli in feces. -A single dose of the phage cocktail reduced dextran sodium sulphate-induced colitis symptoms in mice.	[60]
Colorectal cancer (CRC) and colonic adenoma/humans	71 colorectal cancer patients, 63 adenoma patients, and 91 healthy controls	Metagenomic sequencing of the gut microbiome and microbial interactions in adenoma and colorectal cancer patients	-Uncultured CrAssphage was higher in healthy controls and positively associated with beneficial butyrate-producing bacteria in gut microbiota (GM). -GV was much more dynamic than the GM as the disease progressed.	[52]

Table 2. Cont.

Disease/Model	Subjects	Determination	Main Findings	References
CRC/humans	90 human subjects, (30 healthy controls, 30 of whom had adenomas, and 30 of whom had carcinomas)	Stool samples analyzed by 16S rRNA gene, whole shotgun metagenomics, and purified virus metagenomic sequencing	-The CRC-associated GV consisted primarily of temperate bacteriophages. -Phages influenced cancer by directly modulating the influential bacteria.	[39]
Enteric pathogens/mice	100 C57BL/6J mice	Viruses generated from molecular clones were used to infect cell lines to liberate virions. Subsequently, clones were used to infect mice that were euthanized and investigated for results of viral infections	-Chronic murine astrovirus complements defects in adaptive immunity by elevating cell-intrinsic IFN-λ in the intestinal epithelial barrier in immunodeficient mice. -Elements of the GV can protect against enteric pathogens in an immunodeficient host.	[51]
Alcoholic hepatitis/humans	89 patients with alcoholic hepatitis, 36 with alcohol use disorder, and 17 healthy people as controls	Metagenomic sequencing of virus-like particles from fecal samples, fractionated using differential filtration techniques	-Patients with alcohol use disorder showed increased viral diversity in fecal samples compared to controls and patients with alcoholic hepatitis. -History of antibiotic treatment was associated with higher GV diversity. -Specific viral taxa, such as *Staphylococcus* phages and *Herpesviridae*, were associated with increased hepatic disease severity.	[1]
Viral entities/humans	662 samples from 1-year-old children	Processing of metagenomics and metaviromics datasets	-Viral enrichment during sample processing showed a loss of a significant part of the GV and did not represent integrated bacteria containing dormant phages (prophagues). -Approximately 65–83% of the viral populations in the metavirome were not aligned with the metagenome data.	[61]
Nonalcoholic fatty liver diseases (NAFLD)/humans	73 patients with NAFLD	RNA and DNA virus-like particles from fecal samples	-Patients with NAFLD and cirrhosis showed a significant decrease in intestinal viral diversity compared with controls. -Advanced NAFLD was associated with a reduction in the proportion of phages compared with other intestinal viruses.	[62]
IBD/humans	54 Patients with IBD and 23 healthy controls	Virus-like particles were purified from stool samples and characterized by DNA and RNA sequencing and VLP particle counts	-Viral populations associated with IBD showed perturbations with respect to healthy controls. -*Anelloviridae* showed a higher prevalence in IBD compared to healthy controls, and *Analloviridae* DNA levels were biomarkers of the effectiveness of immunosuppression. -IBD subjects had a higher ratio of *Caudovirales* to *Microviridae* phages compared to healthy controls.	[54]
CRC/humans	80 colorectal primary tumors tissues and corresponding normal colorectal tissues	GV and bacteriome analysis for CRC tissues	-The number of viral species increased whereas bacterial species decreased in CRC tissues compared with healthy ones. -Phages were the most preponderant viral species in CRC tissues, and the main families were *Myoviridae*, *Siphoviridae*, and *Podoviridae*. -Primary CRC tissues were enriched for Enterobacteria, *Bacillus*, *Proteus*, and *Streptococcus* phages, together with their pathogenic hosts in contrast to normal tissues.	[45]
Type 2 diabetes (T2D)/humans	71 T2D patients and 74 healthy controls	Whole-community metagenomic sequencing data of fecal samples	-Significant increase in the number of gut phages in fecal samples was found in the T2D group. -Significant alterations of the gut phageome cannot be explained simply by covariation with the altered bacterial hosts.	[46]

Table 2. *Cont.*

Disease/Model	Subjects	Determination	Main Findings	References
Cognitive maintenance/humans	120 subjects, 60 with obesity and 60 without obesity	Neuropsychological assessment in humans, extraction of fecal genomic DNA and whole-genome shotgun sequencing	-GV was dominated by *Caudovirales* and *Microviridae* phages. -Subjects with increased *Caudovirales* and *Siphoviridae* levels in the gut microbiome performed better cognitive status. -Phages should be considered novel actors in the microbiome–brain axis.	[46]
Cognitive maintenance/mice	11 mice were orally gavaged with saline and fecal material from humans	Behavioral testing in mice and study of gene expression in mouse prefrontal cortex	-Microbiota transplantation from human donors with increased specific *Caudovirales* levels led to increased scores in novel object recognition. -Phages should be considered novel actors in the microbiome–brain axis.	[53]
CRC/humans	74 patients with CRC and 92 healthy controls	Shotgun metagenomic analyses of viromes of fecal samples	-Gut phage community diversity was significantly increased in patients with CRC compared with controls. -GV dysbiosis was associated with early- and late-stage CRC.	[63]
Fructose intake/mice	25 C57BL/6J mice per group were used for phage production, and 36 mice were used for the in vivo dietary crossover study	*Lactobacillus reuteri* survival and phage production during gastrointestinal transit in mice	-Fructose intake activated the Ack pathway, involved in generating acetic acid, which promotes phage production.	[64]
Malnutrition/humans	8 monozygotic and 12 dizygotic twin pairs	Shotgun pyrosequencing of VLP-derived DNA	-Phage plus members of the *Anelloviridae* and *Circoviridae* families of eukaryotic viruses discriminate discordant from concordant healthy pairs.	[43]
Type 1 diabetes (T1D)/humans	103 T1D children and their mothers	Determination of virus antibodies, enterovirus RNA, and enzyme immunoassay analysis	-Autoantibody-positive children had more enterovirus infections than autoantibody-negative children before the appearance of autoantibodies. -Enterovirus infections seem to be associated with the induction of β-cell autoimmunity in young children with increased genetic susceptibility to T1D.	[65]
High-fat diet/mice	12 C57BL/6J pregnant female mice	Mice were administered with subtherapeutic antibiotic dosages or no antibiotic and subsequently analyzed for GV composition and 16S rRNA metagenomics	-High-fat diet significant shift away from the relatively abundant *Siphoviridae*, accompanied by increases in phages from the *Microviridae* family. -Phage structural genes significantly decreased after the transition to a high-fat diet.	[41]
IBD/humans and mice	Fecal samples collected from 3 ulcerative colitis patients in remission and 3 unrelated healthy controls were transferred to C57BL/6 mice	Fecal virus-like particles (VLPs) isolated from ulcerative colitis patients and healthy controls were transferred to mice	-VLPs isolated from ulcerative colitis patients specifically altered the relative abundances of several bacterial taxa involved in IBD progression in mice. -Phages are dynamic regulators of GM and implicate the GV in modulating intestinal inflammation and disease.	[31]
T1D/humans	Fecal samples from 11 children who had developed serum autoantibodies associated with T1D and healthy controls	Detection of phage and eukaryotic viral sequences	-GV of T1D subjects was less diverse than those of controls. Lower phage diversity in cases than in controls. -Specific components of the GV were both directly and inversely associated with the development of human autoimmune disease. -Among eukaryotic viruses, there was a significant enrichment of *Circoviridae*-related sequences in controls in comparison with T1D patients.	[44]
Hypertension/humans	196 samples	Viral and bacterial metagenomic investigation of fecal samples	-Virus could have higher discrimination power than bacteria to differentiate healthy prehypertension samples from hypertension patients	[48]

4.2. Obesity, Diabetes and Malnutrition

Obesity and diabetes are two forms of metabolic diseases that are highly prevalent worldwide [31]. In recent decades, there has been substantial evidence that abnormalities in GM composition can play a major role in the development of both diseases, although most evidence refers to gut bacterial composition and activities [66]. However, recent findings found significant differences in some viral families between obese and diabetic patients with respect to healthy patients in children [43,44] and mouse models [67].

A recent study found that both viral richness and diversity in the GV were lower than those found for lean subjects and in obese patients with T2D compared to lean controls [31]. Surprisingly, these results are contradictory to those previously reported by Ma et al. [45], who found a higher phage richness in T2D patients than in nondiabetic controls, as well as an increased relative abundance of the families *Siphoviridae*, *Podoviridae*, and *Myoviridae* and the unclassified order *Caudovirales* in T2D patients [45]. Previous Enterovirus infection was found to be a risk factor for T1D in children [43]. Afterward, another study showed a higher prevalence of the families *Circoviridae* and *Picornaviridae* in T1D pediatric patients than in healthy children [44].

High-fat-diet-induced obese mice showed a significant reduction in the family *Siphoviriade* and an increase in the virus families *Microviridae*, *Phycodnaviridae*, and *Miniviridae* in the fecal virome [65]. Rasmussen et al. [67] proposed GV modification as a potential therapeutic strategy against T1D and obesity. To verify this hypothesis, VLPs were transferred from slim mice to high-fat diet-induced obese mice, and as a result, weight gain and diabetes symptoms significantly decreased in obese mice [67].

Regarding viral species, 17 were found to have significantly different proportions in obese and diabetic subjects compared with lean subjects [65]. Among them, 4 viral species (*Micromonas pusilla* virus, *Cellulophaga* phage, *Bacteroides* phage, and *Halovirus*, unclassified DNA viruses) were higher in obese and T2D patients, whereas 13 viral species, including Hokovirus, Klosneuvirus, and Catovirus, were lower in obese-plus-T2D subjects with respect to lean controls [31,65].

Malnutrition is a global health problem that affects large numbers of individuals regardless of age, gender, race, social status, and geographic boundaries. It can be defined as an imbalance between energy and nutrient intake and the individual's requirements, which can alter body measurements, compositions, and functions [68]. Children with malnutrition have been reported to have an immature gut GM composition compared to those without malnutrition. This lack of maturity in their GM is characterized by a lower α-diversity of the GM as well as a disproportionate expansion of the phylum Proteobacteria [69]. Similarly, disruption of the GV, including that of intestinal phages and eukaryotic virus members, could increase the risk of severe acute malnutrition [64]. A recent study found that phages of the order *Caudovirales* contributed differentially to stunted growth in malnutrition induced by environmental enteric dysfunction [37]. As the phylum Proteobacteria exists in a higher proportion in the GM with malnutrition relative to that of children without stunting and as *Caudovirales* phages (especially *Siphoviridae*) have Proteobacteria as one of the main bacterial hosts [70] and are also present in greater numbers in malnourished children than in healthy children, there might be a cooccurring phage-bacterial dynamic in the gut of stunted children [14], with both viruses/phages contributing to the severity of malnutrition.

4.3. Liver Diseases

The liver is a very important pivotal organ for host metabolism and maintains bidirectional communication with the gut via the gut–liver axis [61]. Thus, the liver plays a central role in the pathogenesis of several metabolic diseases. Recent works have investigated the potential changes in GV linked to liver diseases such as alcoholic hepatitis [51], NAFLD [61], and bile acid metabolism [50]. Additionally, although it is not a liver disease itself, the potential changes in the GV in response to the high intake of fructose are also important [63]. Beyond its lipogenic effect, fructose intake is also related to hepatic inflammation and cellular stress, such as oxidative and endoplasmic stress, which contributes to the progression of simple steatosis to nonalcoholic fatty liver disease [71].

In the case of NAFLD, patients with a more severe disease showed lower viral diversity than patients with a lower degree of disease or healthy controls [61]. At the same time, the proportion of phages among the total GV was also significantly lower in the case of severe NAFLD patients than in the less severe cases of the controls [61].

Regarding fructose intake, fructose increases the growth of *Lactobacillus reuteri*, a key important bacterial species considered an important lysogen, which are bacterial prophages inserted within their genomes that promote phage production [63]. Due to its higher sweetening power, fructose is one of the most abundant sugars consumed in a Western-style diet and results in more pronounced fructose-mediated phage production by *L. reuteri* than the intake of other sugars [63].

In the case of alcoholic liver disease, disease-specific alterations in the GV were reported, and gut viruses were identified as potent drivers of alcohol-specific liver disease [51]. In contrast to NAFLD, in alcoholic liver disease, increased viral diversity was found in patients with alcoholic liver disease, especially in those with a higher degree of alcoholic hepatitis [51]. Regarding viral proportions, the authors found an increase in eukaryotic viruses such as *Parvoviridae* and *Herpesviridae*, along with increases in intestinal phages such as Enterobacteriaceae phages, *Escherichia* phages, and *Enterococcus* phages in patients with alcoholic liver disease compared to controls [51]. Both *Parvoviridae* and *Herpesviridae* may be found in higher proportions in NAFLD subjects because they may have a depressed immune system or because the medication administered to them indirectly causes increased replication of the viruses in host cells [51]. The latter aspect regarding the relation of GV and hepatic disease is the relation of the activity of the *Bacteroides* phage BV01, a temperate phage integrated into *Bacteroides vulgatus*, a species that can repress the microbial modification of the bile acid pool in the host, which could be linked to beneficial changes in human host metabolism [50].

4.4. Cancer

Although the relationship between the GV and some types of cancer, such as metastatic melanoma [56] or adenoma [60], has been investigated, most works on the relationship between the human GV and cancer have focused on colorectal cancer (CRC) [52–55,60], which is logical since it is the type of cancer that has the most direct contact with the intestinal virome. According to Wong and Yu [72], CRC is related to modifications in the GM, in which some bacterial genera, such as *Roseburia*, are potentially protective taxa, whereas other genera, such as *Bacteroides*, *Escherichia*, *Fusobacterium*, and *Porphyromona*, are considered procarcinogenic agents.

Metagenomic analysis of stool samples from CRC patients revealed an increase in the richness and diversity of the intestinal GV with respect to control patients [53,54,60]. In another case, it was found that the differences between CRC patients and controls were insufficient for identifying specific virome communities between healthy and cancerous states [52]. The fact that phage richness is higher in CRC patients was hypothesized to be due to an increase in intestinal permeability, known as a "leaky gut", caused by this phage, which facilitates the infiltration of pathogens and triggers chronic inflammation [73]. Another study found that phages, especially those from the families *Siphoviridae* and *Myoviridae*, are vital driving factors during the transformation from a healthy intestine to intestinal adenocarcinoma and to CRC [49].

In another work, the families Inovirus and Tunalikerirus were related to the development of CRC due to their capacity to insert random oligonucleotides into the bacterial genome, stimulating the production of bacterial biofilms and thus contributing to the carcinogenesis of the colon [74]. Both families are known to infect gram-negative bacterial hosts, including enterotoxigenic *Bacteroides fragilis*, *Fusobacterium nucleatum*, and genotoxic *Escherichia coli*, bacterial species often implicated in CRC development [53].

Another recent study of the GV in bulk from CRC patients reported significant reductions in Enterobacteria phages and CrAssphages compared to healthy controls [60]. Some viral species were reported to have the potential to act as discriminant markers of CRC; Orthobunyavirus, Tunalikevirus, Phikzlikevirus, Betabaculovirus, and Sp6likevirus were the viral genera with significantly higher abundances in CRC patients than in control patients [53].

Upon investigating primary tumor tissues of CRC, phages were found to be the most preponderant viral species, and the main families were *Myoviridae*, *Siphoviridae*, and *Podoviridae* [54,75]. The most frequently detected eukaryotic viruses include human endogenous Retrovirus K113, human Herpesviruses 7 and 6B, Megavirus chilensis, Cytomegalovirus, and Epstein-Barr virus [54]. A higher relative presence of human papillomavirus was also found in CRC versus non-CRC tissues [76]. Additionally, it was also shown that Epstein-Barr virus infection could contribute to CRC development by inducing mutagenesis in intestinal cells [54].

5. Intestinal Diseases Mediated by Bacteria

One of the earliest applications of phages in human medicine was their use as tools to fight pathogenic or antimicrobial-resistant bacteria. By infecting bacteria, phages can significantly alter the GM, primarily by integrating into bacterial genomes as prophages (lysogeny) or by killing bacteria (lysis). Among these, an increase in phage lytic action is associated with decreased bacterial diversity in IBD [50]. By modulating the intestinal bacteriome, intestinal phages show promising therapeutic potential in several diseases beyond bacterial infections [26] as well as therapeutic options in the treatment of drug-resistant infections in humans [77].

Among digestive tract diseases, IBD is a chronic inflammatory disease that is subdivided into two categories: Ulcerative colitis (UC) and Crohn's disease (CD). Although the exact cause of IBD remains unknown, it was hypothesized that an alteration of the GM is closely related to its pathogenesis and significantly increases the risk of this disease [5]. Previous works found, for both UC and CD patients, an increase in *Caudovirales* content and a reduction in the abundance of *Microviridae*, as well as higher GV richness than those found in control patients [5]. In another recent study, a predominance of temperate virions (mostly Caudoviral taxa) was observed in the GV of IBD patients, suggesting an increased lysogenic conversion of phages [36].

In addition to phages, a recent study also demonstrated that eukaryotic virus populations that inhabit the human intestinal mucosa can be different in IBD patients with respect to healthy controls [42]. At the family level, UC patients showed a higher relative abundance of *Pneumoviridae*, whereas the *Anelloviridae* family was observed in higher proportions in healthy subjects. At the genus level, UC patients showed a higher presence of the Orthopneumovirus genus than healthy controls, whereas they showed lower amounts of the giant viruses Coccolithovirus and Minivirus, as well as the vertebrate-infecting virus Orthopoxvirus [42]. Additionally, other studies also found that the *Anelloviridae* family was more prevalent in IBD mucosal samples than in healthy controls [28,78].

6. Therapies including Transfer of Gut Viruses

The human gut microbiome strongly influences various metabolic processes, such as digestion, the immune system, and endocrine functions [49]. Therefore, GV modification has shown great potential as a disease therapy through fecal microbiota transplantation (FMT), fecal viral transplantation (FVT), and phage therapy (PhT). These therapies provide the first tantalizing evidence that manipulation of the phageome may be an effective therapeutic strategy [79]. There are precedents for the successful use of such therapies in the treatment of antibiotic-induced intestinal dysbiosis [80], IBD [7,78,79,81], obesity [67,82], T2D [67], or even certain types of cancer [55,56] (Table 3).

Table 3. Studies investigating fecal viral transplantation and its relationship with specific diseases.

Indication/Model	Subjects	Dosage and Time of Exposition	Main Findings	Reference
Inflammatory bowel disease (IBD)/humans	5 patients with symptomatic chronic-relapsing *Clostridium difficile* infection	Stool collection and characterization according to fecal microbiota transplantation (FMT) standards	-Fecal filtrate transfer (FFT) eliminated symptoms of *C. difficile* infection for a minimum period of 6 months. -Bacterial components, metabolites, or phages mediate many of the effects of FMT, and FFT might be an alternative approach, particularly for immunocompromised patients.	[79]
IBD/piglets	16 piglets were used to obtain FFT, transferred to 14 piglets by rectal transfer and to 13 by oro-gastric administration	FMT administration by cognate rectal FFT, oro-gastric FFT administration, and saline solutions	-FFT increased viral diversity and reduced Proteobacteria abundance in the ileal mucosa of FFT receiver piglets relative to controls.	[81]
Obesity and type 2 diabetes (T2D) induced by diet/mice	40 C57Bl/&NTac mice	Mice with a high-fat diet plus fecal viral transplantation (FVT) and high-fat diet plus ampicillin plus FVT were compared to controls	-At both 4 and 6 weeks after the first FVT, a significantly lower body weight gain was observed in the high-fat diet + FVT mice and compared to high-fat diet mice. -FVT normalized the blood glucose tolerance in the high-fat + FVT mice. -FVT strongly influences and partly reshapes the gut microbiota composition both with and without ampicillin treatment.	[67]
Phage adherence/in vitro	Bacteriophage T4	T4 phages were serially diluted and used to inoculate plates	-Phage adherence to the mucus model provides immunity applicable to mucosal surfaces. -The symbiotic relationship between phage and hosts provides protection for mucosal surfaces.	[83]
IBD/mice	C57BL/6J and C3H/HeJBir wild-type and Il10 mice kept under special pathogen-free conditions	Norovirus infection and investigation in changes induced in structural and functional intestinal barrier changes	-Norovirus caused epithelial barrier disruption in Il10 mice. -Norovirus might trigger individuals with a nonsymptomatic predisposition for IBD by impairment of the intestinal mucosa.	[78]
Antibiotic disturbance/mice	16 BALB/c mice	Administration of antibiotic treatment in the drinking water for 2 days	-Mice showed a perturbed microbiome because of antibiotic treatment, which was reverted over time similar to the pretreatment one. -Mice that had received FVT maintained gut microbiota (GM) more similar to the original before antibiotic treatment compared to mice that had received nonviable phages.	[80]

Table 3. Cont.

Indication/Model	Subjects	Dosage and Time of Exposition	Main Findings	Reference
Obesity/humans	A total of 87 individuals took part-565 individuals responded to advertisements	Fecal microbiome transfer	-There was no effect of FMT on weight loss in adolescents with obesity, although a reduction in abdominal adiposity was observed.	[82]
Clostridium difficile infection/mice	26 C57BL/6 mice	Comparison of effects of the fecal VLP fraction against conventional FMT on the ileal microbiome	-VLP fraction played a potential role in modifying the gut microbiome during dysbiosis. -In both recipient groups, transplantation of the fecal VLP fraction alone produced the same outcome as that of the whole FMT.	[7]
Melanoma/humans	10 patients with anti-PD-1-refractory metastatic melanoma	Fecal transfer by FMT	-FMT showed favorable effects in immune cell infiltrates and gene expression profiles in both the gut lamina propia and tumor microenvironment. -There were two partial responses and one complete response in melanoma patients after FMT.	[56]
Colorectal cancer/humans	72 patients with colorectal cancer and 52 healthy subjects	Elimination of *F. nucleatum* by phages	-Oral administration of the phage-guided irinotecan-loaded nanoparticles in piglets led to negligible changes in hemocyte counts, immunoglobulin, and histamine levels, as well as liver and renal functions. -Phage-guided nanotechnology for the modulation of the GM might inspire new approaches for the treatment of colorectal cancer.	[55]
Stunting/humans	15 nonstunted and 15 stunted children	Isolation of gut phages, sterilization, and cross-infection of gut bacteria community belonging to other children	-Gut phages can regulate gut bacterial abundance and composition in an age-specific manner. -Proteobacteria from non-stunted children increased in the presence of phages from younger stunted children.	[14]
Leaky gut/rats	5 Wistar rats	Phage cocktail was given to rats for 10 days	-Increased intestinal permeability may be induced by phages that affect GM.	[73]
Obesity and T2D/humans	61 patients	Fecal transfer by FMT from healthy donors	-FMT achieved ≥20% of lean-associated microbiota in obese with T2D patients	[84]

Table 3. Cont.

Indication/Model	Subjects	Dosage and Time of Exposition	Main Findings	Reference
Clostridium difficile infection/humans	24 subjects with Clostridium difficile infection and 20 healthy controls	Ultradeep metagenomic sequencing of virus-like particle preparations and bacterial 16S rRNA sequencing	-Subjects with Clostridium difficile infection showed a significantly higher abundance of Caudovirales and lower Caudovirales diversity, richness, and evenness compared with healthy controls. -FMT decreased the abundance of Caudovirales in Clostridium difficile infection. Symptoms of infections decreased when most Caudovirales came from the donor and not from the recipient.	[42]
Intestinal inflammation and colitis/humans and mice	58 C57Bl/6 and Swiss Webster germfree mice 20 Patients with active ulcerative colitis	Three independent experiments with a total of n = 23 for vehicle-treated animals and n = 21 for bacteriophage-treated animals	-Treating germ-free mice with bacteriophages led to immune cell expansion in the gut. -Increasing bacteriophage levels exacerbated colitis via toll-like receptors 9 and IFN-γ stimulation. -Phages from active ulcerative colitis patients induced more IFN-γ compared to healthy individuals.	[38]

FMT is one of the most effective and accepted approaches to modulating the GM by restoring gut microbiome homeostasis through the reintroduction of beneficial microbes from a healthy donor [20]. The viral mechanism of action contributing to FMT therapies involves tripartite mutualistic interactions among bacteriophages or eukaryotic viruses, bacteria, and the host [20]. This approach has been successfully employed in clinical trials for the treatment of diseases such as IBD [85]. In fact, the efficacy of FMT in the treatment of *C. difficile* infections is approximately 90% and is currently the most promising application of FMT [20]. Additionally, FMT has also been successfully employed as a treatment for other symptoms and diseases, such as in the restoration of dysbiosis originating from severe antimicrobial treatments [80], showing better results than probiotic administration [20]. In addition, FMT was also useful in treating metabolic diseases such as T1D [86], T2D [84], obesity combined with T2D [67], necrotizing enterocolitis, small intestinal bacterial growth, and post-antibiotic microbiome dysbiosis [7,20]. These results, especially those in humans [84,86], suggest that FMT can change the metabolic repertoire of bacterial/mammalian host communities and/or regulate the profile of metabolic gene expression in the bacteriome.

However, the use of FMT presents significant risks to the health of the recipient subject due to the potential presence of pathogens, particularly obligate and opportunistic bacterial pathogens. Thus, an alternative option that avoids this risk is the use of FVT in which both eukaryotic and bacterial cells are removed, whereas the entire viral portion of a fecal sample is provided to another host [79]. In this regard, it was reported that some changes in viral populations could be related to the development of pediatric T1D [43] as well as pediatric and adult inflammatory bowel disease, including the reproducible expansion of *Caudovirales* and the reduction of *Microviridae* [28,35,36,40,42]. Among the methods using filtered fecal transplantation, FVT removes fecal bacteria and thus decreases the risk of bacterial infection associated with FMT, although the recipient maintains certain risks to the recipient due to the potential transfer of unwanted eukaryotic viruses (Figure 2). A seminal study by Ott et al. [79] demonstrated that administration of a sterile fecal filtrate achieved successful remission in patients with *C. difficile* infection. However, it should be considered that although the presence of eukaryotic viruses in the gut is essential for good maintenance of intestinal microbial homeostasis and host immunity [20], the human gut can harbor numerous genera of potentially pathogenic viruses, such as papillomaviruses, herpesviruses, hepatitis viruses, bocaviruses, enteroviruses, rotaviruses, and sapoviruses [87]. Therefore, FVT could be potentially dangerous, particularly for immunocompromised hosts [5]. Thus, especially for these patients, thorough GV monitoring of the donor should be performed to avoid the potential health risks derived from fecal transplantation [5].

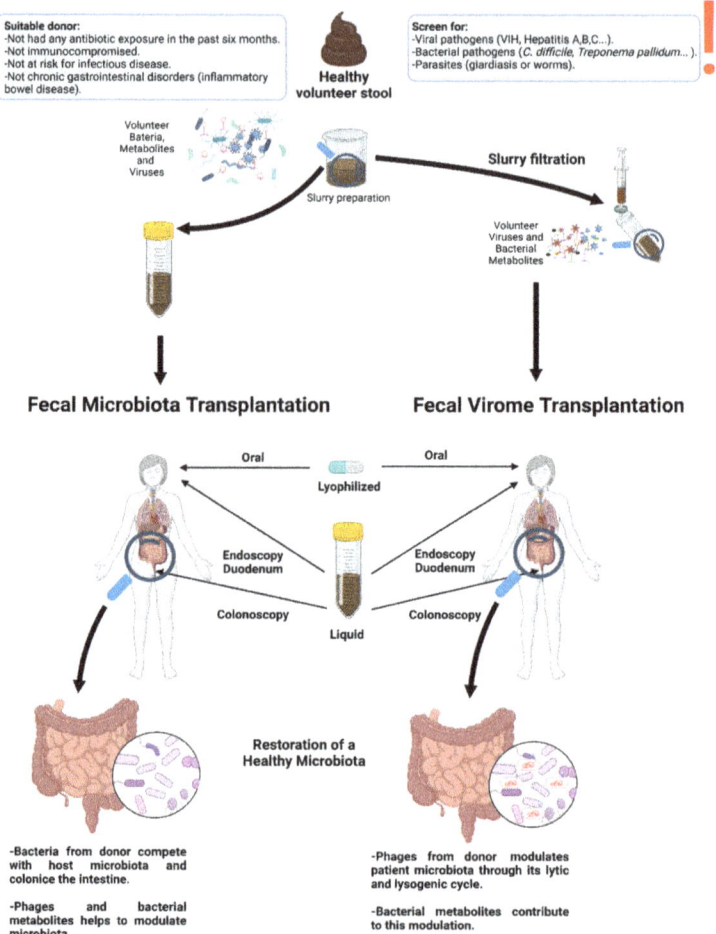

Figure 2. Representation of microbiota and virome transplantation in humans. The first step in this process is the selection of healthy volunteers and the creation of biobanks with stool samples. Volunteers must meet several requirements and have pathogen-free stool to avoid disease transmission to the transplant recipient. Two different strategies have been developed when performing fecal transplants. In fecal microbiota transplantation (FMT), no microorganisms are removed from the samples, whereas in fecal virome transplantation (FVT), the feces are filtered to eliminate the bacteria, molds, and yeasts present in the donor's samples and to keep only the viruses, primarily bacteriophages, present in the fecal samples. Fecal transplants can be administered in a variety of ways, for example, through gastroscopy or colonoscopy. Stool samples can also be lyophilized, and therefore, these transplants can be performed orally, through the administration of a tablet, or through the anal route in the form of a suppository.

Another option is PhT, a method that uses only phages to treat bacterial infections, which has demonstrated advantages in treating pathogenic and/or drug-resistant bacterial infections [5]. Currently, there is evidence that phages can stimulate and modulate the immune system of the host by various mechanisms. Indeed, phages can colonize the intestinal mucus layer, directly bind to mucin glycoproteins via their capsis, and provide the mammalian host with a defense mechanism against bacteria trying to breach the intestinal barrier [83]. Phages can also induce innate defenses from the host against bacterial colonization, stimulating the production of inflammatory cytokines and activating dendritic cells and innate lymphoid cells to produce interferons [20]. Some exploratory studies found a curative role of PhT in the treatment of extraintestinal diseases [5], such as improving diabetes outcomes in mice [64], reducing necrotizing enterocolitis in piglets [82], and reducing *Clostridium difficile* infection symptoms in humans, toward the ability of gut phages to restrict pathobiont growth and to improve the richness of the GM [79].

Both FVT and PhT have been applied to reshape the dysbiotic gut microbiome caused by antibiotic treatments [80], as well as in the treatment of various metabolic diseases, such as metabolic syndrome [82], mental disorders [88], and malignant tumors [56]. The majority of PhT studies are still exploratory and have been conducted in mice, and their results need to be confirmed in humans [5]. However, recent studies revealed that the relationships between phages and bacterial populations might influence growth stunting in children [14,37]. It was found that a combined therapy using phages targeting *Fusobacterium nucleatum* (a tumor-causing bacterium) and irinotecan (an antitumor drug) effectively inhibited the growth of *F. nucleatum* but stimulated the proliferation of the butyrate-producing bacterium *Clostridium butyricum* in mice [55]. In addition, other work showed that administering rats with a bacteriophage cocktail against *Staphylococcus*, *Streptococcus*, *Proteus*, *Pseudomonas*, *Escherichia coli*, *Klebsiella pneumoniae*, and *Salmonella* spp. achieved increased intestinal permeability, weight loss, and reduced pathogen activity [73]. Another recent study showed that phage supplementation with Lactococcal 936 bacteriophage increased memory in flies [46]. The authors attributed this effect to phages of the *Siphoviridae* family, which are positively associated with cognition, suggesting a possible association with poststroke cognitive dysfunction [46].

However, the results from PhT were not positive in all cases. In this sense, it was reported that the transplantation of VLPs from UC patient feces to human microbiota-associated mice aggravated colitis in mice and worsened the bacterial taxa associated with IBD pathogenesis [41,79]. In another work, the administration of a cocktail of Enterobacteriaceae phages belonging to the order *Caudovirales* exacerbated intestinal inflammation and did not induce the lysis of any endogenous microbes [38]. Thus, a better understanding of broad phage activity is necessary prior to proposing this strategy for more widespread use than is currently the case.

7. Conclusions

Although bacteria represent the most abundant population and account for the most DNA in the GM, other populations, such as viruses, are also abundant and can interact with both host and bacteria in various forms. Thus, one of the causes for which prebiotics and/or probiotics sometimes show lower than expected effects, both in intensity and duration, in the correction of intestinal dysbiosis could be the interaction with other microorganisms from the GM, such as viruses. Here, we present the latest scientific evidence that some phages and eukaryotic viruses can affect not only diseases impacting the digestive system but also metabolic diseases such as metabolic syndrome, obesity, T1D and T2D, and even cognitive status. The major barriers to a good understanding of GV composition and functions are the low VLP alignment capability with datasets and bioinformatic tools, as well as the ease of the degradation of RNA viruses from decay during metagenomic sequencing. In addition, DNA viruses do not possess any equivalent to the bacterial 16S rRNA gene, which would allow their rapid identification. However, it is important to avoid barriers that currently limit GV determination. Thus, in the near future, stool metagenomic investigations should include the identification of bacteria and viruses and their correlation networks. With this approach, it would be possible to achieve a better understanding of the action of intestinal viruses on metabolic diseases, as well as the use of fecal or viral transfer tools in the prevention and/or treatment of these pathologies.

Author Contributions: Conceptualization, H.C.A. and J.M.M.; methodology, J.M.M.; writing—original draft preparation, S.E. and A.L.-S.; writing—review and editing, A.L. and A.C.-C. visualization, A.d.C.M.P.; supervision, H.C.A.; project administration, J.M.M.; funding acquisition, J.M.M. All authors have read and agreed to the published version of the manuscript.

Funding: The APC was funded by European Regional Development Funds (FEDER), grant ED431C 2018/05.

Institutional Review Board Statement: Not applicable.

Informed Consent Statement: Not applicable.

Data Availability Statement: Not applicable.

Acknowledgments: The authors thank the European Regional Development Funds (FEDER), grant ED431C 2018/05, and National Institute of Allergy and Infectious Diseases (NIH/ NIAID), grant R01 AI109022, for covering the cost of publication. We also want to thank the Fullbright program of the Spanish Ministerio de Universidades, grant PRX21/00141, for covering the stage of Jose Manuel Miranda Lopez at Cornell University.

Conflicts of Interest: The authors declare no conflict of interest.

References

1. Johansen, J.; Plichta, D.R.; Nissen, J.N.; Jespersen, M.L.; Shah, S.A.; Deng, L.; Stokholm, J.; Bisgaard, H.; Nielsen, D.S.; Sørensen, S.J.; et al. Genome binning of viral entities from bulk metagenomics data. *Nat. Commun.* **2022**, *13*, 965. [CrossRef] [PubMed]
2. Roca-Saavedra, P.; Mendez-Vilabrille, V.; Miranda, J.M.; Nebot, C.; Cardelle-Cobas, A.; Franco, C.M.; Cepeda, A. Food additives, contaminants and other minor components: Effects on human gut microbiota—A review. *J. Physiol. Biochem.* **2018**, *74*, 69–83. [CrossRef] [PubMed]
3. Lopez-Santamarina, A.; Mondragon, A.D.C.; Lamas, A.; Miranda, J.M.; Franco, C.M.; Cepeda, A. Animal-origin prebiotics based on chitin: An alternative for the future? a critical review. *Foods* **2020**, *9*, 782. [CrossRef] [PubMed]
4. Liang, G.; Bushman, F.D. The human virome: Assembly, composition and host interactions. *Nat. Rev. Microbiol.* **2021**, *19*, 514–527. [CrossRef] [PubMed]
5. Cao, Z.; Sugimura, N.; Burgermeister, E.; Ebert, M.P.; Zuo, T.; Lan, P. The gut virome: A new microbiome component in health and disease. *eBioMedicine* **2022**, *81*, 104113. [CrossRef]
6. Kennedy, E.A.; Holtz, L.R. Gut virome in early life: Origins and implications. *Curr. Opin. Virol.* **2022**, *55*, 101233. [CrossRef]
7. Lim, E.S.; Zhou, Y.; Zhao, G.; Bauer, I.K.; Droit, L.; Ndao, I.M.; Warner, B.B.; Tarr, P.I.; Wang, D.; Holtz, L.R. Early life dynamics of the human gut virome and bacterial microbiome in infants. *Nat. Med.* **2015**, *21*, 1228–1234. [CrossRef]
8. Shkoporov, A.N.; Hill, C. Bacteriophages of the human gut: The "known unknown" of the microbiome. *Cell Host Microbe* **2019**, *25*, 195–209. [CrossRef]
9. Yutin, N.; Makarova, K.S.; Gussow, A.B.; Krupovic, M.; Segall, A.; Edwards, R.A.; Koonin, E.V. Discovery of an expansive bacteriophage family that includes the most abundant viruses from the human gut. *Nat. Microbiol.* **2018**, *3*, 38–46. [CrossRef]
10. Shkoporov, A.N.; Clooney, A.G.; Sutton, T.D.S.; Ryan, F.J.; Daly, K.M.; Nolan, J.A.; McDonnell, S.A.; Khokhlova, E.V.; Draper, L.A.; Forde, A.; et al. The human gut virome is highly diverse, stable, and individual specific. *Cell Host Microbe* **2019**, *26*, 527–541.e5. [CrossRef]
11. Dutilh, B.E.; Cassman, N.; McNair, K.; Sanchez, S.E.; Silva, G.G.Z.; Boling, L.; Barr, J.J.; Speth, D.R.; Seguritan, V.; Aziz, R.K.; et al. A highly abundant bacteriophage discovered in the unknown sequences of human faecal metagenomes. *Nat. Commun.* **2014**, *5*, 4498. [CrossRef] [PubMed]
12. Zuo, T.; Sun, Y.; Wan, Y.; Yeoh, Y.K.; Zhang, F.; Cheung, C.P.; Chen, N.; Luo, J.; Wang, W.; Sung, J.J.Y.; et al. Human-gut-DNA virome variations across geography, ethnicity, and urbanization. *Cell Host Microbe* **2020**, *28*, 741–751.e4. [CrossRef] [PubMed]
13. Gregory, A.C.; Zablocki, O.; Zayed, A.A.; Howell, A.; Bolduc, B.; Sullivan, M.B. The gut virome database reveals age-dependent patterns of virome diversity in the human gut. *Cell Host Microbe* **2020**, *28*, 724–740.e8. [CrossRef] [PubMed]
14. Khan Mirzaei, M.; Khan, M.A.A.; Ghosh, P.; Taranu, Z.E.; Taguer, M.; Ru, J.; Chowdhury, R.; Kabir, M.M.; Deng, L.; Mondal, D.; et al. Bacteriophages isolated from stunted children can regulate gut bacterial communities in an age-specific manner. *Cell Host Microbe* **2020**, *27*, 199–212.e5. [CrossRef]
15. Minot, S.; Sinha, R.; Chen, J.; Li, H.; Keilbaugh, S.A.; Wu, G.D.; Lewis, J.D.; Bushman, F.D. The human gut virome: Inter-individual variation and dynamic response to diet. *Genome Res.* **2011**, *21*, 1616–1625. [CrossRef]

16. Hsu, B.B.; Gibson, T.E.; Yeliseyev, V.; Liu, Q.; Lyon, L.; Bry, L.; Silver, P.A.; Gerber, G.K. Dynamic modulation of the gut microbiota and metabolome by bacteriophages in a mouse model. *Cell Host Microbe* **2019**, *25*, 803–814.e5. [CrossRef]
17. Edwards, R.A.; McNair, K.; Faust, K.; Raes, J.; Dutilh, B.E. Computational approaches to predict bacteriophage-host relationships. *FEMS Microbiol. Rev.* **2016**, *40*, 258–272. [CrossRef]
18. Lam, S.; Bai, X.; Shkoporov, A.N.; Park, H.; Wu, X.; Lan, P.; Zuo, T. Roles of the gut virome and mycobiome in faecal microbiota transplantation. *Lancet Gastroenterol. Hepatol.* **2022**, *7*, 472–484. [CrossRef]
19. Łoś, M.; Węgrzyn, G. Pseudolysogeny. *Adv. Virus Res.* **2012**, *82*, 339–349. [CrossRef]
20. Mäntynen, S.; Laanto, E.; Oksanen, H.M.; Poranen, M.M.; Díaz-Muñoz, S.L. Black box of phage–bacterium interactions: Exploring alternative phage infection strategies. *Open Biol.* **2021**, *11*, 210188. [CrossRef]
21. Rascovan, N.; Duraisamy, R.; Desnues, C. Metagenomics and the human virome in asymptomatic individuals. *Annu. Rev. Microbiol.* **2016**, *70*, 17. [CrossRef]
22. Zhang, T.; Breitbart, M.; Lee, W.H.; Run, J.-Q.; Wei, C.L.; Soh, S.W.L.; Hibberd, M.L.; Liu, E.T.; Rohwer, F.; Ruan, Y. RNA viral community in human feces: Prevalence of plant pathogenic viruses. *PLoS Biol.* **2006**, *4*, 108. [CrossRef]
23. Yang, J.Y.; Kim, M.S.; Kim, E.; Cheon, J.H.; Lee, Y.S.; Kim, Y.; Lee, S.H.; Seo, S.U.; Shin, S.H.; Choi, S.S.; et al. Enteric viruses ameliorate gut inflammation via toll-like receptor 3 and toll-like receptor 7-mediated interferon-β production. *Immunity* **2016**, *44*, 889–900. [CrossRef]
24. Chelluboina, B.; Kieft, K.; Breister, A.; Anantharaman, K.; Vemuganti, R. Gut virome dysbiosis following focal cerebral ischemia in mice. *J. Cereb. Blood Flow Metab.* **2022**, *42*, 1597–1602. [CrossRef] [PubMed]
25. Ferrero, D.; Ferrer-Orta, C.; Verdaguer, N. Viral RNA-dependent RNA polymerases: A structural overview. *Subdell Biochem.* **2018**, *88*, 39–71. [CrossRef]
26. Li, J.; Yang, F.; Xiao, M.; Li, A. Advances and challenges in cataloging the human gut virome. *Cell Host Microbe* **2022**, *30*, 908–916. [CrossRef] [PubMed]
27. Gregory, A.C.; Gerhardt, K.; Zhong, Z.-P.; Bolduc, B.; Temperton, B.; Konstantinidis, K.T.; Sullivan, M.B. MetaPop: A pipeline for macro- and microdiversity analyses and visualization of microbial and viral metagenome-derived populations. *Microbiome* **2022**, *10*, 49. [CrossRef]
28. Norman, J.M.; Handley, S.A.; Baldridge, M.T.; Droit, L.; Liu, C.Y.; Keller, B.C.; Kambal, A.; Monaco, C.L.; Zhao, G.; Fleshner, P.; et al. Disease-specific alterations in the enteric virome in inflammatory bowel disease. *Cell* **2015**, *160*, 447–460. [CrossRef]
29. Park, A.; Zhao, G. Mining the virome for insights into type 1 diabetes. *DNA Cell Biol.* **2018**, *37*, 422–425. [CrossRef]
30. Monaco, C.L.; Gootenberg, D.B.; Zhao, G.; Handley, S.A.; Ghebremichael, M.S.; Lim, E.S.; Lankowski, A.; Baldridge, M.T.; Wilen, C.B.; Flagg, M.; et al. Altered virome and bacterial microbiome in human immunodeficiency virus-associated acquired immunodeficiency syndrome. *Cell Host Microbe* **2016**, *19*, 311–322. [CrossRef]
31. Yang, K.; Niu, J.; Zuo, T.; Sun, Y.; Xu, Z.; Tang, W.; Liu, Q.; Zhang, J.; Ng, E.K.W.; Wong, S.K.H.; et al. Alterations in the gut virome in obesity and type 2 diabetes mellitus. *Gastroenterology* **2021**, *161*, 1257–1269.e13. [CrossRef] [PubMed]
32. Tarantino, G.; Citro, V.; Cataldi, M. Findings from studies are congruent with obesity having a viral origin, but what about obesity-related nafld? *Viruses* **2021**, *13*, 1285. [CrossRef] [PubMed]
33. Bajaj, J.S.; Sikaroodi, M.; Shamsaddini, A.; Henseler, Z.; Santiago-Rodriguez, T.; Acharya, C.; Fagan, A.; Hylemon, P.B.; Fuchs, M.; Gavis, E.; et al. Interaction of bacterial metagenome and virome in patients with cirrhosis and hepatic encephalopathy. *Gut* **2021**, *70*, 1162–1173. [CrossRef] [PubMed]
34. Galtier, M.; De Sordi, L.; Sivignon, A.; de Vallée, A.; Maura, D.; Neut, C.; Rahmouni, O.; Wannerberger, K.; Darfeuille-Michaud, A.; Desreumaux, P.; et al. Bacteriophages targeting adherent invasive *Escherichia coli* strains as a promising new treatment for Crohn's disease. *J. Crohn's Colitis* **2017**, *11*, 840–847. [CrossRef]
35. Fernandes, M.A.; Verstraete, S.G.; Phan, T.; Deng, X.; Stekol, E.; Lamere, B.; Lynch, S.V.; Heyman, M.B.; Delwart, E. Enteric virome and bacterial microbiota in children with ulcerative colitis and crohn disease. *J. Pediatr. Gastroenterol. Nutr.* **2019**, *68*, 30–36. [CrossRef]
36. Clooney, A.G.; Sutton, T.D.S.; Shkoporov, A.N.; Holohan, R.K.; Daly, K.M.; O'Regan, O.; Ryan, F.J.; Draper, L.A.; Plevy, S.E.; Ross, R.P.; et al. Whole-virome analysis sheds light on viral dark matter in inflammatory bowel disease. *Cell Host Microbe* **2019**, *26*, 764–778.e5. [CrossRef]
37. Desai, C.; Handley, S.A.; Rodgers, R.; Rodriguez, C.; Ordiz, M.I.; Manary, M.J.; Holtz, L.R. Growth velocity in children with environmental enteric dysfunction is associated with specific bacterial and viral taxa of the gastrointestinal tract in Malawian children. *PLoS Negl. Trop. Dis.* **2020**, *14*, e0008387. [CrossRef]
38. Gogokhia, L.; Buhrke, K.; Bell, R.; Hoffman, B.; Brown, D.G.; Hanke-Gogokhia, C.; Ajami, N.J.; Wong, M.C.; Ghazaryan, A.; Valentine, J.F.; et al. Expansion of bacteriophages is linked to aggravated intestinal inflammation and colitis. *Cell Host Microbe* **2019**, *25*, 285–299.e8. [CrossRef]
39. Ingle, H.; Lee, S.; Ai, T.; Orvedahl, A.; Rodgers, R.; Zhao, G.; Sullender, M.; Peterson, S.T.; Locke, M.; Liu, C.-T.; et al. Viral complementation of immunodeficiency confers protection against enteric pathogens via interferon-λ. *Nat. Microbiol.* **2019**, *4*, 1120–1128. [CrossRef]
40. Liang, W.; Feng, Z.; Rao, S.; Xiao, C.; Xue, X.; Lin, Z.; Zhang, Q.; Qi, W. Diarrhea may be underestimated: A missing link in 2019 novel coronavirus. *Gut* **2020**, *69*, 1141–1143. [CrossRef]

41. Sinha, A.; Li, Y.; Mirzaei, M.K.; Shamash, M.; Samadfam, R.; King, I.L.; Maurice, C.F. Transplantation of bacteriophages from ulcerative colitis patients shifts the gut bacteriome and exacerbates the severity of DSS colitis. *Microbiome* **2022**, *10*, 105. [CrossRef] [PubMed]
42. Zuo, T.; Lu, X.-J.; Zhang, Y.; Cheung, C.P.; Lam, S.; Zhang, F.; Tang, W.; Ching, J.Y.L.; Zhao, R.; Chan, P.K.S.; et al. Gut mucosal virome alterations in ulcerative colitis. *Gut* **2019**, *68*, 1169–1179. [CrossRef] [PubMed]
43. Sadeharju, K.; Hämäläinen, A.-M.; Knip, M.; Lönnrot, M.; Koskela, P.; Virtanen, S.M.; Ilonen, J.; Åkerblom, H.K.; Hyöty, H. Enterovirus infections as a risk factor for type I diabetes: Virus analyses in a dietary intervention trial. *Clin. Exp. Immunol.* **2003**, *132*, 271–277. [CrossRef]
44. Zhao, G.; Vatanen, T.; Droit, L.; Park, A.; Kostic, A.D.; Poon, T.W.; Vlamakis, H.; Siljander, H.; Härkönen, T.; Hämäläinen, A.-M.; et al. Intestinal virome changes precede autoimmunity in type I diabetes-susceptible children. *Proc. Natl. Acad. Sci. USA* **2017**, *114*, E6166–E6175. [CrossRef] [PubMed]
45. Ma, Y.; You, X.; Mai, G.; Tokuyasu, T.; Liu, C. A human gut phage catalog correlates the gut phageome with type 2 diabetes. *Microbiome* **2018**, *6*, 24. [CrossRef] [PubMed]
46. Mayneris-Perxachs, J.; Castells-Nobau, A.; Arnoriaga-Rodríguez, M.; Garre-Olmo, J.; Puig, J.; Ramos, R.; Martínez-Hernández, F.; Burokas, A.; Coll, C.; Moreno-Navarrete, J.M.; et al. Caudovirales bacteriophages are associated with improved executive function and memory in flies, mice, and humans. *Cell Host Microbe* **2022**, *30*, 340–356.e8. [CrossRef]
47. Bikel, S.; López-Leal, G.; Cornejo-Granados, F.; Gallardo-Becerra, L.; García-López, R.; Sánchez, F.; Equihua-Medina, E.; Ochoa-Romo, J.P.; López-Contreras, B.E.; Canizales-Quinteros, S.; et al. Gut dsDNA virome shows diversity and richness alterations associated with childhood obesity and metabolic syndrome. *iScience* **2021**, *24*, 102800. [CrossRef] [PubMed]
48. Han, M.; Yang, P.; Zhong, C.; Ning, K. The Human Gut Virome in Hypertension. *Front. Microbiol.* **2018**, *9*, 3150. [CrossRef]
49. de Jonge, P.A.; Wortelboer, K.; Scheithauer, T.P.M.; van den Born, B.J.H.; Zwinderman, A.H.; Nobrega, F.L.; Dutilh, B.E.; Nieuwdorp, M.; Herrema, H. Gut virome profiling identifies a widespread bacteriophage family associated with metabolic syndrome. *Nat. Commun.* **2022**, *13*, 3594. [CrossRef]
50. Campbell, D.E.; Ly, L.K.; Ridlon, J.M.; Hsiao, A.; Whitaker, R.J.; Degnan, P.H. Infection with bacteroides phage bv01 alters the host transcriptome and bile acid metabolism in a common human gut microbe. *Cell Rep.* **2020**, *32*, 108142. [CrossRef]
51. Jiang, L.; Lang, S.; Duan, Y.; Zhang, X.; Gao, B.; Chopyk, J.; Schwanemann, L.K.; Ventura-Cots, M.; Bataller, R.; Bosques-Padilla, F.; et al. Intestinal virome in patients with alcoholic hepatitis. *Hepatology* **2020**, *72*, 2182–2196. [CrossRef] [PubMed]
52. Hannigan, G.D.; Duhaime, M.B.; Ruffin, M.T., IV; Koumpouras, C.C.; Schloss, P.D. Diagnostic potential and interactive dynamics of the colorectal cancer virome. *mBio* **2018**, *9*, e02248-18. [CrossRef]
53. Nakatsu, G.; Zhou, H.; Wu, W.K.K.; Wong, S.H.; Coker, O.O.; Dai, Z.; Li, X.; Szeto, C.H.; Sugimura, N.; Lam, T.Y.T.; et al. Alterations in enteric virome are associated with colorectal cancer and survival outcomes. *Gastroenterology* **2018**, *155*, 529–541.e5. [CrossRef] [PubMed]
54. Marongiu, L.; Landry, J.J.M.; Rausch, T.; Abba, M.L.; Delecluse, S.; Delecluse, H.J.; Allgayer, H. Metagenomic analysis of primary colorectal carcinomas and their metastases identifies potential microbial risk factors. *Mol. Oncol.* **2021**, *15*, 3363–3384. [CrossRef] [PubMed]
55. Zheng, D.W.; Dong, X.; Pan, P.; Chen, K.W.; Fan, J.X.; Cheng, S.X.; Zhang, X.Z. Phage-guided modulation of the gut microbiota of mouse models of colorectal cancer augments their responses to chemotherapy. *Nat. Biomed. Eng.* **2019**, *3*, 717–728. [CrossRef]
56. Baruch, E.N.; Youngster, I.; Ben-Betzalel, G.; Ortenberg, R.; Lahat, A.; Katz, L.; Adler, K.; Dick-Necula, D.; Raskin, S.; Bloch, N.; et al. Fecal microbiota transplant promotes response in immunotherapy-refractory melanoma patients. *Science* **2021**, *371*, 602–609. [CrossRef]
57. Zuo, T.; Wong, S.H.; Lam, K.; Lui, R.; Cheung, K.; Tang, W.; Ching, J.Y.L.; Chan, P.K.S.; Chan, M.C.W.; Wu, J.C.Y.; et al. Bacteriophage transfer during faecal microbiota transplantation in *Clostridium difficile* infection is associated with treatment outcome. *Gut* **2018**, *67*, 634–643. [CrossRef]
58. Haro, C.; Garcia-Carpintero, S.; Alcala-Diaz, J.F.; Gomez-Delgado, F.; Delgado-Lista, J.; Perez-Martinez, P.; Rangel Zuñiga, O.A.; Quintana-Navarro, G.M.; Landa, B.B.; Clemente, J.C.; et al. The gut microbial community in metabolic syndrome patients is modified by diet. *J. Nutr. Biochem.* **2016**, *27*, 27–31. [CrossRef]
59. Aron-Wisnewsky, J.; Vigliotti, C.; Witjes, J.; Le, P.; Holleboom, A.G.; Verheij, J.; Nieuwdorp, M.; Clément, K. Gut microbiota and human NAFLD: Disentangling microbial signatures from metabolic disorders. *Nat. Rev. Gastroenterol. Hepatol.* **2020**, *17*, 279–297. [CrossRef]
60. Gao, R.; Zhu, Y.; Kong, C.; Xia, K.; Li, H.; Zhu, Y.; Zhang, X.; Liu, Y.; Zhong, H.; Yang, R.; et al. Alterations, interactions, and diagnostic potential of gut bacteria and viruses in colorectal cancer. *Front. Cell. Infect. Microbiol.* **2021**, *11*, 657867. [CrossRef]
61. Lang, S.; Demir, M.; Martin, A.; Jiang, L.; Zhang, X.; Duan, Y.; Gao, B.; Wisplinghoff, H.; Kasper, P.; Roderburg, C.; et al. Intestinal virome signature associated with severity of nonalcoholic fatty liver disease. *Gastroenterology* **2020**, *159*, 1839–1852. [CrossRef] [PubMed]
62. Liang, G.; Conrad, M.A.; Kelsen, J.R.; Kessler, L.R.; Breton, J.; Albenberg, L.G.; Marakos, S.; Galgano, A.; Devas, N.; Erlichman, J.; et al. Dynamics of the stool virome in very early onset inflammatory bowel disease. *J. Crohn's Colitis* **2020**, *14*, 1600–1610. [CrossRef] [PubMed]

63. Oh, J.H.; Alexander, L.M.; Pan, M.; Schueler, K.L.; Keller, M.P.; Attie, A.D.; Walter, J.; van Pijkeren, J.P. Dietary fructose and microbiota-derived short-chain fatty acids promote bacteriophage production in the gut symbiont *Lactobacillus reuteri*. *Cell Host Microbe* **2019**, *25*, 273–284.e6. [CrossRef] [PubMed]
64. Reyes, A.; Blanton, L.V.; Cao, S.; Zhao, G.; Manary, M.; Trehan, I.; Smith, M.I.; Wang, D.; Virgin, H.W.; Rohwer, F.; et al. Gut DNA viromes of Malawian twins discordant for severe acute malnutrition. *Proc. Natl. Acad. Sci. USA* **2015**, *112*, 11941–11946. [CrossRef]
65. Schulfer, A.; Santiago-Rodriguez, T.M.; Ly, M.; Borin, J.M.; Chopyk, J.; Blaser, M.J.; Pride, D.T. Fecal viral community responses to high-fat diet in mice. *mSphere* **2020**, *5*, e00833-19. [CrossRef]
66. Pascale, A.; Marchesi, N.; Govoni, S.; Coppola, A.; Gazzaruso, C. The role of gut microbiota in obesity, diabetes mellitus, and effect of metformin: New insights into old diseases. *Curr. Opin. Pharmacol.* **2019**, *49*, 1–5. [CrossRef]
67. Rasmussen, T.S.; Mentzel, C.M.J.; Kot, W.; Castro-Mejía, J.L.; Zuffa, S.; Swann, J.R.; Hansen, L.H.; Vogensen, F.K.; Hansen, A.K.; Nielsen, D.S. Faecal virome transplantation decreases symptoms of type 2 diabetes and obesity in a murine model. *Gut* **2020**, *69*, 2122–2130. [CrossRef]
68. Khaliq, A.; Wraith, D.; Nambiar, S.; Miller, Y. A review of the prevalence, trends, and determinants of coexisting forms of malnutrition in neonates, infants, and children. *BMC Public Health* **2022**, *22*, 879. [CrossRef]
69. Subramanian, S.; Huq, S.; Yatsunenko, T.; Haque, R.; Mahfuz, M.; Alam, M.A.; Benezra, A.; Destefano, J.; Meier, M.F.; Muegge, B.D.; et al. Persistent gut microbiota immaturity in malnourished Bangladeshi children. *Nature* **2014**, *510*, 417–421. [CrossRef]
70. Low, S.J.; Džunková, M.; Chaumeil, P.A.; Parks, D.H.; Hugenholtz, P. Evaluation of a concatenated protein phylogeny for classification of tailed double-stranded DNA viruses belonging to the order Caudovirales. *Nat. Microbiol.* **2019**, *4*, 1306–1315. [CrossRef]
71. Jegatheesan, P.; De Bandt, J.P. Fructose and NAFLD: The multifaceted aspects of fructose metabolism. *Nutrients* **2017**, *9*, 230. [CrossRef]
72. Wong, S.H.; Yu, J. Gut microbiota in colorectal cancer: Mechanisms of action and clinical applications. *Nat. Rev. Gastroenterol. Hepatol.* **2019**, *16*, 690–704. [CrossRef] [PubMed]
73. Tetz, G.; Tetz, V. Bacteriophage infections of microbiota can lead to leaky gut in an experimental rodent model. *Gut Pathog.* **2016**, *8*, 33. [CrossRef] [PubMed]
74. Johnson, C.H.; Dejea, C.M.; Edler, D.; Hoang, L.T.; Santidrian, A.F.; Felding, B.H.; Ivanisevic, J.; Cho, K.; Wick, E.C.; Hechenbleikner, E.M.; et al. Metabolism links bacterial biofilms and colon carcinogenesis. *Cell Metab.* **2015**, *21*, 891–897. [CrossRef] [PubMed]
75. Cepko, L.C.S.; Garling, E.E.; Dinsdale, M.J.; Scott, W.P.; Bandy, L.; Nice, T.; Faber-Hammond, J.; Mellies, J.L. Myoviridae phage PDX kills enteroaggregative *Escherichia coli* without human microbiome dysbiosis. *J. Med. Microbiol.* **2020**, *69*, 309–323. [CrossRef]
76. Massimino, L.; Lovisa, S.; Antonio Lamparelli, L.; Danese, S.; Ungaro, F. Gut eukaryotic virome in colorectal carcinogenesis: Is that a trigger? *Comput. Struct. Biotechnol. J.* **2021**, *19*, 16–28. [CrossRef]
77. Lin, D.M.; Koskella, B.; Ritz, N.L.; Lin, D.; Carroll-Portillo, A.; Lin, H.C. Transplanting fecal virus-like particles reduces high-fat diet-induced small intestinal bacterial overgrowth in mice. *Front. Cell. Infect. Microbiol.* **2019**, *9*, 348. [CrossRef]
78. Basic, M.; Keubler, L.M.; Buettner, M.; Achard, M.; Breves, G.; Schröder, B.; Smoczek, A.; Jörns, A.; Wedekind, D.; Zschemisch, N.H.; et al. Norovirus triggered microbiota-driven mucosal inflammation in interleukin 10-deficient mice. *Inflamm. Bowel Dis.* **2014**, *20*, 431–443. [CrossRef]
79. Ott, S.J.; Waetzig, G.H.; Rehman, A.; Moltzau-Anderson, J.; Bharti, R.; Grasis, J.A.; Cassidy, L.; Tholey, A.; Fickenscher, H.; Seegert, D.; et al. Efficacy of sterile fecal filtrate transfer for treating patients with *Clostridium difficile* infection. *Gastroenterology* **2017**, *152*, 799–811.e7. [CrossRef]
80. Draper, L.A.; Ryan, F.J.; Dalmasso, M.; Casey, P.G.; McCann, A.; Velayudhan, V.; Ross, R.P.; Hill, C. Autochthonous faecal viral transfer (FVT) impacts the murine microbiome after antibiotic perturbation. *BMC Biol.* **2020**, *18*, 173. [CrossRef]
81. Brunse, A.; Deng, L.; Pan, X.; Hui, Y.; Castro-Mejía, J.L.; Kot, W.; Nguyen, D.N.; Secher, J.B.M.; Nielsen, D.S.; Thymann, T. Fecal filtrate transplantation protects against necrotizing enterocolitis. *ISME J.* **2022**, *16*, 686–694. [CrossRef] [PubMed]
82. Leong, K.S.W.; Jayasinghe, T.N.; Wilson, B.C.; Derraik, J.G.B.; Albert, B.B.; Chiavaroli, V.; Svirskis, D.M.; Beck, K.L.; Conlon, C.A.; Jiang, Y.; et al. Effects of fecal microbiome transfer in adolescents with obesity: The gut bugs randomized controlled trial. *JAMA Netw. Open* **2020**, *3*, e2030415. [CrossRef] [PubMed]
83. Barr, J.J.; Auro, R.; Furlan, M.; Whiteson, K.L.; Erb, M.L.; Pogliano, J.; Stotland, A.; Wolkowicz, R.; Cutting, A.S.; Doran, K.S.; et al. Bacteriophage adhering to mucus provide a nonhost-derived immunity. *Proc. Natl. Acad. Sci. USA* **2013**, *110*, 10771–10776. [CrossRef] [PubMed]
84. Ng, S.C.; Xu, Z.; Mak, J.W.Y.; Yang, K.; Liu, Q.; Zuo, T.; Tang, W.; Lau, L.; Lui, R.N.; Wong, S.H.; et al. Microbiota engraftment after fecal microbiota transplantation in obese subjects with type 2 diabetes: A 24-week, double-blind, randomised controlled trial. *Gut* **2022**, *71*, 716–723. [CrossRef]
85. Schwartz, M.; Gluck, M.; Koon, S. Norovirus gastroenteritis after fecal microbiota transplantation for treatment of *Clostridium difficile* infection despite asymptomatic donors and lack of sick contacts. *Am. J. Gastroenterol.* **2013**, *108*, 1367. [CrossRef]
86. Ianiro, G.; Gasbarrini, A.; Cammarota, G. Autologous faecal microbiota transplantation for type 1 diabetes: A potential mindshift in therapeutic microbiome manipulation? *Gut* **2021**, *70*, 2–3. [CrossRef]

87. Mukhopadhya, I.; Segal, J.P.; Carding, S.R.; Hart, A.L.; Hold, G.L. The gut virome: The 'missing link' between gut bacteria and host immunity? *Ther. Adv. Gastroenterol.* **2019**, *12*, 1756284819836620. [CrossRef]
88. Kelly, J.R.; Borre, Y.; O' Brien, C.; Patterson, E.; El Aidy, S.; Deane, J.; Kennedy, P.J.; Beers, S.; Scott, K.; Moloney, G.; et al. Transferring the blues: Depression-associated gut microbiota induces neurobehavioral changes in the rat. *J. Psychiatr. Res.* **2016**, *82*, 109–118. [CrossRef]

Disclaimer/Publisher's Note: The statements, opinions and data contained in all publications are solely those of the individual author(s) and contributor(s) and not of MDPI and/or the editor(s). MDPI and/or the editor(s) disclaim responsibility for any injury to people or property resulting from any ideas, methods, instructions or products referred to in the content.

MDPI AG
Grosspeteranlage 5
4052 Basel
Switzerland
Tel.: +41 61 683 77 34

Nutrients Editorial Office
E-mail: nutrients@mdpi.com
www.mdpi.com/journal/nutrients

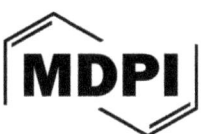

Disclaimer/Publisher's Note: The statements, opinions and data contained in all publications are solely those of the individual author(s) and contributor(s) and not of MDPI and/or the editor(s). MDPI and/or the editor(s) disclaim responsibility for any injury to people or property resulting from any ideas, methods, instructions or products referred to in the content.

www.ingramcontent.com/pod-product-compliance
Lightning Source LLC
LaVergne TN
LVHW070443100526
838202LV00014B/1659